Handbook of
Home Health
Orientation

ABOUT THE AUTHOR

Tina M. Marrelli, MSN, MA, RNC, is the editor and publisher of *Home Care Nurse News* and the President of Marrelli and Associates, Inc., a health care consulting and publishing firm. Ms. Marrelli is the author of *The Handbook of Home Health Standards and Documentation Guidelines for Reimbursement,* also known as "The Little Red Book" (Mosby, 1994), *The Nurse Manager's Survival Guide* (Mosby, 1997), and *The Nursing Documentation Handbook* (Mosby, 1996). She is also the co-author of *Home Health Aide: Guidelines for Care* (Marrelli, 1996), *Home Care and Clinical Paths: Effective Care Planning Across the Continuum* (Mosby, 1996), and *Home Health Aide: Guidelines for Care Instructor Manual* (Marrelli, 1997).

Ms. Marrelli received a Bachelor's degree in Nursing from Duke University School of Nursing in 1976. She has directed various home care programs and has extensive experience in home care, hospice, and hospital settings. In 1984, she received a Master of Arts in Management and Supervision, Health Care Administration. Ms. Marrelli worked at the central office of the Health Care Financing Administration (HCFA) for 4 years in the areas of home care and hospice policy and operations, where she received the Bureau Director's Citation. She is a member of Sigma Theta Tau and is certified by the American Nurses Association (ANA) credentialing center as a home health nurse. Ms. Marrelli is a Clinical Instructor at The Case Western Reserve University Frances Payne Bolton School of Nursing and serves on the National Hospice Organization's Standard and Accreditation Committee. In 1996 she (finally!) completed a Master of Science in Nursing.

Marrelli and Associates, Inc. provides consultative services to hospitals, home health agencies, and hospice programs in the areas of management, accreditation, and other quality initiatives, daily operations, and clinical documentation. Correspondence, including feedback, recommendations, or suggestions about this text may be directed to the author at: Marrelli and Associates, Inc., P.O. Box 629, Boca Grande, FL 33291-0629.

Handbook of Home Health Orientation

Tina M. Marrelli
Home Health Care Consultant
Boca Grande, Florida

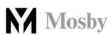 Mosby

St. Louis   Baltimore   Boston
Carlsbad   Chicago   Naples   New York   Philadelphia   Portland
London   Madrid   Mexico City   Singapore   Sydney   Tokyo   Toronto   Wiesbaden

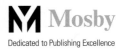
Mosby

Dedicated to Publishing Excellence

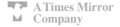
A Times Mirror Company

Vice President and Publisher:
  Nancy L. Coon
Editor: Loren S. Wilson
Developmental Editor: Aimee E. Loewe
Project Manager: Deborah L. Vogel
Project Specialist: Mary E. Drone
Production Editor: Sarah E. Fike
Designer: Pati Pye
Manufacturing Manager: Linda Ierardi
Cover Design: Dave Zielinski

Copyright © 1997 by Mosby–Year Book, Inc.
A Mosby Lifeline imprint of Mosby–Year Book, Inc.

Printed in the United States of America
Composition by Top Graphics
Lithography/color film by Top Graphics
Printing/binding by R.R. Donnelley & Sons

Mosby–Year Book, Inc.
11830 Westline Industrial Drive
St. Louis, Missouri 63146

International Standard Book Number 0-8151-5558-1

97 98 99 00 01 / 9 8 7 6 5 4 3 2 1

CONTRIBUTORS

Marilynn Berendt, RN, BSN, EdM, CD
Director of Infusion
In Home Care Service-West, Inc.
Downers Grove, Illinois

Bonnie Bolinger, RN, CETN
Wound Care Consultant
The Atlanta Consulting Group
Savannah, Georgia

Nikki Coffin, MS, RN
Regional Nurse Consultant
Abbot Infusion Services
Abbot Park, Illinois

Janice Cuzzell, RN, MA, CSN
Wound Care Consultant
The Atlanta Consulting Group
Savannah, Georgia

Dana Ellis, RN, BSN, CCRN
Cardiac Home Care Specialist
Virginia Beach, Virginia

Gail Ohlund, RN
Psychiatric Home Care Consulting Services
San Clemente, California

Christine Pierce, RN, CS, MSN, ANP
Corporate Director
Home Care Services
Mayfield Village, Ohio

Mary Jo Savage, MSN, RN
Pediatric Clinical Specialist
Medical University of South Carolina
Charleston, South Carolina

Carolyn Viall, MSN, RN
Nurse Manager, Pediatrics
Medical University of South Carolina
Charleston, South Carolina

REVIEWERS

Linda Canon, RN
Dublin, Ohio

Dana Ellis, RN, BSN, CCRN
Virginia Beach, Virginia

Laura L. Friend, BSN, RN
Education Coordinator
West Virginia Council of Home Health Agencies
Middlebourne, West Virginia

Lynda S. Hillard, MBA, RN, CNAA
Health and Home Care Consultant
Pleasanton, California

Linda Krulish, MHS, PT
Director of Business Development
Health Care Plus
Columbus, Ohio

Kathy Larsen, RN, MS, CS
Home and Community Health Specialist
Columbus, Ohio

Deb Leasure, RN
Staff Development Coordinator
Buckeye Home Health
Zanesville, Ohio

Kriss Ann Loughman, MSN, RN
Senior Human Resource Development Specialist
Meridia Home Health Care
Cleveland, Ohio

Karen Reese, MS, RN
Faculty
Santa Rosa Junior College
Santa Rosa, California

Anne Rooney, MPH, MS, RN
Home Care Consultant
Oak Park, Illinois

Mary Fran Stulginsky, RN, MS
Consultant and Nurse Educator
Home Health and Hospice
Ellicot City, Maryland

Marilyn Warling, RN, BSN
Medicare Director, External Relations and Benefit Integrity
Wellmark (Blue Cross/Blue Shield of Iowa and South Dakota)
Des Moines, Iowa

Sandy M. Whittier, RNC, BSN
Clinical Coordinator, Nursing and Rehabilitation
Whidden Home Health and Hospice
Everett, Massachusetts

Maureen Williams, RN, C, MEd
Clinical Educator
Visiting Nurses Association of Northern Virginia
Arlington, Virginia

PREFACE

Home care has undergone significant change and incredible growth since I wrote the first edition of the "Little Red Book," the *Handbook of Home Health Standards and Documentation Guidelines for Reimbursement* (edition 3, Mosby, 1998) over 10 years ago. It has been well documented that home care and hospice continue to be two of the fastest growing segments of health care.

This new book, *Handbook of Home Health Orientation,* was written to create a text to assist in helping nurses and other clinicians and managers to make the transition to successful home health practice and operations, as well as to support the continued growth of clinicians already established in home care. Increasing numbers of nurses, therapists, social workers, dietitians, physicians and other specialists and managers are transitioning into home care. These clinicians may be coming from inpatient settings, be transferring from supervisory to home care practice positions, or be experienced home care clinicians who want to increase their knowledge base of new information. Please know that the word "nurse" is primarily used throughout the text, but the text is also directed toward therapists and other clinicians moving into home care who must understand the glossary, standards, and operations unique to this community-based practice setting.

This book is intended to be a resource for reference long after the formal orientation period has been completed, as well as to provide a structure during orientation for the standardization of care and care processes. There is a related companion text, *The Manual of Home Health Practice: Guidance for Effective Clinical Operations,* that was especially designed to be used by the instructor, preceptor, or educator at the organization. Thus there is a handbook for easy retrieval and ready reference of needed information by each clinician; and the larger text, which contains more specificity and exercises for discussion, is the curriculum framework to be used by the instructor or educator during the formal orientation sessions. The two texts were designed to be used together to assist in standardizing care and care processes throughout the organization.

These books support effective daily operations while assisting the practitioner in the delivery of safe and effective client care. Together they integrate the most important components of home care and compliance with various regulators. The care planning, care coordination, reporting, and documentation are provided in a customer service–oriented structure that can be used to meet the unique needs of the organization and the patient populations served.

With the growth of home care, the increasing acuity of patients cared for at home, and the various emerging specialties, it is unrealistic and unsafe to provide new team members with an introductory class or a 2-week (or other shortened time frame) orientation and expect the clinicians to function safely and effectively in daily practice and operations in home care or hospice. This book then becomes a resource long after formal orientation has been completed. Compliance requirements, such as knowledge of the Medicare rules related to coverage and documentation, correct completion of the HCFA 485 forms, performance of a complete and comprehensive patient assessment, and others are areas addressed in depth to improve practice and operations.

Although sometimes the text refers to "home health care," this information is also directed toward hospice workers providing care in the home who must also obtain physician orders in a timely manner, schedule patients based on multifaceted parameters, and meet coverage and documentation requirements to ensure quality, compliance, and payment. Therefore the term *home care* is used throughout the text and refers to any program or organization providing services and care in patients' homes. Similarly, the terms *patient* and *client* are used interchangeably; and the term *patient* is used in the text, except in Chapter 10, which is the psychiatric home care chapter.

It is my hope that clinicians and managers moving into home care receive the information they need "at the front end," at the beginning of their hiring and orientation process so that patients, their families, the clinicians themselves, their communities, and their organizations receive a high-quality level of care demonstrated by achieved outcomes, personal and professional satisfaction, and positive feedback. This text may assist in all these endeavors.

Tina M. Marrelli

ACKNOWLEDGMENT

Thanks to the many nurses and other clinicians and managers who had input into this text and who, over the years, called and wrote to me with tips that "made their lives easier." Special kudos go to Bill and Buddy Glass for humor and items too numerous to list.

CONTENTS

HOME CARE CLINICIAN: OVERVIEW OF AN IMPORTANT ROLE

WELCOME TO HOME CARE: THE HEALTH CARE SETTING OF THE FUTURE

Tina M. Marrelli, MSN, MA, RNC

> *"Home care is exploding in this country. The assumption cannot be made that acute care nurses can simply become home care experts. Nor can the assumption be made that graduates of current nursing programs are prepared to assume complex home health care responsibilities. Home health care nursing is different!"*
>
> *Miller and Daley, 1996*

Home care in the United States is a diverse and rapidly growing industry and continues to be the fastest growing segment of the health care industry. Over 18,500 providers deliver home care services to approximately 7 million individuals who require services (National Association for Home Care, 1996). It has been projected that in the next decade the needs for home care and related services are expected to triple (Lewin-VHI, 1993). The U. S. Bureau of Labor Statistics indicates that when most industries experienced decline because of recession, home care employment increased 19.2%—almost triple the rate for the health care industry generally (National Association for Home Care, 1993). Many factors have contributed to this growth. Many people believe that the American health care system is undergoing a paradigm shift. Numbers and trends such as these have broad implications for nurses as the site of care moves from an inpatient and acute care direction to a more community-based and chronic care focus. These changes focus on lower-cost settings and comfort and privacy in the patient's home. This shift has been phrased as "from helicopter to hospice" or from "cure to care."

For many patients, based on their health problems, home is also the lowest-cost health care setting. One study demonstrated cost savings in home care by studying 30 ventilator-assisted adults; the average annual home care cost was $55,814. Compared to inpatient hospital costs, the savings were estimated to be about $152,000 to $177,000 per patient (Bach, Alba, and Holland, 1992). Significant savings are also seen when terminally ill cancer patients are cared for at home. Carney and Burns (1991) calculated savings of 39% to 51% for patients in home hospice care.

Clearly the scope and breadth of the kinds of patients seen in home care demand strong clinicians with excellent interpersonal assessment and other multifaceted skills. The additional skills needed to function effectively in these holistic and accountable roles sometimes cannot be readily transferred to the specialty of home care nursing. This book provides the information needed to make a successful transition to this new practice. It is an ongoing reference guide that should be used well beyond the defined orientation period and into home care practice. Nurses, other clinicians, and managers must be prepared to meet the challenge of the vision of the future in which most patients will be cared for at home. This chapter discusses the bigger picture contributing to the growth of home care.

FACTORS AFFECTING THE DELIVERY OF HEALTH CARE

Multifaceted forces influence the delivery of health care today and have important implications for managers and clinicians. The following factors impact home care service delivery and set the stage for understanding the current home care environment:

1. Shift from inpatient care to outpatient and community-based care
2. Providers changing and/or combining organizational structures
3. Reimbursement shift from fee-for-service to managed care
4. Diversity in the types and missions of health care providers
5. Continuing communication problems between providers
6. Fragmentation of care and planning due to organizational structures
7. Increasing accreditation and regulatory focus
8. Technological advances
9. Legal and risk management issues
10. Emergence of problematic and difficult ethical issues
11. Cost and quality dilemma
12. Patient as consumer

Shift from Inpatient Care to Outpatient and Community-Based Care

Although the implications of this shift of focus to outpatient and community-based care cannot yet be determined, it is certain that health care will look very different from the current model. Models of care, roles of care team members, and definitions will change significantly. This kind of change can be frightening, but it often holds unique opportunities and creates leaders to assist, manage, and direct through turbulent change.

Providers Changing and/or Combining Organizational Structures

Local community newspapers publish news about hospitals, even those that have been fierce competitors, merging or working together to form alliances or other structures. As health care must change to survive, vertical and horizontal networks are forming to serve patients who are cared for through a managed care contract. These mergers that create "one-stop shopping" for payors and other consumers of care seek to increase efficiency and thereby improve quality.

Reimbursement Shift from Fee-for-Service to Managed Care

Managed care seeks to care for a patient across the life span and across the health care continuum of care settings by incorporating regulation and competition to try to control costs. This shift to the managed care environment has caused significant changes in the home care industry. Managed care has forced all health care providers, including home care and hospice organizations, to define the care provided and account for the cost of all resources and services used.

Diversity of Types and Missions of Health Care Providers

As health care organizations must change to survive, myriad specialty and alternative care settings and services are emerging. This is heralding a change from "business as usual." Emerging specialty areas that include short-stay hospitals, massage therapists, and other alternative care models serving both home care organizations and hospitals are examples of the broadening of the scope of health care as self-care and patient education toward self-management become goals in the new health care model.

Continuing Communication Problems Between Providers

As patients assume more responsibility for their own care, the health care glossary must become a common and understandable language among all providers and health care consumers. For example, nurses, physical therapists, physicians, and occupational therapists use the term *functional* differently. For quality and cost reasons, all providers must be "singing from the same page" and with the same understanding.

Fragmentation of Care and Planning Because of Organizational Structures

Historically hospitals were created for the convenience of the providers. Physicians could go one place to see patients. In addition, other economies of scales were created when patients were grouped together in one setting. However, as reimbursed sources grew, so too did the fragmentation of care from a patient perspective. Discharge planners, case managers, home care nurses, triage nurses, and others who interface with patients at the end of one care site and the beginning of another are well versed in hearing about preventable inefficiencies and redundancies in the marketplace. Examples include patients with no follow-up after hospitalization, patients who call the hospital because they are unsure of the process for drop-off of urine samples, or patients who return to the emergency room for nonemergency care because primary care follow-up was not coordinated at the last care setting.

Increasing Accreditation and Regulatory Focus

Because of the growth in number of patients, the problems with quality in the system, and the continued and spiraling costs, health care, particularly home care and hospice, is coming under increased scrutiny from various perspectives. Federal regulatory bodies include the Centers for Disease Control and Prevention, The Occupational Safety and Health Administration, Medicare law, and related Omnibus Budget Reconciliation Acts (OBRAs) such as OBRA 1990, which relates to advance directive requirements. Accreditation is a labor-intensive process of self-assessment. Achievement of accreditation is a standard for most managed care contracts in home care.

Technological Advances

The rapid increase of technological advances has significantly increased patient diagnoses and treatment in all health care settings. At the same time, in some managed care environments, patients must exhaust their possibilities in the general practitioner's office before being referred for specialist care and/or technology.

Legal and Risk Management Issues

As active consumers of health care, patients appropriately expect care to be provided according to perceived standards of care and practice. Patients want more but do not want to pay more at the same time that hospitals are redesigning and "rightsizing" and nurse-to-patient ratios are decreasing while acuity increases. This trend of doing more with fewer resources will continue. Providers and consumers of care must "weather the storm" until the pendulum swings back.

Emergence of Problematic and Difficult Ethical Issues

The convergence of technology, differing belief systems, cost concerns, and other issues has contributed to the emergence of ethical concerns. Some of these include physician-assisted suicide and rationing of care.

Cost and Quality Dilemma

It is well known that the U.S. health care system pays more for health care than any other country and yet does not have discernible or improved patient outcomes. In fact, some third-world countries have lower infant mortality and morbidity rates than the United States. The U.S. health care system must become outcome focused to be able to demonstrate effective care and quantify activities that are attributable to care.

Patient as Consumer

Patients must assume more responsibility for care. The baby-boomer generation, which accounts for the largest segment of the population, is more self-care educated than any other patient population. This responsibility for self and care expands the role of the health care provider to include the roles of teacher and facilitator. All of these factors together have contributed to the environment of growth in home care.

REASONS FOR THE GROWTH IN HOME CARE

A number of reasons exist for the growth in home care. Seven of the main reasons and their implications for the future of home care are discussed in the following paragraphs. See also Box 1-1.

Health Care Reimbursement System

The health care reimbursement system has fueled the growth of home care. Medicare is the largest payor of home care services and as such has set many of the standards for the home care industry. Medicare is the health reimbursement mechanism or insurance program for the elderly, the disabled, and those patients with end-stage renal disease (ESRD). The expenditures for Medicare have increased steadily since it became law in 1965. The home care sector has *grown faster* than any other sector in the Medicare budget, skyrocketing from $2.5 billion in 1989 to

---

BOX 1-1   THE SHIFT TO HOME CARE: THREE PERSPECTIVES

From the patient, clinician, and payor's perspectives, home care offers the following benefits:

The Patient's and/or Consumer's Perspective
- Only one patient receives care at a time (decreasing risks of medication errors, patient identification problems, and so on).
- Care is provided in the privacy and safety of one's own home.
- Patient's have more control over decision making regarding visitors, clothing, meals, and scheduling.
- The patient and family, by location and choice, form a partnership with home care providers to achieve agreed-on outcomes.

The Payor's Perspective
- Outcomes may be more attributable to care because fewer clinicians are providing care than in inpatient settings.
- The home is generally a lower-cost setting than the hospital.
- Patients are more involved in care and care planning, which reduces costs.

The Clinician's Perspective
- One patient and family receives care at a time, which is the model learned in schools.
- Care is more personalized and individualized.
- Patients are equal partners in care and care choices, including agreed-on outcomes or quantifiable goals of care.

From Marrelli T, Hilliard L: *Home care and clinical paths: effective care planning across the continuum,* St. Louis, 1996, Mosby.

about $16 billion in 1995 (Weiss, 1996). The National Association for Home Care (NAHC) identified a total of 17,561 home care organizations, comprised of approximately 9000 Medicare-certified agencies; almost 2000 Medicare-certified hospices; and more than 7000 agencies, home care aide organizations, and hospices that do not participate in Medicare (NAHC, 1995).

Medicare Hospital Insurance (Part A) currently pays for home care, as well as hospital inpatient care, skilled nursing facility care, and hospice care. The estimated depletion dates for the Medicare Part A Trust Fund vary between the year 2002 and 2005. This estimate is based on probable economic and demographic assumptions.

The government cannot allow health care costs to continue to spiral out of control. As the Medicare outlay increases proportionately, Congress, taxpayers, and consumers are searching for effective reform of the process and system. President Clinton's failed Health Security Act was initiated to address three areas of health care: cost, access, and quality. Clearly, cost is the prime concern. The effects of that failed plan are being felt across the nation, and managed care and health care reform are continuing at the state and regional levels without national legislation.

Just as hospitals shifted from a cost-based reimbursement system to diagnostic-related groups (DRGs) in the early 1980s, home care is shifting from a cost-based reimbursement system to some form of a prospective payment system (PPS) as payors search for more cost-effective ways to provide coverage to their beneficiaries or "covered lives." In parts of the country where there is already significant managed care penetration, managed care payors are the largest reimbursement and referral sources. (Please refer to the glossary for terms related to home care practice and operations.)

Implementation of the Diagnostic-Related Groups

When DRGs were initiated in the early 1980s, hospitals needed to decrease the length of stay for patients because they would be reimbursed on a PPS rather than on a cost-based system. The meteoric growth of home health care from the 1980s into the early 1990s and the subsequent growth of hospital-based home health agencies (HHAs) was a response to the implementation of DRGs. Hospitals realized additional revenues and profits by diversifying into home care, and, as a result, the hospital home care industry grew by more than 500% between 1980 and 1994 (Church, 1996). In addition, hospital home care programs keep patients within their own system while extending care outside the hospital walls and into the community and thus are able to work toward a goal of seamless and integrated care across a continuum.

A simplistic example of the financial impact of the DRG system on a hospital can best be described through a patient example. Two Medicare beneficiaries are admitted through the emergency room of a hospital to the critical care unit to rule out a myocardial infarction. One patient has a noneventful course of care and is discharged 5 days later; the other patient experiences further cardiac problems, resulting in an extended hospitalization (more than 22 days). Notwithstanding additional diagnostic findings resulting in a change in diagnosis and possibly an increase in payment, the hospital would be paid the same amount for both patients. The course of care for the second patient may also include diagnostic cardiac angiography, which would not be reimbursed separately in this scenario. The hospital would have to absorb the cost of this additional, expensive procedure.

Hospitals continue to benefit from increasing admissions under PPS, but need to continue to control and decrease each patient's length of stay to remain viable. Home care is the way this can occur (Marrelli and Hilliard, 1996). To home care nurses, this means that patients with higher acuity levels are being sent home. Home care nurses refer to this as "sicker and quicker." This change immediately has created and increased the need for more home care services and competent clinicians and managers.

Increased Public and Professional Acceptance of Home Care

For many reasons, including nosocomial infection rates and media reports of inpatient drug errors, patients want to go home, and doctors and other health care team members are respecting that choice. The surge of consumerism and customer service in the current health care environment has caused patients to demand to be cared for at home. Home can be perceived as the most patient-centered site to receive health care. Home care nurses must truly respect the individual life-style choices seen during care and support the patient, family members, and friends involved in aspects of the patient's care.

Available Technology for and in the Home

There was a time when portable x-ray machines were too big to fit into most homes and dobutamine was given only in the intensive care unit with the patient hooked up to the electrocardiograph. New technology now allows very ill patients to receive care at home.

Some innovative home care programs are using personal telemedicine (PT) units or televisits. The PTs are about the size of a microwave oven and allow the nurse and patient to communicate and simultaneously see each other on the video monitor. Other programs have personal emergency response systems (PERSs) to enable their frail, elderly, or otherwise at-risk patients to communicate and call for assistance.

Lower Cost Issue

Generally home care continues to be the lower cost setting for health care, but some believe that the fact that home care remains cost-based reimbursement is the main reason for its continued growth. For this reason, the Health Care Financing Administration (HCFA) is conducting demonstration projects for a PPS, and congressional legislation has been introduced for PPSs in home care. Historically, other payors set their visit or care rates based on Medicare or other factors. As managed care penetration continues, this practice is decreasing.

The complexity of reimbursement in home care causes many HHAs to have contracts with different insurers or third party payors, all of whom may have very different administrative and clinical requirements. This can be extremely frustrating to managers and home care nurses as the industry continues to go through tumultuous change.

Emerging and Growing Patient Populations

The following four special patient populations exist in home care:

1. "Baby boomers," the largest segment of the population, who were born in the 1950s and are beginning to need health care services
2. Patients who are cared for at home and rehabilitation centers after shock trauma or head injury and may need hyperalimentation or other care for the rest of their lives
3. Infants, the youngest emerging population, who graduate from the neonatal intensive care unit and need continued services, technology, and care at home after discharge
4. The elderly, who continue to increase in number; for the first time in history, the United States has three generations of elderly

I remember caring for a 67-year-old woman who had to be admitted for an emergency abdominal surgery; however, as the home care nurse, I knew that her 89-year-old bedridden father lived with her and that my patient was his primary caregiver. Arrangements had to be made for the father's care before the daughter could be admitted to the hospital. This scenario is more usual than unusual today and brings complex responsibilities. The detail-oriented, time-consuming care, coordination, and communication needed to facilitate these arrangements can be a part of the home care nurse's role to facilitate patient care.

Growth of Medicare Home Care and Clarification of Medicare Coverage Requirements in 1989

Before 1989, coverage determinations made on home care claims varied from region to region and from intermediary to intermediary. At that time there were over 40 different fiscal intermediaries for home care, and denials were at an all-time high. In the late 1980s home care agencies received drastic increases in the numbers of Medicare denials. A lawsuit, now referred to as the Duggan or Staggers lawsuit, was initiated by NAHC and significantly clarified coverage.

Some believe that this "clarification" expanded or liberalized coverage to such an extent that this has contributed to the increases in Medicare home care outlays and services and further contributed to the growth. For home care nurses and managers the clarification more clearly "explained the rules" of coverage and documentation requirements.

SUMMARY

Care continues to shift to outpatient, home care, and other community-based settings. The three most important reasons for this are cost, quality, and access. This overview of home care shows it to be a complex system comprised of regulation, law, standards, and clinical practice. The home care nurse must effectively integrate and operationalize this information to be an advocate for patients, as well as provide and document high-quality care that allows the home care organization to be paid for covered services. The changing health care environment and the growing and diverse home care industry set the stage for change and opportunity.

REVIEW EXERCISES

1. Identify four factors affecting the delivery of health care.
2. List five reasons for the continued growth of home care.
3. Explain the DRG system through a patient example.
4. Define one benefit of home care from:
   a. A patient's perspective
   b. A payor's perspective
   c. A clinician's perspective
5. List four regulatory bodies involved in home care.

REFERENCES

Bach JR, Alba AS, Holland IE: The ventilator-assisted individual: cost analysis of institutional vs. rehabilitation and in-home management, *Chest* 101: 26-30, 1992.

Carney K, Burns N: Economics of hospice care, *Oncol Nurs Forum* 18:761-786, 1991.

Church L: The new rules of home health, *Health System Review,* January/February 1996.

Lewin: *VHI analysis of NMES data: the heavy burden of home care,* Washington, DC, 1993, Families USA.

Marrelli T, Hilliard L: *Home care and clinical paths: effective care planning across the continuum,* St. Louis, 1996, Mosby.

Miller M, Daley B: Home health nursing: there is a difference, *Home Health Care Management Pract* 8(4):64-70, 1996.

National Association for Home Care: *Basic statistics about home care,* Washington, DC, 1996, National Association for Home Care.

National Association for Home Care: *Basic statistics about home care 1996,* Washington, DC, 1996, National Association for Home Care.

Weiss H: Manager's corner: budget negotiators put Medicare on chopping block, *Home Care Nurse News* 3(2)3-4, 1996.

chapter

2

HOME CARE NURSING: A HISTORICAL PERSPECTIVE

Nikki Coffin, MS, RN

> *"The most important practical lesson that can be given to nurses is to teach them what to observe—how to observe—what symptoms indicate improvement—what the reverse—which are of importance. . . . All this is what ought to make part, and an essential part, of the training of every nurse."*
>
> *Florence Nightingale*

The nursing care of people in their home environment has strong roots in history and is important information for home care nurses today. As far back as the eleventh century and through Florence Nightingale's era of practice, providing health-related services for people in their place of residence has been reported (Wiles, 1984). In more recent times and as discussed in the preceding chapter, the legislation of Medicare and Medicaid (health care for the poor) in 1965 has been a powerful influence on the growth and structure of home care. In fact, in 1963, 3 years before Medicare became law, there were only 1100 home care programs. The federally financed home health care program under Medicare became the basis for financial support and provided for the availability of the full gamut of health care services to a segment of society previously not served. Expansion of services to meet this enlarged client base dramatically increased health care costs. Multiple efforts to control these costs resulted in systems of prospective payment and incentives for acute care settings to find alternative care arenas (Albrecht, 1992). Advanced technology and client preference have been additional factors nurturing the provision of care for people in their home environment.

The continuing expansion of home health care will be a challenge for the clinical professions. The increasing patient acuity and complexity of patient care influenced by restructuring and reform in the health care system requires clinicians who are skillful, theoretically sound, and guided by research-based standards of practice.

HOME CARE DEFINITIONS

In an attempt to describe and clarify home care practice, several professional health care groups have presented their definitions and interpretations. The American Medical Association (AMA), the American College of Physicians (ACP), the American Hospital Association (AHA), the American Nurses Association (ANA), the National Association for Home Care (NAHC), and the Public Health Service (PHS) of the Department of Health and Human Services (HHS) have each put forth descriptions.

The AMA interprets all home care activities as those that are a logical extension of physician services, whereas the ACP perceives home care as the provision of care in a patient's home rather than an institution or office. The AHA provides a list that includes such items as medical care and supervision, social work services, nursing and pharmaceutical services, and transportation and equipment (Humphrey, 1988).

The ANA describes the scope and distinguishing characteristics of home health in its effort to define the practice. According to the ANA (1986), home health care practice is the application of nursing to manage a health deficit in a client's place of residence. Clients and caregivers are the focus of care. The goal is to initiate, manage, and evaluate resources necessary to promote an optimal level of well-being.

The NAHC definition includes services to people who are recovering, disabled, chronically ill, or who may be in danger of abuse or neglect. Generally it defines care that cannot be easily or effectively provided by informal caregivers for any length of time (Humphrey, 1988).

The definition put forth by the PHS is perhaps the most comprehensive and states that home health care is "that component of a continuum of comprehensive health care whereby health services are provided to individuals and families in their places of residence for the purpose of promoting, maintaining or restoring health, or maximizing the level of independence, while minimizing the effects of disability and illness, including terminal illness. Services appropriate to the needs of the individual patient and family are planned, coordinated, and made available by providers organized for the delivery of home care through the use of employed staff, contractual arrangements, or a combination of the two patterns" (Warhola, 1980).

Home health care practice is a synthesis of community health nursing and skills from other specialty nursing practices (ANA, 1992; Marrelli, 1993). Home health care is focused on individuals in collaboration with a caregiver (Humphrey, 1988). Practice centers on secondary prevention, assistance to families/caregivers, and direct treatment and coordination of community resources (Marrelli, 1993). It requires technical and comprehensive clinical decision-making in both autonomous and interdependent modes; complete physical, psychosocial, and environmental assessments; the inclusion of family dynamics and the home environment; and the awareness of the unique circumstances of being a guest in the home. As a generalist focusing on the client, family, or caregiver or as a specialist with additional advanced practice expectations, it has become obvious that home health nursing practice is more than just basic nursing performed outside of an acute setting.

THE DEVELOPMENT OF HOME CARE

As far back as the New Testament in the Bible, discussions are presented of Phoebe as a person who visited the sick in their homes to provide care. Later, during the eleventh century, military nursing orders developed and eventually became visiting nurse services (Stanhope, 1989). Credit for founding the first public health nursing association goes to William Rathbone of Liverpool, England. After a prolonged experience of having a nurse care for his wife in their home, Mr. Rathbone supported the further development of nurses and home care services in England. It was Rathbone's work and writings that inspired Florence Nightingale to write recommendations for nursing care in the home (Kalish and Kalish, 1986).

Home care development in the United States began in the early 1800s. The Buffalo District Nursing Association begun by Elizabeth Marshall is credited with establishing the first Visiting Nurses Association (VNA) in 1885. The New York City Mission, established in 1877, is described as the precursor of modern home care; and Frances Root, a member of the first class graduated from Bellevue Hospital, was the first home care nurse (Stanhope, 1989).

By 1890, 21 VNAs existed in the United States. In 1883 Lillian Wald and Mary Brewster, nursing colleagues, founded the Henry Street Settlement in New York City, a highly organized enterprise that provided services to all. The model for existing home care agencies today, the Henry Street Settlement provided health education, care for the sick, and communication and referral to patients and physicians. Personnel assisted with arrangements for hospitalization, as well as daily comforts, and kept data on all the work they accomplished. In addition to the nursing staff, other persons were employed to manage various social and civic efforts.

In 1909, following an initial experience with Lillian Wald, the Metropolitan Life Insurance Co. began to offer home nursing to its policy holders. From this introduction of payment for home care services, the provision of services to persons other than the poor developed (Kalish and Kalish, 1986).

In 1912 a small group of 3000 visiting nurses in the United States requested that the ANA and the National League for Nursing consider means to standardize public health nursing. The National Organization for Public Health Nursing was developed out of that effort, with Lillian Wald serving as the first president. The organization provided for standards of quality, collection and analysis of data, advisory services to colleagues and universities, and advisory and placement services for nurses (Stanhope, 1989).

The model of modern home care is one that includes the provision of medical, nursing, therapy, personal care, laboratory, pharmacy, equipment, nutrition and social services. Following the 1965 introduction of Medicare and Medicaid law and guidelines for the operation and financing of these services, many changes and revisions occurred. With amendments of the 1970s and 1980s, the number of home care days reimbursed was increased, and eligibility extended (Albrecht, 1992).

In 1982 the Tax Equity and Fiscal Responsibility Act (TEFRA) was enacted in an effort to control the cost resulting from the greater number of services that were needed. TEFRA directed the prospective payment system for reimbursing hospitals, which in turn, as described in the previous chapter, further increased the demand for home care. Today there are approximately 18,500 home care entities providing various types of home care services and products, with about one half being Medicare certified.

CURRENT STRUCTURES OF HOME CARE ORGANIZATIONS

Home care agencies can generally be divided into five categories based on their mission, vision, and administrative and organizational framework. As mergers and coalitions are responding to the managed care environment, some agencies are a blend of these structures. For example, a VNA may be the hospital's home care agency, or a proprietary agency may merge with a nonprofit entity to work together to provide care across a defined geographic area.

Official

Official, or public, agencies usually offer very comprehensive types of community services related to health promotion and disease prevention. As nonprofit entities, the support of public funding, in addition to funds from Medicare, Medicaid, and private payors, allows for those functions. An example would be a county or other municipal health department.

Voluntary and Private Nonprofit

Voluntary and private nonprofit agencies are supported by charities such as United Way, as well as Medicaid, Medicare, and private funds. Typically these are VNAs governed by boards of directors.

Combination

Agencies can be a combination of the official and the voluntary.

Hospital-Based

Hospital-based or facility-based home care organizations differ in that they have established boards of directors and accessible inpatient services that can provide for continuity across the continuum of care. Revenue generated by home care provides a source of income for the institution.

Proprietary

The proprietary or privately owned or held agencies are not eligible for tax exemption and usually operate for a profit. The owners of the proprietary agencies are responsible for their governing.

HOME CARE TODAY

We know that home care is primarily a nursing-driven business. The nurse creates the plan of care, based on the physician's initial referring orders and the in-home assessment, which is then signed by the physician. The philosophy and mission, the structure, and even the pay scale for nurses vary among the home care organizations across the country.

The increasing need for and competition in home health care can be positive forces. They also call for increased diligence in monitoring and valuing the humanitarian aspects of home care. To survive in this competitive arena, providing quality care must be balanced with cost-effectiveness and accountability. Regardless of the type or structure of the organization providing home care, the primary goal is to meet the health care needs of people in a safe, quality-driven manner.

QUALITY IMPROVEMENT IN HOME CARE

Before the introduction of Medicare as coverage for home care in 1965, the major emphasis relating to quality involved field supervision of team members, an annual agency evaluation, the collection of a modicum of statistical data, and nursing education requirements. The Medicare conditions of participation introduced eligibility requirements and some quality assurance criteria to home care. The emphasis was on structure and process, but there was no standardization of quality assurance (Stanhope, 1989).

Many believe that quality is truly about the way care is provided every day and the qualifications and competency of the caregivers. With this basic tenet, it is more important than ever that clinicians in home care strive to provide the best quality of care and demonstrate that quality through quantifiable means. Home care must standardize care and care processes to continually assure quality and be able to collect standard information for comparison and research because internal mechanisms to monitor and continually improve performance are vital to any quality initiative. Accreditation bodies such as the Joint Commission for Accreditation of Health Care Organizations (JCAHO) and the National League for Nursing's Community Health Assessment Program (CHAP) are two examples of entities that assist in assuring quality by conferring accreditation on organizations that have achieved identified and measurable standards.

HOME CARE NURSING TODAY: THE ROLE OF THE HOME CARE NURSE

About the time that Medicare was introduced, the ANA was developing its Division of Practice, which eventually led to the publication of the ANA's *Standards of Home Health Nursing Practice* in 1992.

Model of Home Care Nursing

The complex nature of home health services uses all the skills of clinicians and managers caring for patients. The nurse's own philosophy, a chosen structural or theoretical framework for practice, and adherence to the standards and policies create the basis for safe and effective patient care.

Figure 2-1 shows a model for application of home care nursing. This model integrates the varied and overlapping roles with the skills needed to function effectively in the home care environment.

SUMMARY

Home care nursing has a long history of providing care and support to patients and their families. The best of home care nursing practice integrates multifaceted skills and creates a workable plan that is implemented by the care team and the patient and family in their unique home

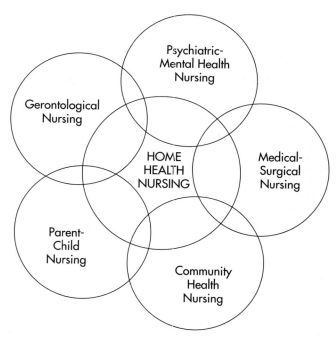

FIGURE 2-1   Conceptual model of home health nursing. (From *A statement on the scope of home health nursing practice,* Washington, DC, ANA.)

environment. This collaborative effort toward the ultimate goals of self-care and education for safe care at home become the guiding forces for clinicians practicing in home care.

REVIEW EXERCISES
1. Describe the history of home care nursing.
2. Define home health care versus home care nursing.
3. List the five structures of home care organizations.
4. Identify the nurse who is commonly referred to as the mother of home care nursing in the United States.
5. Discuss the first insurer who is credited with employing home care nurses to provide home visits to policyholders.
6. Define the two main accreditation bodies in home health care.

REFERENCES

Albrecht MN: The community health nurse in home health and hospice care. In Lancaster J, Stanhope M: *Community health nursing process and practice for promoting health,* ed 3, St. Louis, 1992, Mosby.

American Nurses Association: *A Statement on the scope of home health nursing practice,* Washington, DC, 1992, American Nurses Association.

Humphrey JC: The home as a setting for care: clarifying the boundaries of practice, *Nurs Clin North Am* 23(2):305-314, 1988.

Kalish BJ, Kalish P: *The advance of American nursing,* ed 2, Boston, 1986, Little, Brown, pp 1-53.

Marrelli TM: *The nurse manager's survival guide,* St. Louis, 1997, Mosby.

Nightingale F: *Notes on nursing: what it is, and what it is not,* Philadelphia, 1992, JB Lippincott, p 59.

Stanhope MK: Home care: past perspectives and implications for the present and future. In Meisenheimer CG: *Quality assurance for home health care,* Maryland, 1989, Aspen, pp 3-12.

Warhola C: Planning for home health services: a resource handbook, DHHS Publ. No. (HRA) 80-14017, Washington DC, 1980, US Public Health Service, Department of Health and Human Services.

Wiles E: Home health care nursing. In Stanhope M, Lancaster J: *Community health nursing: process and practice,* St. Louis, 1984, Mosby, pp 780-801.

3

HOME CARE: ITS OWN SPECIALTY

Tina M. Marrelli, MSN, MA, RNC

"She must have the necessary humanitarian impulses, and must be educated to the social viewpoint. It is difficult, but possible to produce such a high type of nurse for this important work. Certain it is that hosts of nurses must undertake it if we are to meet the pressing problems of the day."

Minnie Hoodnow, 1937

The American Nurses Association (ANA) standards provide the structural, theoretical framework for home care practice. In addition to these and other standards, the following components provide information about the "nuts and bolts" of home care practice.

SKILLS AND KNOWLEDGE NEEDED IN HOME CARE: MULTIFACETED ROLE
Basic Rules and Standards

Knowledge of administrative and clinical rules and standards of home care is necessary. For Medicare-certified agencies this includes an in-depth knowledge and understanding of the following:

1. Medicare Conditions of Participation
2. The home health agency (HHA) manual related to Medicare coverage and documentation requirements
3. Correct completion of the Health Care Financing Administration (HCFA) 485 Series forms

It is important to note that payors other than Medicare may also request that the HCFA form 485 be used for their patients.

Although home care generally is a more regulated environment than an inpatient setting in which the patients are in one building and can be supervised, because of the increasing costs and resources attributed to home care and its growth there is much regulatory oversight. Frail and elderly patients in their own homes who are dependent on someone for care may be vulnerable to unscrupulous caregivers.

Home care regulations include Medicare; any state licensure for home care (about half the states have licensure for home care); accreditation bodies; and any applicable laws or regulations, either national or local. Home care clinicians need to be aware of these rules, since the home care nurse is in the pivotal role of documenting care, and many times reimbursement hinges on the documentation.

For all home care clinicians, an in-depth, clinical base of knowledge is needed that is particularly related to observation and physical assessment skills; problem solving; effective communication with physicians, patients, and other team members; and detailed documentation of care and care planning.

Customer Service and Patient-Centered Interpersonal Skills

In home care, simply put, the patients call the shots. Other customers in home care include family members, caregivers, peers, physicians, social workers, managed care nurses, and others who interface with the clinician toward reaching the patient's goals. More and more, customer service and quality are being (re)defined by patient and customer satisfaction.

Unlike many inpatient facilities, where the structure defines the services, in home care, because the patient is at home, patient needs are the criteria that drive the program. The customer-service skills home care clinicians use go a long way in effectively caring for patients and creating good will in the local community. A smile, a kind word, and finding ways to do things better or improve care for patients contribute to customer service for any organization.

Attention to Detail

The ability to pay incredible attention to detail is also a valuable skill that is needed both in documenting and in addressing complex patient needs. Details range from correctly completing all the data elements on the HCFA 485 form and the nursing assessment sheet and following up with verbal orders after speaking with the physician about a change in the plan of care (Form 485) to checking through each medication in a shoebox that may be handed to you during admissions. It has been said that excellence is in the details—this is very true in home care.

Flexibility

Home care agencies value clinicians who possess multifaceted skills accompanied by flexibility. It is the home care clinician who must "bend" or renegotiate, based on the patient's needs and desires, to meet patient-centered outcomes. Obviously flexibility plays an important role in scheduling visiting times, but it is also necessary to be flexible about other aspects of care that center around accommodating patient and caregiver needs. The home care clinician must be prepared for the unexpected (e.g., a snow storm, the supplier delivering the wrong size catheter, or the patient forgetting to tell you that the house numbering system on their street has been changed). She or he should try to always have additional catheters or supplies that are needed for individual patients, because there will be days where what can go wrong does. Be prepared!

Reliable Car and Effective Driving Skills

The home care clinician must have a reliable car and safe, effective driving skills; must like (or at least not mind) to drive (even in inclement weather); have a good sense of direction (or a map); and be willing to take risks (everyone takes wrong turns sometimes or gets lost).

Assumption of Responsibility: Case Management

Home care case managers must be willing and able to assume responsibility for the patient and the patient's plan of care. This total patient management function, with its associated prioritizing and complex decision making, renders home care nursing unique. Sick or at-risk patients depend on the home care clinician as the team member who coordinates and plans continued care.

Case management is an effective tool in home care. From the initial admitting assessment, beginning with the identification and use of nursing or other diagnoses through documentation to discharge, it is the home care nurse who plans, coordinates, and follows through on planned care. The home care nurse or therapist is the team member who identifies when goals are achieved or when progress has occurred and communicates these findings to the other team members for their input and follow-up. The team members directly provide and thus impact the care and see the results of the care provided. Because of the small number of team members involved in care (as opposed to the inpatient setting), outcomes may be more directly attributable to care rendered. In this true case or care management role, the nurse ensures that "everyone on the team is on the same page" in relation to patient care and outcome achievement.

Note that in practice, many in home care receive a great deal of personal and job satisfaction from the simple positive patient and family outcomes and feedback.

Strong Clinical Skills

The experience gained through inpatient clinical care has implications for the transition to becoming an effective home care practitioner. The clinical skills that are very helpful include observation; assessment; teaching; technical skills such as catheterization, infusions, and other medication administrations; critical thinking; documentation; care coordination; analysis of clinical data; knowledge of admitting processes; and discharge planning.

Ability to Function as a Generalist and Specialist

Home care clinicians must possess the ability to function as both a generalist and specialist. This means that, although the home care clinician may be able to competently and proficiently care for a wide range of patients and clinical problems, she or he usually has an additional area of expertise (e.g., specialized clinical practice area, orientation of new staff, information resource).

Home care clinicians care for patients of all ages and health problems. Care needs can vary from day to day or from visit to visit. In home care, even though each clinician may care for a defined patient caseload, the wide range of clinical problems and nursing diagnoses demand that she or he be a resource. Sometimes home care can feel like a solitary practice. Thus peers are often sought out for their input into solutions to patient problems. Other resources are other discipline team members, preceptors, and managers. This team support is very important in making a successful and long-term transition to home care.

Expertise such as maternal-child care or being a certified infusion nurse is also important as new nurses are introduced to home care. (See Chapter 18 for information about certifications and other opportunities for professional growth in home care.)

Self-Direction and Independence

Although resources are available, self-direction and the ability to function autonomously in a nonstructured atmosphere are vital. The transition is huge from an inpatient area such as an intensive care unit (ICU) where the nurse must tell someone if she or he leaves the unit and where there are protocols and standing orders for contingency plans to a large geographic territory where one nurse cares for patients and may call in two times a day to a manager. For this reason, many nurses new to home care may find the transition difficult. Being aware of this change, processing it to one's comfort level, and speaking with the manager can help.

Self-direction involves initiating and following through on patient needs and clinical responsibilities. This includes having well-developed time management skills to address the many detailed aspects of home care, including visit schedules, timely completion of required documentation, and detail-oriented administrative- or visit-related activities such as completing plans of care, making phone calls, and communicating with other team members.

Continued Education

The desire to continue to learn and to be open to new information and clinical skills is necessary. Home care providers must always be learning. New technologies, research, and other information come from many sources. In the mid-1980s, patients receiving dobutamine for severe cardiac failure were in the ICU. Now patients receive this care at home from proficient home care nurses. Other patients that remain home now include patients needing blood or blood component therapies and ventilator care (see Chapter 17).

Sincere Appreciation of and for People

Home care clinicians must enjoy interacting with patients and caregivers. This includes interacting positively with and being empathetic toward patients, families, and caregivers who are most often in the midst of crisis. The feelings of loss, grief, or helplessness that accompany illness or disability are clearly seen by home care clinicians as patients experience these feelings and perhaps their frustrations, in their own environment; the nurse just happens to be there. This supportive role of helper and listener goes a long way in assisting patients in adapting to these changes.

Since many traditional caregivers continue to work outside the home, professional team members use their teaching and training skills to maintain patients safely in their homes. This teaching or consulting role brings satisfaction to the clinicians as well as comfort and security to their families.

Open-Mindedness and Acceptance of Others

Home care team members need to be open and sincerely accepting of each person's unique and chosen life-style and of the associated effects that these life-style choices have on their health. Many clinicians have cared for patients who have had throat or neck cancer from smoking, yet continue to smoke through their stomas even after radical surgery and a tracheostomy. Judgments about life-style, the presence or absence of family support, and the choices patients make with which team members may not agree must be voiced diplomatically and carefully and only when appropriate.

In home care, staff care for diverse patient populations who may have cultural beliefs and traditions that they may personally disagree with or even find offensive. It is important to be able to be objective and professional while caring for all patients and patient problems. Your supervisor may be able to assist you with patients that are difficult for you to care for or those that present ethical dilemmas.

Ability to Balance Clinical and Administrative Responsibilities

The awareness and acceptance of the constant balance between clinical and administrative responsibilities is important. Home care clinicians must have the knowledge that both demands are equally important, but in different ways and for different reasons.

Sense of Humor

A kind sense of humor can help patients and peers get through rough days. Humor is being officially recognized for its healing power. When used appropriately with colleagues, patients, and others, it can convey kindness and an appreciation of life and its sometimes humorous situations.

Ability to Acknowledge that Change is Difficult

Change can be difficult. The home care culture and structure can be very different for nurses making the transition to home care. Although the "down the hall" camaraderie and the daily on-site supervision of inpatient areas are missing, that support and those resources may be just a phone call away or a matter of getting together with home care colleagues after scheduled patient "visiting hours."

Time-Management Skills

Successful mastery of time management and delegation skills is essential to daily operations in home care. These skills will be needed throughout a home care (or any other) career. Clinicians must be able to manage scheduling visits, documentation, and other administrative support activities related to patient care. For example, the tracking of 485s or recertification, verbal orders, projection of schedules, and adherence to the plan of care demand professionals who are detail-oriented and even value that detail. *Mastering the management of many details is key to long-term success for staff making the transition to home care.*

COMMUNITY HEALTH AND HOME CARE ROLES: THE INTERFACE

It is important to note that any nurse practicing in the home setting, including hospice nurses, public health nurses, and other community-based home visitors, must have the skills that have been discussed.

Home health nursing is a synthesis of community health nursing and selected technical skills from other specialty practices. With a basis in community health nursing, the best home care integrates health promotion and disease prevention with the goals of self-care into its practice. Home care then is a complex integration of hands-on care and technical skills with higher level assessment and analysis skills that take into account the patients' care setting, as well as the family and other caregivers and the realistic setting of common goals. In home care the patients and their caregivers are the focus of care as they will continue the plan after home care has withdrawn. Home care at its best truly plans for discharge on admission and has a contract with patients and caregivers to facilitate the achievement of common and predetermined goals and outcomes to identify when discharge is appropriate.

There have been attempts to differentiate or define the relationship between home care nursing and community health nursing practice. This is important to know as reimbursement systems are changing and home care begins to look more like community health (Figure 3-1). In essence, managed care, of which capitation is one model, is a method that incorporates regulation and competition to try and control costs. When capitated reimbursement is fully operationalized, the payors may cover more traditional community health practices, with the knowledge that prevention can save resources. An example is the frail, 84-year-old woman who has chronic obstructive pulmonary disease (COPD). When the heat, humidity, and pollen count are high, she has traditionally had an exacerbation of the COPD, has come into the emergency room, and has been admitted into the high-cost ICU. Nurses who have practiced in community health before home health know that, when they bring and install an air conditioner at her home, teach her about the need to increase fluids, caution her to stay indoors with the air conditioner on, and increase her bronchodilators after speaking with the doctor, she stays well throughout the summer, or at least does not go into the ICU. These patient education– and self-care–directed functions will only increase as payors cover care for patients across the continuum, and the bulk of it will be provided at home. Some states such as California require additional training before a nurse can practice or be a manager in home or community health.

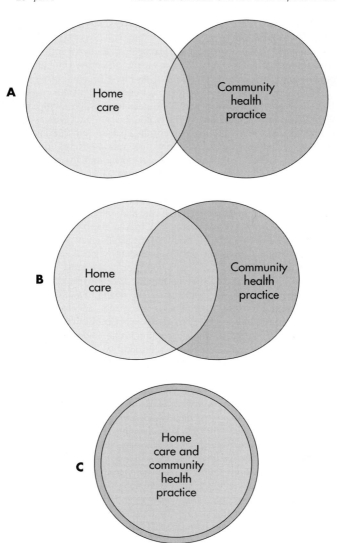

FIGURE 3-1 Interaction of home care and community health practice. **A,** Present. **B** and **C,** Future.

Home care nursing at its best is needed to establish and maintain boundaries strengthened by practice standards. Increased levels of education, advanced skill, research, and commitment to collaborative functioning by all professionals involved are factors nurturing home care growth with positive outcomes.

THE MOST COMMON PROBLEMS CARED FOR IN HOME CARE

With the increasing acuity level of patients being cared for at home, it is easy to see why research-based standards must be adhered to and why there must be standardization of patient care and care processes. Patients needing home care have varied health problems. Georgetown University School of Nursing conducted an HCFA-sponsored study and reported the following as the most common medical diagnoses found in the Medicare home care patient population (Saba and Coopey, 1991):

- Congestive heart failure
- Cerebral vascular accident
- Chronic obstructive pulmonary disease
- Pneumonia
- Hypertension

Other diagnoses included pressure ulcers, diabetes mellitus, cancers, and myocardial infarctions.

ACCREDITATION IN HOME CARE

Over the past decade there has been increasing pressure to decrease costs in health care. Home care, because it is seen as the lowest-cost setting for health care, is receiving increased pressure to demonstrate quality in care and services. When care is given compassionately, competently, and efficiently, it costs less. This satisfies consumers or customers of care (i.e., the patients/clients and the insurance payors).

The emphasis on quality and performance improvement are important factors in health care practice and operations. Quality improvement initiatives are credited as being the method that rebuilt and revitalized the Japanese manufacturing industry. Accreditation is one way to initiate the processes of continuous quality and performance improvement in home care. Accreditation helps home care organizations measure their performance in relation to nationally accepted standards. The actual labor-intensive, lengthy process of accreditation promotes the coordination and integration of quality health care delivery by all team members involved in care. There are two main accreditation bodies in home care. They are the Community Health Accreditation Program (CHAP) and the Joint Commission on Accreditation of Healthcare Organizations (JCAHO). Both have developed standards and have measured home care providers against these standards. Accreditation is usually required by managed care organizations before contracting with home care organizations. Home care programs may choose to seek accreditation for the purpose of stimulating continuous improvement in patient care and services.

Quality improvement is a proactive approach that minimizes the potential for future errors rather than focusing on their resolution after the problems occur. This is another way of ensuring that quality is designed into the product and services.

Accreditation brings an additional level of recognition to a home care organization. Home care accreditation demands continuous quality and performance improvement, as it is an ongoing process and an investment in the improvement of services. In addition, accreditation demonstrates a home care organization's commitment and accountability to patients/clients, payors, regulators, and others.

In summary, accreditation is not an overlay to practice and care provided in the home; rather, it is the belief that services or interventions should be provided in the right way at the right time. To this end and whenever possible, this book is set up along functional lines, and applicable accreditation standards are integrated into the information provided.

SUMMARY

The structure and rules of home care practice may have changed, but the roots of home care are well-defined in history. Home care nursing practice is exciting, dynamic, independent, challenging, and rewarding. It is nursing at its best. Its basis should be scientific theory and research, and its practice boundaries determined by professional standards.

Throughout the many changes and the tumultuous growth in home care, one factor has remained constant: the essential and predominant component of home health care is nursing care. Reviewing the information found in Box 3-1 and revisiting these same questions and your responses in the months to come may be helpful as the transition to home care continues.

REVIEW EXERCISES

1. Identify three of the top diagnoses cared for in home care.
2. List four differences between inpatient and home care practice.
3. Describe the interface between community health and home care nursing.

BOX 3-1   **MAKING THE LEAP: 10 QUESTIONS FOR CONSIDERATION**

The following 10 questions are directed toward clinicians who are considering making the change to home care. Although they are phrased as yes or no questions, there are no right or wrong answers. The questions are cues to start thoughtful consideration of the depth and breadth of the change in practice and setting that occurs when the care setting is the home.

1. Do you like to work alone primarily?

Considerations: And although you may work alone, can you make the needed and added efforts to communicate and care-conference with other team members? The care coordination that occurs many times is not face-to-face and requires multiple phone calls, voice mails, and paper trails to meet patient care needs, as well as regulatory requirements.

2. Do you believe that *all* team members make equally important contributions to patients and outcomes?

Considerations: They do in home care.

3. Do you know the unique skills and treatment modalities that others bring to the team and the patients?

Considerations: In home care the therapists, social workers, home health aides, dietitians, and others have specified activities that the case manager must readily identify to consult with these specialists.

4. Do you like to drive, even at night?

Considerations: Patient care is 24 hours a day, and on-call nurses and primary care clinicians may make visits at all hours. Some patients may live in very remote or inaccessible areas; others live in rural, urban, or suburban settings. The distance that must be traveled to provide care requires that team members like to drive.

5. Do you value and pay attention to detail?

Considerations: In home care excellence is in the details of daily operations, scheduling, documenting, reporting, and the myriad other facets that contribute to quality patient care with predetermined and positive outcomes.

6. Are you considered an expert or excellent clinician who has strong assessment skills and critical thinking skills?

continued

BOX 3-1   **MAKING THE LEAP: 10 QUESTIONS FOR**
           CONSIDERATION—cont'd

Considerations: The clinical skills and strengths brought to home care are key to making a successful transition. Other areas addressed during the orientation (e.g., documentation, time management in a two- or three-county area) take so much of the focus that when the clinical skills are already strong, the new clinician makes the transition more efficiently. In addition, unlike the inpatient setting, where we can find another clinician for a second opinion, the clinical skills in home care demand strength, depth, and experience in assessment and other skills.

7. Generally, can you talk to anyone about anything?

Considerations: In home care, that's just what happens. As a guest in a patient and family's home, we begin a very personal relationship with boundaries that are sometimes more difficult to maintain because of this very personal contact.

8. In your other work experiences, was it hard for you personally when patients and caregivers had very different life-styles and made choices about care that you may not have agreed with?

Considerations: In home care, clinicians care for patients in the middle of a chosen life-style and values that may be very different from our own. But these very differences are also what make home care such a unique and sometimes inspiring setting in which to work.

9. Are you aware of personal and car safety generally?

Considerations: In home care nurses practice in the community, and crime and theft may be a part of some communities. This awareness of ourselves and property is a real part of providing home care. It can be very frightening when the clinician pulls up to a curb in an urban area and everyone is sitting outside watching her or his every move. Similarly, night visits when it is snowing and icy, quiet, and dark can make the home care nurse feel very alone.

10. Do you want to work in the health care setting in which patients and their families are equal partners in care and care planning and make their own choices and the clinicians are facilitators for teaching and self-care?

Considerations: Then you have chosen home care, the health care setting of the future.

4. Autonomy in practice, clinical assessment, and time management are three important competencies that must be achieved by the clinician entering into home care practice. True or False?
5. List five of the skills and knowledge areas that a clinician must have to be successful in home care.

REFERENCE

Saba VK, Coopey M: *Develop and demonstrate a method for classifying home health patients to predict resource requirements and to measure outcomes,* Home Health Care Classification Project, Georgetown University School of Nursing, HCFA Co-operative Agreement No. 17-C-98983/3-01, February 1991, Table 8.50, p 138.

FOR FURTHER READING

American Nurses Association: *Standards of home health nursing practice,* Washington, DC, 1986, American Nurses Association.

American Nurses Association: *A statement on the scope of home health nursing practice,* Washington, DC, 1992, American Nurses Association.

Applegate V: Moving from the operating room to home care, *Orthopedic Nursing,* 14(2):30-31, 1995.

Murray T: Switching from hospital-based practice to home care, *Home Care Provider* 1(2):79-82, 1996.

Nightingale F: *Notes on nursing: what it is and what it is not,* Commemorative Edition, Philadelphia, 1992, Lippincott.

Sherry D: The incredible f-l-e-x-i-b-l-e nurse, *Nursing 85,* December, 1985, p 72.

Stulginsky M: Nurses' home health experience. Part I. The practice setting, *Nursing Health Care* 14(8):402-407, 1993.

Stulginsky M: Nurses' home health experience. Part II. The unique demands of home visits, *Nursing Health Care* 14(9):476-485, 1993.

4

ORIENTATION CONSIDERATIONS

Tina M. Marrelli, MSN, MA, RNC

"Nurses who would laugh at the idea of learning a specialty such as oncology in a 2-week orientation somehow expect that hospital nurses will learn home health care in that length of time and are disappointed when the hospital nurses fail."

Carr, 1991

Everyone knows how exciting and difficult it can be to leave what one seems to know intrinsically to learn new skills in a foreign environment. But the challenge is worth the work. Welcome to home care! Even though, as stated in the opening quotation, there is much to learn in home care and the process appropriately takes much longer than the length of the official orientation period, no nurse new to home care should care for patients without an effective orientation. Orientation periods range in scope, depth, and span, depending on the organization. The information in this chapter provides a framework for review and reference as the nurse makes the transition to home care. Because this book is organized functionally, this chapter provides information about the nuts and bolts of the orientation process.

THE DIFFERENCE: MORE THAN THE ENVIRONMENT

In home care, which is at some level the antithesis of inpatient care, the patient has control and calls the shots. This alone can be frightening. Because the goals of care are focused on patient education and ultimately on self-care and independence, home care patients must be very knowledgeable about their health history and problems. In home care the nurse assists and supports patients with their choices and care.

Unlike the hospital, there are no set visiting hours and no limits on the ages of visitors. Patients wear what they want, keep the hours they choose, eat when and what they want, and make choices about other facets of life-style. Home care staff are truly in an assistive role in home care, with the focus directed toward discharging the patient back to the community, either caring for self or with a trained caregiver.

Many patients in the community have caregivers who have been trained by home care nurses to administer injections, including B_{12}, insulin, or Calcimar, as well as to ensure that wounds that may never heal are kept clean and to change urinary catheters.

Orientation is perhaps the most important period in the role transformation to home care clinician, and the initial information presented may set the stage for future growth and professional development. The orientation period is the time designated to hone clinical skills, find answers, and develop new relationships with peers and managers. It has been said that excellence "is in the details," and this is very true in home care. During orientation, information is provided about documentation, detailed assessments, thoughtful data analysis, and the importance of clear communications to other team members. These are the kinds of details that contribute to safe and effective home care. Perhaps most important, orientation is the time to be detail-oriented and provided with information that constitutes the "practical wisdom" of home care.

AN OVERVIEW OF THE MARKET SEGMENTS

There are different and specialty home care entities within the home care industry, and professional clinicians may join and work in any of these segments. All of these market segments are considered "home care." In addition, some home care companies may provide all, or just one of these segments directly, and all of these kinds of home care businesses can be accredited.

Durable Medical/Home Medical Equipment Company

The durable medical/home medical equipment companies are comprised of distributors and manufacturers that primarily supply and deliver equipment such as wheelchairs, walkers, and oxygen to patients in their homes. Nurses and/or respiratory therapists may be employed to facilitate patient teaching, create educational materials, provide assessments, and market their services.

Home Infusion Therapy Company

Home infusion companies provide for the delivery and administration of infusion services to patients. These services can include parenteral and enteral nutrients, the delivery and administration of blood or blood products, dobutamine therapy, intravenous antibiotics or chemotherapy, and hyperalimentation. This market has had significant growth through the 1980s and 1990s, and it continues to change due to regulatory and reimbursement changes. Still, it is usually more cost-effective to provide these services at home than in an inpatient setting. For an in-depth review of this specialty area for home care nurses, refer to Chapter 17.

Private Duty or Personal Care Company

These agencies provide care to patients in their homes. They are the traditional "staffing" agencies that provide shifts or 24-hour care to patients, based on their needs and ability to pay. Services include nurses, home health aides, live-in attendants, companions or sitters, and homemakers. Services may be paid by the patient or family or, if they are skilled, reimbursed by insurers.

Home Health Agency

The home health agency (HHA) is the largest segment of home care and provides skilled services. This segment of the industry employs the most clinicians. For this reason, this text will focus on this component of home care practice, although the information provided helps ensure quality, regardless of the type of home care service, organization, or product offered.

Community-Based Hospice Providers

Hospice care is growing at an unprecedented rate. Hospice care focuses on quality and making each day the best it can be for patients who have a limited life expectancy. The true team concept in hospice care assists patients and their families and friends through care, death, and bereavement programs. Some hospices may be specialized, such as a pediatric hospice program. Hospice care is a philosophy and not a care site; however, most hospice care is provided at home. Hospices may be hospital-based, freestanding community-based, an inpatient specialty area, a home health organization, or other models. The Medicare hospice benefit is a managed care benefit, and the hospice team case manages the hospice patient across care sites (see Chapter 16).

DEFINING HOME HEALTH AGENCY ORIENTATION

Figure 4-1 illustrates the percent of agencies that provide home care services. Skilled nursing is the most common service provided, followed by personal care, and then physical therapy. The scope of services provided by an HHA include skilled nursing services, physical and occupational therapy, speech-language pathology services, medical social services, and home health aides, based on patient needs and the

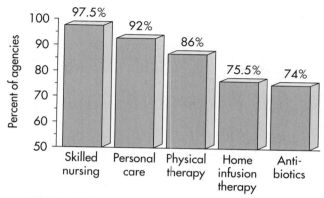

FIGURE 4-1 The services most often offered in home care. *(Redrawn with permission of Marion Merrell Dow Inc Managed Care Digest Series, Institutional Digest, 1995; data from SMG Marketing Group Inc, 1995.)*

unique mission of the home care organization. (The home care team and their roles is discussed later in this chapter.)

There are many aspects of home care that must be covered in the limited official orientation period. There will be several overall behavioral outcomes or goals for the transitioning home care clinician:

1. Completes the orientation within the time allocated
2. Identifies key staff members and customers (defined by the organization)
3. Describes and explains new patient assignment processes
4. Demonstrates clinical competence in the home setting
5. Adheres to policies and procedures as observed/monitored
6. Knows where to go for questions or challenges related to practice and operations
7. Others, as defined by the individual organization

One of Webster's dictionary definitions for orient is "to acquaint with the existing situation or environment." In health care generally there is so much occurring in the external environment that in home care orientation the focus is on the internal organizational environment. The first part of this text provided the environmental framework of health care and its current impact on home care. The American Nurses Association (ANA) defines orientation as "the means by which new staff members are introduced

---

BOX 4-1   **ABSORBING IT ALL: FIVE TIPS FOR ORIENTEES**

1. Complete assessment questions (or weekly evaluation forms) completely and accurately. This assists you and your manager/instructor/preceptor in goal revision.
2. Take notes. Voluminous and important information is provided, and it is sometimes difficult at the beginning to see the bigger picture. These notes can refresh your memory.
3. Ask questions. Others may have the same questions and not ask them. Questions clarify and may inspire additional explanations that may help you remember certain information, as well as address any confusing issues.
4. Actively listen. The depth and breadth of information demands this level of participation.
5. At the conclusion or after a defined time period, whenever the evaluation process occurs, complete evaluation forms and provide comments to assist the organization in the ongoing efforts to improve the orientation program and related processes.

Reprinted with permission from Marrelli and Associates: *Home Care Nurse News,* vol. 3, No. 8, 1996.

to the philosophy, goals, policies, procedures, role expectation, physical facilities, and special services in a specific work setting" (Box 4-1).

COMPETENCY ASSESSMENT AND VALIDATION

Nurses new to home care can expect that their new or perspective home care employer will check their references and have them complete a self-assessment tool or checklist. These checklists identify specific skills or areas of knowledge and education. Figure 4-2 shows an example of a skills checklist. The checklist is a way for employers to identify areas the nurse may need to review or to be observed. It is also a way to validate competency, which is a hallmark of quality in home care practice. This process of identifying educational and orientation needs is a way the home care program ensures that it hires qualified team members. The checklist provides an example and may be used for self-assessment.

It is important to note that some organizations identify their own list of high-risk, low-volume skills and may have all nurses new to home care demonstrate these skills. Examples include tracheostomy care and specialty assessments. A preceptor may accompany the new nurse in the field for certain skills, again to ensure safe and effective patient care.

Text continued on p. 45.

Home Care Nurse Competency Assessment Form

Tasks	Self Assessment (√/—Needs Review)	Competency Demonstrated (Date)	Preceptor or Supervisor Signature

General Home Care Issues:
 	
RN can demonstrate an understanding of:
 	
• Medicare regulations
  • Homebound status
  • Intermittent
  • Skilled need
  • Physician orders			

• Managed care or other payer requirements
  • Authorization status/contact
  • Visit frequencies
  • Supplies/equipment
  • Communication and documentation			

• Organizational mission and philosophy
  • Types of services
  • Conflict resolution
  • Ethical issue resolution			

• Personnel issues
  • Staff scheduling requirements
  • Sick call protocols
  • Time off requests
  • Pay periods and submission of time slips
  • Conflict resolution
  • Dress code and name badges			

FIGURE 4-2 Form used to assess nursing skills in home care.

continued

Tasks	Self Assessment (✓/—Needs Review)	Competency Demonstrated (Date)	Preceptor or Supervisor Signature
• Time management and visit scheduling • Scheduling visits • Contacting patients for visits/delays • Obtaining supplies • Content of visits • Communication with team members • Travel issues			
• Documentation • Submission time frames • Completeness and accuracy guidelines • Clinical documentation issues • Activity logs—visits and mileage			
• Roles of interdisciplinary team members • Registered physical therapist • Occupational therapist • Speech-language pathologist • Medical social worker • Home health aide • Dietitian • Enterostomal therapy nurse • Other clinical specialists			
• Clinical protocols/clinical pathways or others • Specific patients • Guidelines for use			

• Meetings
  • Team meetings (case conferences)
  • Staff meetings
  • Others, as defined by agency					

• Emergencies in home
  • After hours on-call status
  • How to access supervisor
  • Patient teaching—number to call					

• Customer service skills
  • Identifying types of customers
  • Telephone etiquette
  • Handling difficult patients/families					

• Safety
  • Personal role in agency safety plan
  • Driving safely
  • Personal "street" safety
  • Fire and emergency—preparedness
  • Hazard communication plan
  • Reporting accidents					

• Infection control policies
  • Universal precautions
  • Nursing bag technique
  • Care of transportable equipment
  • Disposal of wastes in home
  • Patient/family teaching					

• Process improvement/QA program
  • Role of employee
  • Interaction with staff					

FIGURE 4-2, cont'd Form used to assess nursing skills in home care.

continued

Tasks	Self Assessment (√—Needs Review)	Competency Demonstrated (Date)	Preceptor or Supervisor Signature

• Risk management program
    • Legal liabilities
    • Reporting of unusual occurrences			

• Other areas as defined by organization			
ROLE RESPONSIBILITIES: Generalist RN can demonstrate understanding of:			
• The organization's admission criteria			

• Admission process, including all elements to be completed with patient and/or family
    • Rights and responsibilities
    • Consent for treatment
    • Advance directives
    • Financial/insurance information forms
    • Involvement of patient/family in care planning
    • Initiating patient visit calendar
    • Environmental/safety checklist			

• Completion of admission assessment and related documentation
    • Data base/nursing assessment (age, cultural, gender specific)
    • Clinical note
    • Nursing care plan
    • Medication profile
    • Environmental/safety care assessment and plan
    • Supplemental orders			

• Communication with attending physician • Verbal orders for services/supplies			

• Referral to other disciplines—documentation
  • Criteria for PT, OT, SLP, MSW, dietitian
  • Coordination of care and services
  • Criteria for home health aide
    • Development of HHA care plan
    • Plotting and scheduling of supervisory visits
    • Performing supervisory visits			

• Clinical assessment criteria • By system			
• Clinical procedure(s) • As documented on skills checklist			

• Cultural diversity issues
  • Identify diverse population groups in agency service area
  • List at least two issues that are specific to that cultural group and could impact the delivery of care			

• Access to community resources • Identify local resources			

• Managed care utilization processes
  • Approval points in plan of care
  • Services/equipment/supplies authorization			

FIGURE 4-2, cont'd Form used to assess nursing skills in home care.

continued

Tasks	Self Assessment (✓—Needs Review)	Competency Demonstrated (Date)	Preceptor or Supervisor Signature
Specialist RN can demonstrate understanding of:			
IV Nurse functions			
ET Nurse functions			
Cardiac nurse specialist			
Gerontological nurse specialist			
Maternal/child specialist			
Oncology nurse specialist			
Others as defined by organization			

FIGURE 4-2, cont'd   Form used to assess nursing skills in home care.

ORGANIZATIONAL ORIENTATION TOPICS

The topics that may be addressed by the organizational orientation cover a broad range of content. This information is prioritized in order of importance and emphasizes the regulatory aspects that interface with clinical patient care that must be understood to function safely in home care. This chapter lists topics and areas that should be addressed for quality, safety, practice, and accreditation reasons.

It is important to note that, although this looks like voluminous information, it will all make sense over the months to come. In fact, colleagues who successfully made the transition to home care may have said that "about 6 months into this, it all came together and made sense!" This information is presented in a functional format to make sense to clinicians and managers making this important transition. There are numerous policies in home care, but the listed policies and their associated process/outcomes provide the practical application of the home care specialty. Other policies are incorporated directly into the sections of the text in which they are actually used in home care practice (such as admission visit). Your orientation may initially include other team members such as therapists, pharmacists, home health aides, intake coordinators, home care staff, and clinical managers or educators. This is a great way to meet new colleagues and team members in your new organization. From the beginning, you will see that home care is truly a team effort and that "everyone should be on the same page."

As health care moves to the standardization of care and care processes for quality purposes, nurses see the need for the same information provided across and among the team. Some organizations provide an orientation that is standard for all new employees initially and then as the information becomes more specific, such as for nursing or therapy, the orientation then continues with only those specialized team members.

Mission, Vision, and Values

Home care programs and their managers or owners have unique missions. Simply put, the mission is the bottom line of what the organization does and the reason the organization exists. When the company has a vision or values, the mission statement can be short (e.g., less then one sentence or a few sentences). Examples of missions or mission statements include: "XYZ Home Care provides the best care at the best price with the most competent staff," or "St. Elsewhere Home Care follows the mission of St. Elsewhere Hospital into the community, where we provide comprehensive and high-quality health care."

Process/Outcome

The orientee may receive a copy of the mission statement in his or her orientation packet, along with the history of the organization. Sometimes the mission statement is written on the front or back of the identification/name badge. This mission may also be printed on the agency brochure. It is important that all team members work together, and the mission can help in this quest. On completion of the orientation, the new orientee should be able to state or describe the organization's mission statement and goals.

Organization Brochure

The home care organization's brochure provides important information about the services provided. This is the information shared with patients, discharge planners, and other customers who may be interested in home care services. This brochure lists if the organization is Medicare certified and/or accredited, how patients reach the organization, the on-call system and how to access care after regular business hours, what services are provided through the program, and any specialty programs or other information. Usually the brochure is provided during or before the application process. However, it may be given during the formal orientation as part of the packet of materials for new team members. The geographical areas covered by the organization may also be listed in the brochure or provided as a policy.

Process/Outcome

This information is initially also provided and explained by the nurse during the admitting visit and reinforced on subsequent visits. The new orientee should be able to list and describe the services and other information listed in the brochure about the organization.

Organizational Chart

Where the new employee fits in the organization is very important for reporting, operational, and communication reasons. The organizational chart or table of organization clearly shows the lines of communication and the manager to whom the new team member will report. Keep in mind that in some organizations the new clinician in home care may spend more time with the preceptor or instructor than with her or his immediate supervisor, particularly during orientation, depending on the size and organizational structure of the organization.

Process/Outcome

The new team member in orientation is able to identify managers, peers, and in office support team members to facilitate patient care and organizational operations.

Office Information

This includes the business hours of operations that the office is open, time card and payroll processes, beeper or pager acquisition, car phone and/or allowance, equipment and supply closet/acquisition process, mileage reimbursement, nurse bag sign-out or purchase procedure, schedule of staff meetings, and other processes and details.

Process/Outcome

The new team member can obtain needed supplies or equipment using the standard process provided in the orientation and knows whom to call with a question or for assistance related to these important processes.

Personnel or Human Resource Information

The personnel staff are very important to making a successful transition. As in the hospital, important details must be addressed such as the physical examination, any required laboratory tests, tuberculosis testing, hepatitis vaccine or declination statement, benefit information, CPR certification, professional liability policy, dress code, safety training, standards of conduct, and the organizational grievance process. Background checks, car insurance, and a valid driver's license may also be requested by human resources. Many of these requirements are based on the individual state and organizational policies.

Position Description

The orientee usually receives and may sign a copy of his or her position description and contract, if applicable. An example of a home care nurse position description is shown in Figure 4-3.

Process/Outcome

There may be an evaluation tool with or as a part of the position description for clinicians who are new to home care. Identify what is valued at the organization and work toward achieving high scores on the behaviors and skills listed on the performance appraisal tool.

Important Policies and Procedures

There are numerous but important policies and procedures that the orientee will review and may be asked to sign. In addition, the team member may be given an organization orientation manual that contains the specific and applicable home care clinical and administrative policies.

Process/Outcome

It is very important that the nurse review, be able to describe, and adhere to these policies from accreditation, state survey, and risk management perspectives. The policies include patient rights and responsibilities,

Text continued on p. 53.

JOB DESCRIPTION: HOME HEALTH NURSE-RN

TITLE: Home Health Nurse-RN

DIRECTLY
SUPERVISED BY: Director of Nurses (or designee)

STATUS: Part-Time/Full-Time: Nonexempt

POSITION DESCRIPTION

Provides skilled nursing care, including skilled assessment and instruction for newborn, pediatric, adult, and geriatric patients guided by physician orders and in accordance with established nursing standards and practices.

QUALIFICATIONS AND REQUIREMENTS

Graduate of an accredited school of nursing with current and active state-specific RN license. BSN/PHN preferred.

Minimum 1 year recent acute care or home care experience; with demonstrated competency in 90% of clinical standards within 90 days of hire.

Current CPR certification.

Valid state-specific Driver's License, current automobile insurance, and ready access to a reliable automobile.

A tuberculin skin test (PPD) or chest x-ray and preplacement physical exam at date of hire. Annual tuberculin skin test and a physical exam as required by organization.

Ability to work collaboratively with other clinical and administrative team members.

MARGINAL DUTIES AND RESPONSIBILITIES: Performs other duties as assigned by manager.

PHYSICAL DEMANDS

The physical demands described are those needed for an employee to successfully perform the essential functions of this job. Reasonable accommodations may be made to enable individuals with disabilities to perform the essential functions.

The employee is regularly required to stand; walk; use hands and fingers to examine patients; write; use medical supplies; handle or feel objects, medical and other equipment, and controls; drive; reach with hands and arms; and talk and hear. The employee is frequently required to sit and stoop, kneel, and bend.

The employee must regularly lift and/or move up to 25 pounds, frequently lift and/or move up to 50 pounds, and occasionally lift and/or move more than 100 pounds. Specific vision abilities required by this job include close vision, distance vision, color vision, peripheral vision, depth perception, and the ability to adjust focus.

WORK ENVIRONMENT

The work environment characteristics described here are representative of those an employee encounters while performing the essential functions of this job. In performing this job, the employee regularly travels to patient homes in a variety of weather conditions. The employee occasionally provides skilled nursing care to patients in confined spaces. The noise level in the work environment is usually moderate.

FIGURE 4-3   Sample of a job description for a home care nurse position.

continued

PERFORMANCE EVALUATION: HOME HEALTH NURSE-RN

POSITION TITLE: HOME HEALTH NURSE

PERFORMANCE STANDARD	1	2	3	4
Assesses patient care needs at time of admission and thereafter on an ongoing basis, as patient condition and diagnosis dictate.				
1. Consistently demonstrates knowledge of and adherence to Agency policies and federal/state regulations in assessing patient care needs.				
2. Consistently demonstrates knowledge of and application of principles of the nursing process in the development, implementation, and evaluation of plan of care.				
3. Consistently evaluates nursing plan of care for appropriateness to patient condition, communicates with the physician and other health care team members, and makes referrals as necessary.				
Plans, implements, and evaluates skilled care according to established nursing standards and based on age-specific requirements for newborn, pediatric, adult, and geriatric patients and makes revisions as required, under the physician's plan of treatment.				
1. Consistently uses the principles of the nursing process in care development.				
2. Coordinates care of patient with other care providers, using community resources as appropriate.				
Uses developmental-stage appropriate interventions in planning care for newborn, pediatric, adult, and geriatric patients.				
1. Consistently uses developmental-stage appropriate interventions in planning care for newborn, pediatric, adult, and geriatric patients.				

continued

Consistently notifies physician and other appropriate clinical team members of pertinent changes in the patient's condition.

1. Consistently communicates pertinent changes in the patient's condition to the physician within 4 hours or organizationally mandated time frames.
2. Reports changes in the patient's condition and/or demographic status to the appropriate clinical supervisor and/or other agency staff as appropriate.

Consistently instructs and supervises nursing personnel regarding the needs of the home care patient.

1. Communicates with other members of the team regarding patient care needs as evidenced by attendance at team conferences or other care planning sessions.

Consistently instructs and counsels patient and family regarding patient care needs and community resources, based on age-specific criteria.

1. Uses appropriate communication skills to instruct and counsel patient and family regarding care at home based on age-specific criteria.

Demonstrates knowledge regarding community resources and ability to communicate knowledge to patient and family based on age-specific criteria.

At orientation and annually, thereafter, meets organizational competency requirements for area of specialty.

1. Meets agency competency requirements for area of specialty.

Consistently documents patient assessment, reassessments, interventions, and ongoing care concisely according to organizational policy.

1. Consistently documents care clearly using accepted standards of documentation.
2. Consistently and accurately prepares admission and assessment forms, plan of treatment forms, clinical and progress notes, and other appropriate forms according to organizational policies.
3. Meets all established documentation timelines.

RATING SCALE: Below standard, 1; needs improvement, 2; meets standard, 3; exceeds standard, 4.

FIGURE 4-3, cont'd   Sample of a job description for a home care nurse position.

PERFORMANCE EVALUATION SUMMARY

Total Number of "Exceeds"	× 15 =	(a)
Total Number of "Meets"	× 10 =	(b)
Total Number of "Needs Improvement"	× 5 =	(c)
Total Number of "Below"		(d)
Total Ratings [add (a) + (b) + (c) + (d)]		(e)
Total Number of "Responsibilities"		(f)
Divide (e) by (f)		(g)
RESPONSIBILITIES RATING [Multiply (g) by 1]		(h)
OVERALL RATING (Rating ranges: 1-2.9, Below standard; 3-9.4, needs improvement; 9.5-13.9, meets standard; 14-15, exceeds standard):		

FIGURE 4-3, cont'd　　Sample of a job description for a home care nurse position.

infection control, self-determination/advance directives, community resources, and emergency preparedness.

Patient's Rights and Responsibilities

This policy is listed first because it is a requirement of and is listed as the first of the Medicare Conditions of Participation (COPs). This information is usually explained to the patient or read if the patient needs assistance or has visual problems, and the nurse provides the patient with written notice of his or her rights as a home care patient.

An example of a patient rights and responsibilities form is shown in Figure 4-4. The following five components of the bill of rights may be the most important:

1. The patient is given a signed copy of the notice of rights.
2. The rights explain the respect that the organization will have for the patient and her or his belongings and property.
3. The patient is notified that confidentiality of medical record information is upheld by organization team members.
4. The patient is kept apprised of financial arrangements related to care and coverage and informed that changes are communicated to patients per the rights and responsibility document.
5. The patient/caregiver is made aware of the home health hotline toll-free phone number in each state that patients can use for complaints related to care and/or advance directives.

Process/Outcome

The intent of this process is that patients understand their rights and that team members at all times respect patient choices and decisions. Attitude is essential. The nurse needs to enter the home knowing that she or he is a guest with services to offer that clients are free to accept or reject (Stulginsky, 1993). On completion the nurse will be able to describe the intent and the process at the organization for explaining the patient rights and responsibilities.

Infection Control

There are very specific infection control processes unique to caring for patients in the home environment. The Occupational Safety and Health Administration (OSHA) is the department of the government that is responsible for defining occupational safety for workers. In home care as in the inpatient setting, universal precautions are used as the standard approach to infection control, and the protection and prevention guidelines related to bloodborne pathogens are outlined by OSHA. There are

**HOME CARE PATIENT/CLIENT
RIGHTS AND RESPONSIBILITIES**

As a home care patient/client, you have the right to be informed of your rights and responsibilities before
the initiation of care/service. If/When a patient/client has been judged incompetent, the patient's/client's
family or guardian may exercise these rights as described below. As they relate to:

PATIENT/CLIENT RIGHTS, you have the right:

1. To receive services appropriate to your needs and expect the home care organization to provide safe,
   professional care at the level of intensity needed, without unlawful restriction by reason of age, sex,
   race, creed, color, national origin, religion or disability.
2. To have access to necessary professional services 24 hours a day, 7 days a week.
3. To be informed of services available.
4. To be informed of the ownership and control of the organization.
5. To be told on request if the organization's liability insurance will cover injuries to employees when they
   are in your home, and if it will cover theft or property damage that occurs while you are being treated.

PATIENT/CLIENT CARE, you have the right:

1. To be involved in your care planning, including education of the same, from admission to discharge,
   and to be informed in a reasonable time of anticipated termination and/or transfer of service.
2. To receive reasonable continuity of care.
3. To be informed of your rights and responsibilities in advance concerning care and treatment you will
   receive, including any changes, the frequency of care/service and by whom (disciplines) services will
   be provided.
4. To be informed of the nature and purpose of any technical procedure that will be performed, including information about the potential benefits and burdens as well as who will perform the procedure.
5. To receive care/service from staff who are qualified through education and/or experience to carry
   out the duties for which they are assigned.
6. To be referred to other agencies and/or organizations when appropriate and be informed of any
   financial benefit to the referring agency.

RESPECT AND CONFIDENTIALITY, you have the right:

1. To be treated with consideration, respect, and dignity, including the provision of privacy during care.
2. To have your property treated with respect.
3. To have staff communicate in a language or form you can reasonably be expected to understand and
   when possible, the organization assists with or may provide special devices, interpreters, or other aids
   to facilitate communication.
4. To maintain confidentiality of your clinical records in accordance with legal requirements and to anticipate the organization will release information only with your authorization or as required by law.
5. To be informed of the organization's policies and procedures for disclosure of your clinical record.

FINANCIAL ASPECTS OF CARE, you have the right:

1. To be informed of the extent to which payment for the home care services may be expected from
   Medicare, Medicaid or any other payer.
2. To be informed of charges not covered by Medicare and/or responsibility for any payment(s) that you
   may have to make.
3. To receive this information orally and in writing before care is initiated and within 30 calendar days of
   the date the organization becomes aware of any changes.

Form 3531 © 1994 Briggs Corporation, Des Moines, IA 50306   **RIGHTS AND RESPONSIBILITIES**
To order, phone 1-800-247-2343 PRINTED IN U.S.A.   **Continued on Reverse**

2446 p1 f1 part one

FIGURE 4-4   Example of a patient rights and responsibilities form.
*(Reprinted with permission of Briggs Health Care Products, Des
Moines, Iowa.)*

SELF-DETERMINATION, you have the right:

1. To refuse all or part of your care/treatment to the extent permitted by law and to be informed of the expected consequences of said action.
2. To be informed in writing of rights under state law to formulate advance directives.
3. To have the organization comply with advance directives as permitted by state law and state requirements.
4. To be informed of the organization's policies and procedures for implementing advance directives.
5. To receive care whether or not you have an advance directive(s) in place, as well as not to be discriminated against whether or not you have executed an advance directive(s).
6. To be informed regarding the organization's policies for withholding of resuscitative services and the withdrawal of life-sustaining treatment, as appropriate.
7. To not participate in research or not receive experimental treatment unless you give documented, voluntary informed consent.
8. To be informed of what to do in an emergency.
9. To participate in consideration of ethical issues that may arise in your care.

COMPLAINTS, you have the right:

1. To voice complaints/grievances about treatment or care that is (or fails to be) furnished, or regarding lack of respect for property without reprisal or discrimination for same and be informed of the procedure to voice complaints/grievances with the home care organization. Complaints or questions may be registered with _____
   Define individual(s)
   by phone, in person or in writing. The address and phone are _____

   _____

   The organization investigates the complaint and resolution of same.

2. To be informed of the State Hotline. The _____ also has a State Hotline for complaints
   Define entity
   or questions about local home care agencies as well as to voice concerns regarding advance directives.

   The State Hotline number is **1-800-**_____.

   and the days/hours of operation are _____

PATIENT/CLIENT RESPONSIBILITIES

As a home care patient/client, you have the responsibility:

1. To provide complete and accurate information about illness, hospitalizations, medications, and other matters pertinent to your health; any changes in address, phone or insurance/payment information; and changes made to advance directives.
2. To inform the organization when you will not be able to keep your home care appointment.
3. To treat the staff with respect.
4. To participate in and follow your plan of care.
5. To provide a safe environment for care to be given.
6. To cooperate with staff and ask questions if you do not understand instruction or information given to you.
7. To assist the organization with billing and/or payment issues to help with processing third party payment.
8. To inform the organization of any problems or dissatisfaction with services.

RIGHTS AND RESPONSIBILITIES

2446   p2 f1   part two

FIGURE 4-4, cont'd   For legend see opposite page.

policies addressing the identification, handling, and disposal of biohazardous wastes in home care. Various policies related to the resurgence, prevention, and screening for tuberculosis; the disinfection of supplies; and aspects of infection control, including reporting and identification, will also be provided by the organization.

Process/Outcome

The home care organization should always have proper personal protective equipment available to staff. This equipment includes disposable latex gloves, masks, aprons or other coverings, mouthpieces for cardiopulmonary resuscitation (CPR), and other equipment as necessary. The CPR mask should be on the home care nurse's person (i.e., not in the car parked in front of the patient's home).

Infection control related to the nurse bag and equipment must be maintained. The contents and equipment must be kept from being contaminated, particularly as they could be a source of cross-contamination. Review the organizational policies related to the cleaning of supplies and the frequency of these cleanings. Some organizations have designated "bag check" days, when an inventory of the contents and the process for retrieval and storage of equipment are reviewed.

Effective and regular handwashing in the home is critical to the provision of high quality care. Organizations provide paper towels and soap and/or foam soap, should patients not have running water for the nurse to wash his or her hands. In addition, paper towels (never the patient's cloth towels unless the nurse knows that the towels are clean) and only liquid soap (not bar soap) should be used in the patient's home. It is important to note that infection control and adherence to related policies are heavily weighted standards by accreditation surveyors.

On completion of the orientation, the orientee must be able to describe infection control practices in home care (as specified by the organization) and verbalize and correctly demonstrate bag technique and effective handwashing skills.

Self-Determination/Advance Directives

The Federal Patient Self-Determination Act of 1990 was designed for patients to decide in advance what health care decisions are to be made should the patient lose his or her capacity to do so. All Medicare participating entities, such as hospices and home care agencies, must comply with the advance directive provisions of the Omnibus Budget Reconciliation Act (OBRA). This policy is usually distributed to clinicians during orientation. Because the law requires that organizations inform patients in writing of its policies regarding the implementation of advance directives, as well as educate staff and the community on issues concerning advance directives, most organizations also have the admitting nurse provide this information to the patient on admission to home care *(Home Health Agency Manual—Pub. 11, 132.1* [HCFA]).

Process/Outcome

Many times patients who have come out of the hospital are aware of advance directives and may have thought about and/or discussed them with their family members or physician. The clinician's role is usually to provide an informational flyer of resources should the patient wish more information. On completion of orientation the nurse orientee should be able to describe the intent of the self-determination law and the nurse's role in implementing this requirement in the organization.

Community Resources

A list of available community resources may be given during orientation. This list should provide linkage to services in the community and may include such educational resources as the local cancer society, podiatrists who make home visits, and the area office on aging.

Process/Outcome

The home care nurse usually functions in the case manager role and coordinates care for the patient across health care settings, and patients are notified of services available. Linkage and rapport with community resources assist in ensuring communication with resources after formal home care service is withdrawn. It is important to remember that the ultimate goal of home care is self-care and/or education of family and caregivers and that the nurse is pivotal in the educational process and in helping to identify and follow up on these community connections. On completion the nurse orientee should be able to reference and identify possible resources based on examples or patient cases discussed during orientation.

Emergency Preparedness

The home care organization has a process should an emergency occur during which the normal operations of the agency or office may be shut down. Examples include fire, hurricanes, ice storms and blizzards, floods, power outages that affect local phone service, and earthquakes. The organization has a plan that is practiced should such a disaster occur. This is why many clinicians and managers have cellular phones as a backup system for emergencies.

Process/Outcome

Patient care continues, patients are prioritized based on their needs, and nurses and other team members know their roles and activities in the process. Cellular phones, telephone trees for communications, a listing

---

BOX 4-2   HOME CARE POLICIES

Management/Governance

Agency mission, philosophy,
    and objectives
Conflict of interest policy
Agency scope of services
Agency availability
Organizational relationships
    Governing body list
    Agency organizational chart
Code of organizational ethics
Designated line of authority
Financial management policy
Professional advisory committee
Program evaluation committee
Utilization review committee
Professional staff privileges
Medical advisor role responsi-
    bility
Physician responsibilities in
    home health care
Personnel policies
Staff credentialing
Orientation of new employees
Staff education
Contract services
General office policies
Others

Patient Rights

Patient/client rights and re-
    sponsibilities
Advance directive policy
Patient Self-Determination Act

Ethical issues in home care
Consents policy
Others

Patient Care Policies

Patient admission criteria
Patient referral policy
Patient assignment and sched-
    uling policy
Coordination of home health
    services
Discharge, transfer, or termina-
    tion of service guidelines
Withholding/withdrawal of life
    sustenance/do not resusci-
    tate policy
Refusal of services policy
Care of the terminally ill patient
Others

Home Health Services

Psychiatric home care program
    Handling a suicide crisis
Maternal/child health program
Physical therapy assistant pro-
    tocol
Standards of home care prac-
    tice
Plan of care (treatment) HCFA
    485
Discipline-specific plans of care
Team/case conference policy
    Patient and family education

---

of the patients with an assigned priority number in the on-call book, as well as mock fire or other drills all relate to an emergency preparedness and safety plan that works should this occur.

A list of policies that may be discussed or provided to the new home care nurse follows for review. Some organizations may have a scavenger hunt related to location and identification of these policies and procedures (Box 4-2).

BOX 4-2   HOME CARE POLICIES—cont'd

Home Health Services—cont'd
  Medical administration policy
  Intravenous drug therapy
    and venipuncture policy
  Medical emergency in the
    home
  Response to adverse reac-
    tions policy
  Restricted nursing proce-
    dures and treatments
  Supervision of home health
    services
  Resuscitation policy
  On-call
  Beeper policy
  Clinical laboratory services
  Reporting child, adult, and
    elder abuse
  Guidelines of equipment or
    medical device problems,
    failures, or user errors
  Death of a patient in the
    home
  Others

Infection Control
Infection control policy

Universal precautions policy/
  procedure
Others

Personal Care Services
Home health aide services policy
Others

Home Care Record
Patient clinical records and doc-
  umentation guidelines
List of acceptable abbreviations
Others

Safety Management
Safety management program
  policy
Emergency preparedness plan
OSHA program
Fire safety plan
General office safety
Staff safety protocol
Patient safety
Others

Quality Management Plan
Performance improvement policy
Competency program
Reporting mechanisms

THE HOME CARE TEAM

Home care is a team effort. To work effectively and meet patient goals, as well as to ensure smooth operations, there must be clear and positive communication among and between team members. Case conferencing or team conferences should occur on an ongoing basis and per the organizational policy. Therapists, nurses, and other personnel involved with a particular home care patient all participate in developing the plan of care (POC). It goes without saying that the patient and his or her family or designated caregivers are the focus of the other team members (i.e., the player around whom the others revolve). This ensures that the care is client-centered and directed.

All team members furnishing services must maintain liaison to ensure that their efforts are coordinated effectively and support the objectives outlined in the POC and that the patient's clinical record or minutes of care conferences establish that effective interchange, reporting, and coordination of patient care occurs.

The following paragraphs introduce the members of the home care team. The first six services are those traditionally covered by Medicare. (For discussion of the hospice team, see Chapter 16.)

Nursing

In home care, *skilled nursing* is the term used to convey the use of professional skills or services that require the expertise of a nurse. These services are also referred to as a *skilled nursing visit* or *SNV*. Skilled nursing occurs when knowledge as a professional nurse is used to execute skills, render judgments, and evaluate information. According to Medicare or any other payor paying for skilled nursing, if a nonprofessional can perform a particular task or function, it probably is not skilled. Teaching and training, assessment and observation, and hands-on care are some of the many areas of expertise that comprise skilled care. Skilled nursing services must be furnished in accordance with or under a POC. Just as in the hospital (even more so), there must be physician orders for all care or changes to the plan of care. Under the general category of home care nursing there are nurses who are specialists. These include the enterostomal therapy (ET) nurse or therapist; the infusion specialist; the psychiatric nurse; the diabetes educator specialist; or the cardiac, oncology, hospice, or maternal-child health clinician or specialist. These nurses may have master's degrees or additional training, education, and certification for their areas of specialization. These specialties are addressed in later chapters of this text. (For information about certification for home care nurses, see Chapter 18.)

The Medicare standards for the duties of the registered nurse (RN) are as follows:

1. Makes the initial evaluation visit
2. Regularly reevaluates the patient's nursing needs
3. Initiates the POC and necessary revisions
4. Furnishes nursing services requiring substantial and specialized nursing skill
5. Initiates appropriate preventive and rehabilitative nursing procedures
6. Prepares clinical documentation, coordinates services, and informs the physician and other personnel of changes in the patient's condition and needs

7. Counsels the patient and family in meeting nursing and related needs
8. Participates in in-service programs and supervises and teaches other nursing personnel

Examples of the kinds of patients that an RN would care for include the patient with a complex wound; an unstable congestive heart failure patient for whom the nurse is providing observation and assessment through different data sources (e.g., weight, pedal edema, patient history and input, shortness of breath, respirations), monitoring status, and reporting to the physician; or an elderly caregiver who must be taught to care for his or her spouse's new ostomy.

The Medicare standards for the role of the licensed practical (LPN) or vocational nurse (LVN) are:

1. Furnishes service in accordance with agency policies
2. Prepares clinical documentation
3. Assists the physician and the RN in performing specialized procedures
4. Prepares equipment and materials for treatments, observing aseptic technique as required
5. Assists the patient in learning appropriate self-care activities

Examples of the kinds of tasks that the LPN or LVN might perform include giving insulin injections to the stable, homebound person with diabetes and working with the RN case manager on the wound care patient and providing one of the daily wound care visits.

The role of the nurse in home care is complex, variable and based on multifaceted patient needs and will be described throughout this text. All nurses in home care must practice within the scope of the state Nurse Practice Act, perform their responsibilities in compliance with the home care POC, and have appropriate qualifications for services that require specialized nursing skills and knowledge. Some of the multifaceted roles of the home care nurse are highlighted in Box 4-3.

Physical Therapy

Physical therapy (PT) services are sometimes called licensed physical therapists (LPTs). There are also physical therapist assistants (PTAs) who work in some organizations. As in nursing, much of the state law and practice standards define the therapist's specific roles.

All members of the rehabilitation team have very important roles in home care. PT in home care is based on the patient's problems, and

---

BOX 4-3   THE AMAZING HOME CARE NURSE

Teacher
Displays the patience of Job in educating new staff on Medicare procedures.

Benefactor
More money can never pay for the unflagging concern and attention given freely to staff and patients alike.

Microbiologist
Eradicates megamillions of microbes at a superhuman pace.

World Class Athlete
Covers 20 yards in an effortless bound, stops on a dime, stays on feet 25 hr/day in unending errands of mercy to patients.

Sponsor
Eagle-eye ability to spot special assignments for protegés.

Manager
Master coordinator of a few co-workers and equipment, producing the output of a staff of thousands on a budget of next to nothing.

Researcher
Einsteinlike mind allows incredible understanding of most recent medical advances and Medicare regulations.

Clairvoyant
Uncanny ability to sense and solve problems before they happen.

Accountant
Mighty overseer of travel log, requiring computer-like mind and juggler's hands.

Safety Engineer
Eternally watchful in keeping staff aware of multitudinous and ever-new hazards in environment.

Medical Professional
Nerves of steel give ability to assist in referrals of the most difficult and complicated nature.

Mother
Angel-like ability to soothe nerves of harassed doctors and nurses day in and day out.

Lawyer
Has mind-boggling ability to interpret complicated legalities of reimbursement.

Mentor
Possesses gargantuan generosity, compassion, and empathy in helping protegés learn the many-knotted ropes of home care.

Coach
Gives unflagging guidance and counsel, helping nurse locate patient.

Psychologist
Acts to mitigate stressful patient load of staff, thereby preventing burnout.

Data from Acme United Corp., Fairfield CT.

BOX 4-3 THE AMAZING HOME CARE NURSE—cont'd

Pharmacologist

Extraordinary ability to maintain patient medication sheet, without confusion, complications, or side effects.

Efficiency Expert

Helps case load flow for agency by keeping patient visits on split-second schedule.

Purchasing Agent

Super negotiator with thundering herds of salesmen, thereby procuring lowest prices for best equipment.

Real Human Being

Bountiful, warm, and understanding. A truly giving person. How can such dedication and perseverance exist in the face of superhuman duties and responsibilities? We wish we knew. We can only stand back and admire the Amazing Home Care Nurse. And offer unending congratulations.

---

goals are usually directed toward safety or rehabilitation. Common kinds of patients needing home care PT services include patients after joint replacement surgery, fractured hip repairs, patient status post cerebrovascular accident (S/P CVA) with hemiparesis or paralysis, and acute exacerbations of osteoarthritis. One of the primary skills of the LPT is teaching the family or caregivers the home exercise program. The Medicare standards for the LPT are as follows:

1. Therapy services are provided by a qualified LPT or by a qualified PTA under the supervision of a qualified therapist and in accordance with the POC
2. Qualified LPT assists the physician in evaluating level of function, helps develop the POC (revising as necessary)
3. Prepares clinical documentation
4. Advises and consults with the patient's family and other organization personnel
5. Participates in in-service programs

Occupational Therapy

Occupational therapy (OT) or occupational therapy assistants (OTAs) assist the patient to attain the maximum level of physical and psychosocial independence. Areas of expertise include fine motor coordination, perceptual-motor skills, sensory testing, adaptive/assistive devices, activities of daily living (ADLs), and specialized upper extremity/hand therapies. The kinds of problems frequently seen in home care that require OT intervention include patients with CVAs, amputations, and lung processes (such as chronic obstructive pulmonary disease) for conservation of energy skills.

The Medicare standards for the OT include the following:

1. The OT services are provided by a qualified OT or by a qualified OTA under the supervision of the OT and in accordance with the plan of care
2. The OT assists the physician in evaluating the level of function and helps develop the POC (revising as necessary)
3. Prepares clinical documentation
4. Advises and consults with the patient's family and other agency personnel
5. Participates in in-service programs

Speech-Language Pathology

Speech language pathology (SLP) services are furnished only by a qualified speech language pathologist or audiologist in home care. They are an important rehabilitative service indicated for various speech problems. Patients that usually need SLP in home care include those with a CVA, tracheostomy, laryngectomy, swallowing difficulties and various neuromuscular diseases such as amyotrophic lateral sclerosis. Like all the team members, the SLP creates clinical documentation and provides input into the POC and case conferences about the patient's status and progress on a regular basis for care coordination.

Medical Social Services

Medical social services (MSS) is also called medical social work (MSW) in home care. There are also social work assistants (SWA) in home care who work under the supervision of the masters-prepared social worker. The social services provided in home care are directly related to the treatment of the patient's medical problems. For example, if the patient has multiple medications on the POC, but cannot afford to purchase them, this will clearly impede the successful implementation of the POC. In these instances, in which there is a financial or other impediment to the POC, the MSS is very helpful in meeting the goals of the patient and team.

The Medicare standards for MSS are as follows:

1. The medical social worker or the SWA under the supervision of the qualified MSW and in accordance with the POC, assists the physician and other team members in understanding the significant social and emotional factors related to the health problems
2. Participates in the development of the POC
3. Prepares clinical documentation
4. Works with the family
5. Uses appropriate community resources
6. Participates in discharge planning and in-service programs
7. Acts as a consultant to other agency personnel

Some of the social problems seen in home care include complicated family dynamics and financial, housing, and caregiver concerns.

Home Health Aide Services

Home health aide services are probably the most important service for many patients in home care. They often visit the patient most frequently and provide personal care and ADL assistance to patients. This role and these functions are crucial in the determination if patients can remain at home. The home health aide usually spends more time with the patient and family than any other team member. The home health aide's contribution is invaluable to both the team process and in achieving patient satisfaction and positive outcomes. Home health aides are the "eyes and ears" in home care and hospice.

The Medicare standards for home health aides mandate that they be specially trained. Home health aides are selected on the basis of such factors as a sympathetic attitude toward the care of the sick; the ability to read, write, and carry out directions; and maturity and ability to deal effectively with the demands of the job. Home health aides must be proficient or competent in the following subject areas:

1. Communication skills
2. Observation, reporting and documentation of patient status, and the care or service furnished
3. Reading and recording temperature, pulse, respiration
4. Basic infection control procedures
5. Basic elements of body functioning and changes in body function that must be reported to the aide's supervisor
6. Maintenance of a clean, safe, and healthy environment

7. Recognizing emergencies and knowledge of emergency procedures
8. The physical, emotional, and developmental needs of and ways to work with the populations served by the organization, including the need for respect for the patient, his or her privacy, and his or her property
9. Appropriate and safe techniques in personal hygiene and grooming that include bed bath; sponge, tub, or shower bath; sink, tub, or bed shampoo; nail and skin care; oral hygiene; and toileting and elimination
10. Safe transfer techniques and ambulation
11. Normal range of motion and positioning
12. Adequate nutrition, and fluid intake
13. Any other task that the agency may choose to have the home health aide perform

Home health aides are closely supervised by the RN to ensure their competence in providing patient care.

Pharmaceutical Services

The role of the pharmacist in home care is a growing and very important role as the complexities of drug/drug, drug/disease, and drug/food adverse reactions increase. In home care, nurses are acutely aware of many patients who are inappropriately or overmedicated. Traditionally most home care patients are elderly and have multiple risk factors for therapeutic misadventures secondary to drug therapy. They may have multiple pathologies and different prescribers, exhibit polypharmacy (both prescription and nonprescription medications), and be at greater risk for adverse effects from medications due to altered physiology secondary to aging and disabilities (e.g., poor eyesight, impaired hearing, arthritic fingers).

The nurse in the community sees the whole picture and the many medications given to patients from multiple physicians. The nurse addresses safety concerns related to medications, acts as the patient advocate to clarify medication and orders, and consults with the pharmacists who can effectively evaluate the multiple medication regimens. Traditionally the pharmacist has been considered the provider of a product, drugs. Although this is certainly true and one of the roles, there are many other services that the pharmacist can offer to the home care team. These include specialty monitoring and assessment of the therapeutic or toxic effect of drugs, ongoing in-servicing and provision of detailed information related to drugs, case conferencing, and active participation in home care/hospice rounds.

The pharmacist can do much more than provide drugs; he or she is a drug expert in an excellent position to review medication regimens, screen for incorrect doses or dosage forms, and recommend alternatives. The pharmacist can also suggest simplifying the patient's medication regimen by altering drug delivery systems, scheduling medication administration, or suggesting how to monitor and assess the therapeutic or toxic effect of drugs.

Dietitian Services

The role of the professional, registered dietitian in home care is expanding as more patients are cared for at home. Many home care and hospice programs have dietitians available to make home visits and provide consulting services to promote optimal nutrition. Nurses in home care assess patients for being at risk and in need of nutritional services or intervention (e.g., cachexia, weight loss, or no food in the refrigerator). For accreditation, there are specific standards on which the patient's nutritional status is assessed, ensuring that interdisciplinary nutritional care planning is performed, that there is evidence of counseling or nutrition intervention, and that appropriately qualified staff members are designated to coordinate services. Home care has traditionally relied on home care nurses to identify, coordinate, and implement nutrition-related services. Home care organizations may need the dietician for diet modification and counseling, use of oral supplements, and/or recommendations related to enteral and parenteral nutrition therapies. Other services include teaching (e.g., complex diets), identifying educational materials for use with patient teaching, and serving as in-service educator and resource on nutrition services.

Physician Services

The physician plays an important role in home care services. Because Medicare and other insurers are medical health insurance plans and cover or pay for medically necessary care, they require that the physician certify that the patient needs the services and then sign the POC supporting the care. The HCFA form 485 meets both the certification and POC requirements on one form; hence it is called "The Home Health Certification and Plan of Care." Medicare law requires that payment for services can only be made if a physician certifies the needs for services and establishes a POC. All care and changes in the POC, as well as changes in the patient's condition, must be reported to the physician and documented in the patient's clinical record by the home care nurse. Verbal orders or any changes must be obtained and placed in writing and sent to the physician for signature. The home care organization will have policies related to the forms and process for receiving and documenting verbal and other physician orders. From legal and standards of practice perspectives, it is very important that the home care nurse communicate and coordinate care with the patient's physician(s).

Many home care and hospice organizations also have a medical director. The medical director plays an important role and has numerous responsibilities, including acting as a resource to the organization's management and clinical team members and providing direction related to clinical services. Although specific roles, programs, and practices may vary, the following are some of the important responsibilities of the home care medical director:

1. Provides guidance about the development of new or revised policies and procedures
2. Serves on the home care advisory committee or other boards or committees
3. Collaborates and consults with the managers and facilitates problem solving toward meeting patient needs
4. Participates in educational conferences
5. Serves as the liaison between the home care organization and physician members of the medical community
6. Supports the home care organization through teaching and public relations endeavors, educates physicians about home care (e.g., who's appropriate, need for physician's orders, communications) in the community
7. Assists in the resolution of difficulties that may arise between members of the team and community physicians
8. Acts as a role model by making home visits, when possible, attending scheduled team and other meetings, and participating in other activities that support the mission of the home care organization

Physicians look to the experienced home care nurse for recommendations and solutions to care for their patients.

Administrative, Clerical, Coordinators, and Billing Services

These important people are the glue that holds home care organizations together! Filing clinical records, scheduling team members, and myriad other responsibilities are extremely important tasks and cannot be overstated.

Other Services and Team Members

Other services and team members are based on the home care organization's mission and specialty programs. These may include hospice team members (see Chapter 16), respiratory therapy, and chaplain services.

Although there is a team very involved with every patient's care, usually visits are made by the home care nurse in the community.

SAFETY IN HOME CARE

Personal safety is an appropriate concern in home care, as it is in any community or home. It is particularly important to home care nurses who enter geographical areas with which they may not be familiar and at unusual hours.

The home care clinician should review any protocols her or his organization has related to staff safety and home visits. Beepers, pagers, car phones, and calling in one's schedule to coordinators or other organizational procedures may all assist in staff safety. Some organizations have a local law enforcement person who provides training and education related to home visiting and safety. The information shared is valuable to the nurse both in home care and as a member of a community.

Personal safety starts with the clinician's own awareness of surroundings. Well-honed skills of observation and assessment are essential to maximize safety.

Personal Safety Tips

Whenever going anywhere for the first time, get specific, detailed, and correct directions to the patient's home and have them validated by the patient or caregiver. Whenever possible, carry a detailed map of your community with you in your car.

If you are unsure of a neighborhood or have heard about problems, talk with your supervisor who may contact the local police who know the communities and the problems the best and can work with the home care team for solutions.

Organizations may have contracts with security staff. Your supervisor would know of such arrangements and the process for their use. Be especially mindful of the following personal safety tips:

- Know the community. As you are driving, always be aware of your surroundings.
- You may want to call patients so they can be watching for you. Ask about parking.
- Lock the car doors and keep any valuables such as purse, supplies, and any patient information out of sight.

- Place your equipment where it is not visible as you drive.
- Wear seatbelts while driving.
- When nearing the home, look for the landmarks that have been described and address numbers on houses.
- Keep maps out of sight when possible and try to avoid looking as though you are unfamiliar with the area.
- Try to park in well-lit areas and in front of the home or as close as possible. Lock the car, identifying your route to the front door.
- Be cautious when boarding elevators.
- When making evening or night visits, let your family know where you are going and when you expect to return.
- When walking to your car, have your keys out, ready to unlock the car. Many of the newer car models have "keyless entry" that works with a computer chip that opens the door when the mechanism is directed toward the car and pressed.
- Before unlocking the car, check the back seat and floor areas.
- If you feel unsafe, you probably are. Trust your feelings.
- Speak with your supervisor about your organization's unique policies related to home visiting safety.

Car Safety Tips

Car safety is also very important in home care. It begins with a knowledge of the strengths and weaknesses of your car. Successful and safe clinicians in home care have good driving records and reliable cars that are usually not gas guzzlers; having a small car can also make it easier to find a spot on snowy streets or downtown metropolitan areas. Always make sure you have enough gas. Some home care nurses make it a habit to never let the gas tank get below one-half full/empty. Note the following car safety tips:

- Carry 1 gallon of water, a blanket, and a first aid kit.
- Lock all car doors when entering or leaving the car.
- Carry sand, rug mats, or kitty litter to assist you out of ice and snow.
- If your organization gives you a sign that identifies you as a health care worker, use it per program policies. Sometimes these signs help you to obtain and keep a spot in front of the hospital or laboratory.
- Consider obtaining gas credit cards and joining an automobile club for assistance in emergencies such as running out of gasoline or fuel and dead batteries.
- Take care of your car, winterize it if you live where it is cold, and maintain it well.

- Have the oil and fluid levels and air in your tires checked regularly.
- Make sure your spare tire is in good condition and is inflated.

Map Reading Skills

A skill needed for all home care team members is map reading. Many organizations have a large and diverse catchment area that may cover urban, suburban, and rural areas. You cannot know every side street or bridge in a given area. The ability to navigate and read maps has been sorely tested by experienced home care clinicians. In communities where there is rapid growth, sometimes the newer roads and access routes may not even be on the map. For that reason, the large county book maps that are updated fairly frequently seem to work well. When taking directions from patients or their family members or caregivers, it is most helpful to write down landmarks such as schools, playgrounds, trash dumps, marinas, or shopping centers that confirm that you are on the right track.

Personal safety is enhanced when you can get from one patient's home to the next most easily. Your supervisor or experienced home care team members will know the nuances of any community that can plague a home care clinician's planned day. These include when and where streets are cleaned and parking is prohibited, snow emergency routes, or streets that change direction during rush hours to accommodate the traffic. These challenges can tax the most experienced home care nurse. Be prepared!

SUMMARY

Orientation is an important period in a new home care team member's tenure. Orientation is the time when the organization standards and other information is provided. Orientation itself varies among organizations, and the orientation may set the precedent for and establish the value of standardization of care and education that the organization espouses. Everyone comes into home care with different skills and competencies; orientation is the time to identify areas for improvement and provide needed education and information. Part IV describes the nuts and bolts of home care and clinical practice.

REVIEW EXERCISES

1. List the five segments of the home care industry.
2. Describe the goals or outcomes of the orientation period.
3. Identify five members of the home care team and their roles.
4. Briefly describe the role of the medical director.
5. Discuss personal and car safety tips.
6. List five subject areas that will be covered when new to home care.

RESOURCES

American Medical Association: *Guidelines for the medical management of the home care patient,* Chicago, 1994, American Medical Association.

The American Physical Therapy Association (APTA), Section on Community Home Health publishes *Guidelines for the Provision of Physical Therapy in the Home, 1-703-684-2782.*

Dantone J: *Bridging the gap: procedure and instructional manual for dietary and nursing interventions,* 1996, 1-601-226-3250.

Marrelli T, Friend L: *Home health aide: guidelines for care instructor manual,* Boca Grande, Fla, 1997, Marrelli and Associates, 1-800-993-6397.

Marrelli T, Whittier S: *Home health aide: guidelines for care,* Boca Grande, Fla, Marrelli and Associates, 1996, 1-800-993-6397.

Redus K: A literature review of competency-based orientation for nurses, *J Staff Dev* 10:(5):239-243, 1994.

Home Care Nurse News is a monthly clinically focused newsletter for clinicians and managers in home care and hospice. To review a copy, call 1-800-993-NEWS.

Home Health Aide Digest is a subscription newsletter dedicated to nurturing the occupational and professional growth of home health aides. To review a copy, call Stonerock & Associates at 1-616-344-4593.

The National Association of Social Workers publishes *NASW Clinical Indicators for Social Work and Psychosocial Services in Home Health Care, 1-202-408-8600.*

REFERENCES

Health Care Financing Administration: *Home Health Agency Manual—Publication* 11, 132.1, Washington, DC, Health and Human Services, Revision 277, 1996.

Stulginsky M: Nurses Home Health Experience. Part 1. Practice Setting, *Nursing Health Care* 14:8, 1993.

PATIENT CARE PLANNING AND HOME CARE: THE NUTS AND BOLTS

5

MEDICARE HOME CARE

Tina M. Marrelli, MSN, MA, RNC

> *"When I was a home care and hospice nurse and then went to work at HCFA on issues related to home care and hospice coverage and operations, I did not understand about the Medicare program, even though in 1988 I had written the first edition of the* Handbook of Home Health Standards and Documentation Guidelines for Reimbursement. *Working at HFCA really made me understand Medicare's complexity and what the rules mean to practicing clinicians and their managers."*
>
> *Tina M. Marrelli*

This chapter explains how the Medicare system works and assists in making Medicare make sense to clinicians. It is important that home care staff know the Medicare rules and adhere to them religiously. The many reasons clinicians need to understand Medicare will be explained in this chapter and in Chapter 6. This chapter also provides the information to make the program make sense and understand more fully the role of the Health Care Financing Administration (HCFA) and the regional home health intermediaries (RHHIs).

WHAT IS MEDICARE?

Medicare, authorized under Title XVIII of the Social Security Act, is a nationwide health insurance program that was enacted in 1965 and consists of two parts—parts A and B. Medicare is a law, and it is a federal program for people who are 65 years old and older, or disabled, or have end-stage renal disease (ESRD). Medicare is the world's largest health insurance program, covering more than 37 million beneficiaries, and, as with all insurers, there are coverage rules and exclusions to coverage and eligibility; there must be medical necessity since it is a *medical* insurance program. Medicare has set many of the standards related to home care and home care clinical practice. This chapter describes the Medicare home care program and explains the rules.

THE ROLE OF THE HEALTH CARE FINANCING ADMINISTRATION

The HCFA is a governmental agency within the Department of Health and Human Services. All Medicare and Medicaid (the state program for health care coverage for the poor) programs are administered by HCFA, including hospitals, home care, and hospice programs.

According to Medicare, the population of Medicare beneficiaries is growing older faster and is more disabled than the general population. People older than age 85, the disabled, and those with ESRD have been the fastest growing categories of beneficiaries. In addition, nearly twice as many beneficiaries are women older than age 85. More than half of female beneficiaries have difficulties with three or more activities of daily living (ADLs) such as eating, bathing, dressing; and more than one quarter of all beneficiaries live alone. These facts have implications for home care nursing.

Medicare Part A

Medicare A provides the bulk of the funding for covered inpatient hospital and skilled nursing facility (SNF) stays, with the patient having some financial responsibility for a deductible. Medicare A also pays for home health and hospice services, although there has been discussion of making this traditionally Part A benefit Part B.

Individuals eligible for Social Security are automatically entitled to Medicare when they reach age 65. Individuals who are younger than age 65 and eligible for Social Security disability must have been disabled for at least 2 years. Medicare A, sometimes referred to as "Hospital Insurance," is financed through payroll contribution taxes on workers and their employers (FICA tax). Part A is the part of the Medicare program that is projected to be bankrupt in the near future.

The home health care services that can be provided and covered under Medicare A include skilled nursing, home health aide, physical or occupational therapy, speech-language pathology, and medical social services. This knowledge about Medicare or any other insurer assists in the nursing advocate role of the home care nurse when patients have questions about benefits, coverage, and care.

Of these Part A programs, currently only home care and SNFs remain on a cost-based reimbursement system; the others, such as hospitals, have diagnostic-related groups, which is a prospective payment system (PPS). In fact, for both home care and SNFs the HCFA has PPS demonstration projects to ascertain more effective ways to pay for care. This is important to the home care nurse because the move toward prospective payment or another managed care mechanism demands that home care rethink operations and care directed toward cost-effectiveness.

Medicare Part B

Medicare Part B is voluntary, and enrollment is open to individuals age 65 and older or those already entitled to Part A benefits. The beneficiary pays a monthly premium for Part B coverage. Medicare Part B provides coverage for physician services, some home care related to home medical equipment and supplies, home care services for those without Part A, ambulance services, total parenteral nutrition and some chemotherapy and radiation, and kidney dialysis and transplants. The benefit also covers the full cost of some medical supplies and 80% of the approved amount for durable or home medical equipment such as wheelchairs, hospital beds, oxygen supplies, and walkers. Most Part B benefits have a co-payment that the beneficiary or an additional insurance such as Medigap pays.

It is very important that the home care clinician know about Medicare and other insurers and their health policies. As one of her or his roles (see Chapter 4), the home care team member identifies the correct payor and verifies this information with the patient or caregiver.

On becoming a Medicare beneficiary, patients with Medicare are sent a Medicare card (Figure 5-1). The card is white with a red and blue strip and lists the patient's name and Medicare number, also called the Health Insurance Claim Number. The Medicare card also states whether

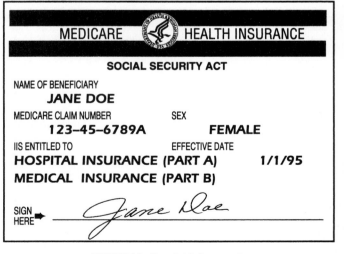

FIGURE 5-1   Sample Medicare card.

or not the patient has Part A and/or Part B. According to the 1996 HCFA Medicare Handbook, "Medicare Part A (or Part B if the patient does not have Part A) pays the entire bill for covered services as long as they are medically reasonable and necessary."

MEDICARE CONDITIONS OF PARTICIPATION

The Medicare Conditions of Participation (COPs) implemented the statutory requirements of the Medicare law that home care and hospice providers must meet on an ongoing basis to participate in the Medicare program (i.e., they must be Medicare certified or have Medicare certification). Home care, hospice or other health care organizations apply for Medicare certification. The HCFA contracts with the state departments of health to perform the actual on-site survey and review for the Medicare certification process.

The initial Medicare certification process is a labor-intensive and lengthy process for the home care organization. Nurse surveyors review all the various components of the Medicare COPs. To perform this review thoroughly, the clinician must read and understand the *Interpretive Guidelines,* a 70-plus–page document that explains the Medicare COPs for home care. Home visits are made, patients and team members are interviewed, and clinical and administrative policies and procedures are reviewed. Once the home health organization receives Medicare certification, which means they have achieved these standards, they can then bill Medicare and other payors for home care services provided to their patients.

Surveys also occur thereafter to determine that a program continues to meet the standards defined in the Medicare COPs. These are usually unannounced and may be a part of the routine surveying process or triggered as a result of a complaint. The survey consists of clinical record reviews, home visits, and review of human resources records. Again the purpose is to ensure the organization's compliance with patient rights and federal, state, and local laws and regulations; acceptance of patients and the plan of care (POC); home health aide supervision and care; and other parameters defined in the COPs.

HCFA contracts with insurance companies to process and adjudicate or make payment determination decisions on Medicare claims or bills that come in from home care and hospices. These specialized insurance companies are called the regional home health intermediaries (RHHIs) because they have responsibility for different geographic regions (Table 5-1). (Home health agencies that are part of a chain may have one RHHI because they have centralized billing in one location).

TABLE 5-1 STATE ASSIGNMENTS TO REGIONAL HOME HEALTH INTERMEDIARIES (RHHIs)

RHHI	STATES
Associated Hospital Services of Maine	Connecticut, Maine, Massachusetts, Rhode Island, Vermont
Blue Cross and Blue Shield of Wisconsin	Michigan, Minnesota, New Jersey, New York, Puerto Rico, Virgin Islands, Wisconsin
Blue Cross and Blue Shield of South Carolina (Palmetto)	Alabama, Arkansas, Florida, Georgia, Kentucky, Louisiana, Mississippi, New Mexico, North Carolina, Oklahoma, South Carolina, Tennessee, Texas
Wellmark, formerly known as IASD Health Services Corp.	Colorado, Delaware, District of Columbia, Iowa, Kansas, Maryland, Missouri, Montana, Nebraska, North Dakota, Pennsylvania, South Dakota, Utah, Virginia, West Virginia, Wyoming
Blue Cross of California	Alaska, Arizona, California, Hawaii, Idaho, Nevada, Oregon, Washington
Health Care Service Corp (Blue Cross of Illinois)	Illinois, Indiana, Ohio

By law, the RHHIs can only pay for covered and necessary Medicare services. That is why it is so important, when admitting patients to home care or hospice, to ensure that all eligibility requirements are met and that the home care documentation clearly supports the eligibility criteria (e.g., homebound) and covered care. Covered care with examples is specified in the *Home Health Agency (HHA) Manual—Pub. 11* (HCFA). (For your own copy of the full text of Medicare covered services please refer to the *Handbook of Home Health Standards and Documentation Guidelines for Reimbursement* [Marrelli, 1998]). Documentation then becomes an important component for payment of Medicare home care services.

BOX 5-1   MEDICARE CONDITIONS OF PARTICIPATION

Patient Rights (42 CFR 484.10)
- Notice of rights
- Exercise of rights and respect for property and person
- Right to be informed and to participate in planning care and treatment
- Confidentiality of medical records
- Patient liability for payment
- Home health hotline

Compliance with Federal, State, and Local Laws; Disclosure and Ownership Information; and Compliance with Accepted Professional Standards and Principles (42 CFR 484.12)
- Compliance with laws and regulations
- Disclosure of ownership and management information
- Compliance with accepted professional standards and principles

Organization, Services, and Administration (42 CFR 484.14)
- Services furnished
- Governing body
- Administrator, supervising physician, or registered nurse
- Personnel policies
- Personnel contracts
- Coordination of patient services
- Services under arrangements
- Institutional planning—capital expenditure plan
- Preparation and annual review of plan and budget
- Laboratory services

Group of Professional Personnel (42 CFR 484.16)
- Advisory and evaluation function

Acceptance of Patients, Plan of Care, Medical Supervision (42 CFR 484.18)
- Plan of care
- Periodic review of plan of care
- Conformance with physician orders

Skilled Nursing Services (42 CFR 484.30)
- Duties of the registered nurse
- Duties of the licensed practical nurse

Therapy Services (42 CFR 484.32)
- Supervision of physical therapist assistant and occupational therapy assistant
- Supervision of speech therapy services

continued

BOX 5-1	MEDICARE CONDITIONS OF PARTICIPATION—cont'd

Medical Social Services (42 CFR 484.34)

Home Health Aide Services (42 CFR 484.36)
- Home health aide training
- Competency evaluation and in-service training
- Assignment and duties of the home health aide
- Supervision of home health aides

Qualifying to Furnish Outpatient Physical Therapy or Speech-Language Pathology Services (42 CFR 484.38)

Clinical Records (42 CFR 484.48)
- Retention of records
- Protection of records

Evaluation of the Agency's Program (42 CFR 484. 52)
- Policy and administrative review
- Clinical record review

The Medicare COPs, as listed in Box 5-1, are the structure or framework of the Medicare law that supports the Medicare program. From a home care clinician perspective, effective patient care and daily organizational activities support the COPs. The large topic headings are the actual COPs, and the topics listed below are the standards that support the COPs that must also be in compliance. It is most important that home care organizations adhere to the policies to which they ascribe. Surveyors may cite deficiencies for the agencies' failure to adhere to their own policies, as well as failure to comply with state or federal regulations. The references below to "CFR" refer to the citation in the law, the Code of Federal Regulations.

The model shown in Figure 5-2 shows how all aspects of home care practice and operations should support the Medicare COPs.

THE NUTS AND BOLTS OF MEDICARE HOME CARE COVERAGE

The main criteria that must be met for patients to be appropriate for and covered under the Medicare home care model generally include the following:

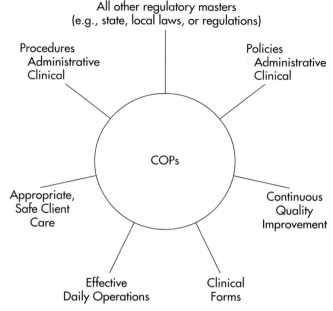

FIGURE 5-2 COPs Model for compliance. All aspects of home care practice and operations should support the Medicare COPs. COPs, Conditions of participation. (Modified with permission from Marrelli and Associates, Inc.)

1. Medicare-certified agency
2. Homebound patient
3. Eligible Medicare beneficiary and appropriate payor
4. Coverable services
5. Covered skilled nursing service
6. Physician-approved POC
7. Documentation supports care covered

Medicare-Certified Home Health Agency

The organization is Medicare certified (i.e., surveyed and approved by state surveyors). Medicare certification is the process of approval for Medicare participation. Medicare nurse surveyors arrive from the state department of health at the home care (or hospice) organization. HCFA contracts with the states for this work.

The surveyors review the overall organization, with the Medicare COPs being the standard for measurement. This includes a review of the clinical and administrative policies and procedures, home visits, and patient interviews. For example, a nurse surveyor will read the patient's POC and check that it is filled out completely; look at the frequency of services and count the visit notes; review the specific physician's orders on the POC and determine if the POC is being followed; and check and count the medications on the 485 and verify that the medication sheet matches exactly and that allergies are addressed consistently. These are the details that contribute to the provision of high-quality care.

Medicare certification surveys are usually performed:

1. On becoming a new Medicare-participating organization
2. On an ongoing basis through the life of the organization
3. When the state believes that patient safety may be compromised

State surveyors are usually specially trained in home care; their role is to protect the welfare and safety of patients who are receiving reimbursement from the federal government (Medicare) for services.

Homebound Patient

Being homebound is one of the eligibility criteria for admission to the home care program. For a Medicare beneficiary to be eligible to receive covered home health services, the law requires that the beneficiary be homebound. The term *homebound* is synonymous with confined to the home, as for medical reasons. In practical language this means that "an individual does not have to be bedridden to be considered as confined to home. However, the condition of these patients should be such that there exists a normal inability to leave home and, consequently, leaving their homes requires a considerable and taxing effort." The full text of the Medicare definition of homebound is listed in Box 5-2. After information has been reviewed and the patient has been assessed, patients are generally classified as homebound or not homebound.

Eligible Medicare Beneficiary and Appropriate Payor

The patient must be an eligible Medicare beneficiary, and Medicare is the appropriate payor. This means that the patient meets the homebound requirements and is a Medicare beneficiary, Medicare is the appropriate

BOX 5-2   MEDICARE DEFINITION OF HOMEBOUND

204. 1 *Confined to the home.*
A. *Patient Confined to The Home.* In order for the patient to be eligible to receive covered home health services under both Part A and Part B, the law requires that a physician certify in all cases that the patient is confined to his or her home. An individual does not have to be bedridden to be considered as confined to the home. However, the condition of these patients should be such that there exists a normal inability to leave home and, consequently, leaving home would require a considerable and taxing effort. If the patient does in fact leave the home, the patient may nevertheless be considered homebound if the absences from the home are infrequent or for periods of relatively short duration or are attributable to the need to receive medical treatment. Absences to need to receive medical treatment include attendance at adult day center to receive medical care, ongoing receipt of outpatient kidney dialysis, and the receipt of outpatient chemotherapy or radiation therapy. It is expected in most instances, absences from the home that occur will be for the purpose of receiving medical treatment. However, occasional absences from the home for nonmedical purposes (e.g., an occasional trip to the barber, a walk around the block, or a drive) would not necessitate a finding that the patient is not homebound if the absences from the home are undertaken on an infrequent basis or are of relatively short duration and do not indicate that the patient has the capacity to obtain the health care provided outside rather than in the home.

Generally speaking, a patient will be considered to be homebound if he or she has a condition due to an illness or injury that restricts his or her ability to leave his or her place of residence except with the aid of supportive device such as crutches, canes, wheelchairs, and walkers, the use of special transportation, or the assistance of another person or if leaving home is medically contraindicated. Some examples of homebound patients that illustrate the factors used to determine whether a homebound condition exists would be: (1) a patient who is paralyzed from a stroke who is confined to a wheelchair or requires the aid of crutches in order to walk; (2) a patient who is blind or senile and requires the assistance of another person to leave his or her residence; (3) a patient who has lost the use of his or her upper extremities and therefore is unable to open doors, use handrails on stairways, etc., and requires the assistance of another individual to leave his or her residence; (4) a patient who has just returned from a hospital stay involving surgery suffering from resultant weakness and pain and, therefore, his or her actions

From *HCFA: HHA Manual— Pub. 11,* Revision 227 (HCFA).

continued

BOX 5-2 **MEDICARE DEFINITION OF HOMEBOUND
—cont'd**

may be restricted by his or her physician to certain specified and limited activities such as getting out of bed only for a specified period of time, walking stairs only once a day, etc.; (5) a patient with arteriosclerotic heart disease of such severity that he or she must avoid all stress and physical activity; and (6) a patient with a psychiatric problem if the illness is manifested in part by a refusal to leave home or is of such a nature that it would not be considered safe to leave the home unattended, even if he or she has no physical limitations.

payor for the home care services, the patient must need the skilled nursing services, and the services are covered (Box 5-3).

We know that many people continue to work full-time well into their 70s. For example, when President Reagan was in the White House, since he was working full-time, Medicare would not have been his primary insurer. Medicare would have been the "secondary payor." In this example, he would not meet the eligibility requirements because Medicare was not the correct payor. These concepts comprise the information that must be elicited by the home care nurse to determine the patient's insurance (see Chapter 6).

Coverable Services

The services must be coverable under the home health benefit, reasonable, and necessary based on the patient's unique medical condition. Medicare is a medical insurance program, and as such the care provided must be medically reasonable and necessary to treat the patient's particular illness, injury, or diagnosis within the context of the patient's unique medical condition. Reasonable and necessary also connotes that it is standard and acceptable medical practice. To be considered reasonable and necessary for the diagnoses or treatment of the patient's illness or injury, the service must be consistent with the nature and severity of the illness or injury, his or her particular medical needs, and accepted standards of medical and nursing practice. An example is a bedridden, status post cerebrovascular accident patient whom the physician refers to home care for monthly B_{12} injections for pernicious anemia. The admitting diagnosis is pernicious anemia. This would be covered care because the patient is homebound and has Medicare, and it is the appropriate payor and because pernicious anemia is listed in the *HHA Manual—Pub. 11* (HCFA)

BOX 5-3   HOMEBOUND CASE EXAMPLES

Answer Yes or No

1. Mrs. Roberts is a 72-year-old lady who had a left hip pinning. In addition, she has had a recent exacerbation of chronic heart failure and diabetes. She requires the assistance of someone to ambulate and is dyspneic after ambulating 35 feet. Visits are needed to assess her condition, do medication and diet teaching, assess her accu-checks, and report the findings to her physician. Mrs. Roberts is receiving physical therapy. Her physician and physical therapist have determined that she needs to use equipment that wouldn't be able to be brought to the home. Mr. Roberts will drive her to the hospital three times a week.

Is Mrs. Roberts homebound?   _____ YES _____ NO

Answer: Yes. Mrs. Roberts is considered homebound. An individual is considered homebound when he or she leaves the home for medical reasons and the documentation shows it requires a considerable and taxing effort to leave. Mrs. Roberts is receiving services that normally cannot be provided in the home.

2. Mr. Newton is a 35-year-old quadriplegic. The home health aide comes in twice a day to bathe, dress, get him up to his motorized wheelchair in the morning, and put him to bed in the evening. A skilled nurse visits him three times a week for disimpaction. Mr. Newton travels daily in a handicapped van to attend classes at a local university.

Is Mr. Newton homebound?   _____ YES _____ NO

No. Mr. Newton would not be considered homebound. Even though he requires assistance, he is leaving his home daily for nonmedical reasons.

3. Mr. Williams is a slightly confused 88-year-old man who needs a skilled nurse to draw a monthly digoxin level. He uses the assistance of a walker to ambulate. A neighbor comes by each evening to drive Mr. Williams to a local cafe. The skilled nurse thinks this may be the only meal Mr. Williams has each day.

Is Mr. Williams considered homebound?   _____ YES _____ NO

From Wellmark, formerly known as IASD Health Services Corp., Federal Intermediary and Carrier, Des Moines, IA.

continued

BOX 5-3   **HOMEBOUND CASE EXAMPLES—cont'd**

No. When an individual leaves his or her home on a frequent basis for nonmedical reasons, he or she will not be considered homebound. (Note: The skilled nurse could arrange for Meals on Wheels.)

4. Mrs. Cruse is an 85-year-old lady who needs the skilled nurse to administer her calcitonin three times a week for treatment of her osteoporosis. Mrs. Cruse is unable to self-administer the drug because of severe arthritis in her hands. On Sundays, church members transport her to church. She requires the assistance of one person to leave church.

Does Mrs. Cruse meet the homebound
criteria as described by Medicare?   _____ YES _____ NO

Yes. Mrs. Cruse would still meet the homebound criteria, since she is leaving her home on an infrequent basis for nonmedical reasons and the documentation shows it requires a considerable and taxing effort for her to leave.

---

as one of the diagnoses for which B_{12} is reasonable, necessary, and standard treatment. Conversely, if a local medical doctor thinks that all patients over age 65 should receive B_{12} injections just because they're over age 65, the care would not be covered. The treatment, care, and service has to be specific, reasonable, and necessary for that condition and be standard treatment as defined in the *HHA Manual—Pub. 11* (HCFA).

Covered Skilled Nursing Service

The ordered nursing care is a covered skilled nursing service (or other skilled services as defined by the *HHA Manual—Pub. 11*, Section 205.1 [HCFA]). When documentation supports covered care (Box 5-4) and services are provided under the POC, Medicare covers the following skilled nursing services:

1. Observation and assessment of the patient's condition
2. Management and evaluation of a patient care plan
3. Teaching and training activities
4. Administration of medications
5. Tube feedings

BOX 5-4   **GENERAL PRINCIPLES GOVERNING
REASONABLE AND NECESSARY
SKILLED NURSING CARE**

When determining whether a service requires the skills of a nurse:
1. Consider the inherent complexity of the service. For example, certain services are complex enough that they are considered skilled. Examples include infusion or urinary catheter insertion, intravenous or intramuscular injections, and venipuncture.
2. Consider the unique condition of the patient. A patient's condition may be such that a service that normally would be classified as unskilled can only be safely and effectively provided by a skilled person. An example in the *Medicare HHA Manual* is of a patient recovering from bowel surgery from irritable bowel syndrome; although an enema is not usually a skilled service, because of this patient's history and recent surgery, the enema could only be given safely and effectively by a nurse. In addition, the enema is needed to treat the illness and injury and therefore is reasonable and necessary covered skilled nursing care.
3 Consider the accepted standards of practice.
4. Remember that a service is not "skilled" just because it is performed by a nurse. If the service can be provided by a non-medical person (i.e., not a nurse), without special training, it is probably not skilled, even if performed by a nurse. Similarly, an unskilled service does not become skilled because no one in the home is competent to perform the service.
5. A skilled nursing service that is taught to a patient or caregiver does not become unskilled. It is still considered skilled when performed by the nurse. The classic example is the patient needing BID dressing changes for a pressure ulcer for 3 weeks. Mr. Jones has been sent home from St. Elsewhere General Medical Center with an open, draining wound that requires irrigation, packing, and dressing twice a day. The agency nurse has taught the family to provide the PM dressing change, but the home care nurse continues the daily morning wound care visits when the family is not available, able, and willing to provide the care. The wound care continues to be skilled nursing care, not withstanding the fact that the family provides it part of the time, and the care may be covered as long as it is required by the patient.
6. The skilled nursing service must be reasonable and necessary to the diagnosis and treatment of the beneficiary's illness or injury within the context of the beneficiary's unique medical condition.

continued

BOX 5-4   **GENERAL PRINCIPLES GOVERNING
REASONABLE AND NECESSARY
SKILLED NURSING CARE—cont'd**

7. Diagnosis should never be the sole factor in determining medical necessity and coverage.
8. Determination of the medical necessity of services should be based on the patient's unique medical condition and individual needs, without regard for whether the condition is acute, chronic, terminal, expected to continue over a long period of time, or in some cases stable (such as the long-term Foley catheter patient who is homebound).

---

    6. Nasopharyngeal and tracheostomy aspiration
    7. Catheters
    8. Wound care
    9. Ostomy care
  10. Heat treatments
  11. Medical gasses
  12. Rehabilitation nursing
  13. Venipuncture
  14. Student nurse visits
  15. Psychiatric evaluation, therapy, and teaching

The *HHA manual—Pub. 11* (HCFA) includes additional examples and provides the rationale for, as well as information about, the clinical documentation that supports coverage for the skilled nursing service provided.

Observation and Assessment of the Patient's Condition
Coverage Considerations
- There is a likelihood of a change in the patient's condition. This is usually based on the patient's past medical history.
- There is evaluation of the patient's need for changes in the treatment. This skill particularly uses the professional nurse's skills of observation, taking a physical history, assessment of findings, critical thinking related to the data, creation of the plan, and communication of findings to the physicians.
- There is a reasonable potential for complications and/or further acute episodes or changes.

- The patient can be admitted for a 3-week observation and assessment period.
- Long-standing patterns where there is no attempt to change the treatment plan would not be reasonable and necessary and therefore not covered.

Patient Example

A frail, 85-year-old man was hospitalized for pneumonia. The infection was resolved, but the patient, who had previously maintained adequate nutrition, will not eat or eats poorly. The patient is discharged to home care for monitoring of fluid and nutrient intake and assessment of the need for tube feeding. Observation and monitoring by licensed nurses of the patient's oral intake, output, and hydration status is required to determine what further treatment or other intervention is needed.

Documentation Considerations

In this example the patient's fluid, food, and/or supplemental intake would be reported in the documentation, as well as observation of signs of dehydration and weight loss. Lung sounds and further signs of pneumonia resolution or worsening (such as chest congestion, cough, fever) would also be observed, assessed, and documented. The reason this patient would be homebound is his immobility and weakness. The initial admitting note should list the reasons the patient is at risk and needs observation and assessment. The documentation should specify the findings and history that support the need for observation and assessment (e.g., the reasons for the likelihood of change in the patient's condition such as abnormal laboratory values, weight changes, edema, or drug toxicity) and should be clearly noted in the clinical record.

Standards of Practice for Excellence

Observation and assessment skills should be used every visit, regardless of the patient problem. These skills are key contributors to the plan created through the use of the nursing process in home care nursing. They include assessment of vital signs of temperature, pulse, respiration, and blood pressure, as well as the other vital sign, pain, every visit. Observation and assessment of a patient with a cardiac or other fluid problem or potential for this problem would include weighing the patient. Along with the patient's history and other physical findings, the nurse or therapist creates the POC in collaboration with the patient and the patient's physician. Based on the findings of observation and assessment, the nurse communicates with the physician about any findings and recommendations for changes to the POC. These communications (e.g., concerning medication or visit frequency changes) are then written as verbal or telephone orders and sent to the physician for signature. There must be specific and current physician orders for all care provided in home care.

Management and Evaluation of a Patient Care Plan

Coverage Considerations

- There are underlying clinical conditions that only a registered nurse (RN) can monitor to ensure that essential nonskilled care is achieving its purpose.
- The unskilled services are complex.
- The involvement of skilled nursing is needed to promote recovery and ensure safety.
- When visits by a nurse are not needed to observe and assess the effects of the nonskilled services being provided to treat the illness or injury, skilled nursing care would not be considered reasonable and necessary to treat it.

Patient Example

An elderly patient with a history of mild dementia is recovering from pneumonia, which has been treated at home. The patient has had an increase in disorientation, has residual chest congestion and a decreased appetite, and has remained in bed, immobile, throughout the episode with pneumonia. Although the residual chest congestion and recovery from pneumonia alone would not represent a high risk factor, the patient's immobility and increase in confusion would create a high probability of relapse. Skilled oversight of the nonskilled services would be reasonable and necessary, pending the elimination of the chest congestion and resolution of the persistent disorientation to ensure the patient's medical recovery. The clinical documentation should focus on the complexity of the overall POC and the underlying clinical conditions of the patient. The documentation should include care coordination conferences and other communications with any community resources assisting the agency to stabilize the patient. Usually these patients have multiple medical problems, as shown in the example, and have multiple medications or may have a history of abuse or noncompliance.

Documentation Considerations

In this example the documentation should show that the RN *actively* manages the POC. Observation alone does not support the need for this service; thus the entries should identify the relationships between symptoms and conditions that create the complexity for "skilled management" to be covered. Document the reason the patient is homebound. For this patient, reasons could include dementia, shortness of breath, immobility, and need for assistance to leave home safely.

Identify the patient's medical problems, the interventions initiated to resolve and/or avoid further medical complications, changes in the POC to maintain the health and medical safety of the patient, efforts related to teaching and training of caregivers, communications with services in the community and any linkages for further care and support, and the response of the caregivers providing the nonskilled care and the goals for care. Some of the factors that may require intervention or direction from the RN include mental status problems, functional limitations, high-risk concerns related to safety of the patient, and medication problems related to abuse or compliance. Documentation should also be directed toward the efforts by the RN to stabilize the POC. Document any deficits in the support system such as language barriers, abuse, unsafe home environment, or no food in home. Document the clinical and social problems that have brought this patient to home care and the progress made to date toward stabilization (Box 5-5).

Standards of Practice for Excellence

Care coordination and communication are very important for these patients and all patients cared for in home care. Community resources, the

---

BOX 5-5   CHECKLIST FOR MANAGEMENT AND EVALUATION OF THE CARE PLAN

Is this a skilled management and evaluation case?
✔ Multiple medical problems
✔ Multiple medications—abuse or noncompliant
✔ Multiple or restrictive functional limitations
✔ ADL deficits caused by physical, mental, emotional problems
✔ Deficits in thought processes
✔ Emotional problems
✔ Nutritional and/or hydration problems
✔ Health-risking behaviors—chemically dependent, noncompliant
✔ Deficits in support system—e.g., abuse, unsafe environment
✔ Multiple community resources
✔ Difficulty in obtaining community resources
✔ History of frequent hospitalizations or emergency room visits related to functional deficits:
   Falls
   Dehydration
   Malnutrition
   Pressure ulcers
✔ Long-term medical problems:
   AIDS
   Cancer
   Transplants

From Wellmark, formerly known as ISAD Health Services Corp., Federal Intermediary and Carrier, Des Moines, Iowa.

physician, the nonskilled caregivers, and families who are often far away or unable or unwilling to be caregivers all contribute to the need for clear communications and the documentation of the communications and plan. The role of the nurse with these patients is primarily that of care coordinator and case manager.

Teaching and Training Activities
Coverage Considerations
- The skills of a nurse are required.
- The test of skill relates to the skill needed to teach; not to what is being taught.
- Must be directed toward the patient's functional loss, illness, or injury.
- If the patient or caregiver cannot or will not be taught or learn (after a reasonable amount of time), further teaching is not reasonable and will not be covered.
- When determining the visit frequency and duration, consider if this is initial instruction or reinforcement. Again, base the plan on the patient's unique condition.
- Three reasons for reteaching or retraining:
  1. Change in procedure
  2. Change in patient condition
  3. Change in caregiver
- There is no requirement that the patient, family, or other caregiver be taught to provide a service if they cannot or choose not to provide the care.
- Eighteen teaching and training activities are listed in the HHA Manual, although the activities are not limited only to those listed.

Patient Example
A physician has ordered skilled nursing care for teaching a diabetic patient who has recently become insulin dependent. The physician has ordered teaching of self-injection and management of insulin, signs and symptoms of insulin shock, and actions to take in emergencies. The teaching services would be reasonable and necessary to the treatment of the illness of injury.

Documentation Considerations
In this example, document in each note the teaching and training occurring at each visit and the patient's response to teaching. This includes the assessment of the patient's baseline knowledge of the information, task, or process to be taught. This patient may be homebound because of activity restrictions, blindness, status post above- or below-knee amputation, paralysis, need for maximum assistance to ambulate from pulmonary vascular disease, neuropathies, and other reasons, based on the patient's unique medical condition identified on admission.

The clinical record must document the reason reteaching or retraining is required (listed previously under Coverage Considerations). On all notes, state the teaching provided, the patient or caregiver demonstration or verbalization of understanding, progress toward predetermined goals for teaching, and other information that supports covered care. When training is not successful, the reasons for its lack of success to date should be documented in the clinical record. In instances of reteaching or retraining (e.g., when a patient loses the use of the dominant hand and must be taught to self-inject with the other hand), the documentation in the clinical record should note the reason that the reteaching or retraining is required.

Standards of Practice for Excellence

In determining the reasonable and necessary number of teaching and training visits, consideration must be given to whether the teaching and training was provided previously in an inpatient setting and constitutes reinforcement or whether it is the initial instruction. (Because of the decreased stays in some hospitals, patients barely receive survival or emergency teaching.)

Patient education is an important and large part of home care practice. Education should occur each visit, since self-care is the ultimate outcome for many home care patients. In addition, nurses must teach caregivers to assume the care in longer-term and chronic care situations. Nurses do not help their patients by making them dependent on daily nursing care or services. Proficient home care nurses are excellent educators. Assessing learner readiness and skill levels, dealing with challenging patients or caregivers, and handling compliance problems are all part of teaching. A review of adult learning principles, as well as classic texts on patient education, will assist in providing this important information. When a nurse transitions from the inpatient setting to home care, not only does the educational style or theoretical framework for patient education change because of the environment and the self-care emphasis, but, more important, the basis of care in home care is education which may be significantly different from that of the inpatient setting.

Patient education materials are an important part of standardizing care and care processes for your organization. Some organizations have patient education committees within which they work toward consensus to design patient education materials for their most common patient problems. This initiative may be a part of the organization's quality or performance improvement process. Other organizations identify a day annually on which team members bring in their patient educational materials (aka trunk files) and a work group revises and distributes updated materials. Most home care organizations have these tools available in the home care library of resources for easy review and retrieval.

Administration of Medications

Medicare covers the services of a licensed nurse to administer medications safely and effectively; it does not cover the drugs. In fact, drugs and biologicals are specifically excluded from coverage by the statute 1861 (m) (5) of the Social Security Act. There are very few exceptions.

The home care nurse plays a large role in moving patients toward self-care related to insulin-dependent diabetes mellitus. Role modeling, time, support, and presence may all help the patient integrate the care of the disease into daily care regimens.

Medicare states that insulin customarily is self-injected by patients or injected by their families. This is why prefilling of syringes is usually not covered care and is not considered a skilled nursing service.

When determining if the patient is unable or unwilling to self-inject, observation and assessment are very important. If a patient is capable of but refuses to perform injections, he or she does not automatically meet the condition of physical or mental inability for coverage purposes. Experienced home care nurses have all had patients who initially state that they "can never give this shot" but who change their minds because of the nurse's education, persistence, and support. Keep in mind that fear may be behind the refusal to self-inject.

Coverage Considerations

- Intravenous, intramuscular, and subcutaneous injections and infusions require the skills of a nurse to administer safely and effectively.
- Must be reasonable and necessary to the treatment of the illness or injury and acceptable standards of medical practice.
- Must be a medical reason the medication cannot be taken orally.
- Frequency and duration of the medication must be within accepted standards of medical practice.

  B_{12}

- Vitamin B_{12}: the patient must have one of the listed diagnoses to be covered, and the frequency must be within accepted standards, unless there is documentation supporting the need for increased or additional dosages.
- Specified anemias: pernicious anemia, megaloblastic anemias, macrocytic anemias, or fish tapeworm anemia.
- Specified gastrointestinal disorders: gastrectomy, malabsorption syndromes such as sprue and idiopathic steatorrhea, surgical and mechanical disorders such as resection of the small intestine, strictures, anastomosis, or blind loop syndrome.
- Certain neuropathies: postlateral sclerosis, other neuropathies associated with pernicious anemia, during the acute phase or acute exacerbation of a neuropathy due to malnutrition and alcoholism.
- Acceptable reasonable and necessary dosage and frequency schedule.

Insulin Injections

- Insulin injections: covered for daily care when the patient is either physically or mentally unable to self-inject and there is no able or willing caregiver (which must be clearly documented in the clinical record).
- Daily insulin visits are the exception to the daily intermittent rule.
- Prefilling of syringes is covered when state law precludes home health aide from filling and the patient otherwise needs skilled care.

Oral Medications

- Oral medications are usually not covered care, (not reasonable, and skilled nursing care unnecessary), except in certain situations.
- Would be based on the complexity of the patient's condition and the number of drugs the patient is taking for evaluation of side effects or reactions. The documentation must show the specific complexities and unique condition requiring skilled observations.

Eyedrops and Topical Ointments

- Do not require the skills of a nurse.
- Even if the patient cannot self-administer and there is no one to administer them, administration is not covered as skilled nursing services.
- Associated observation and assessment needs are covered (the first skilled nursing service), and these could be performed only incidental to the covered skilled nursing service.

Patient Example

An elderly man lives alone and has severe arthritis in his hands. He has been maintained on oral hypoglycemic medications for years, and the physician recently ordered the home care organization to begin daily injections of insulin. The patient also has swollen legs, neuropathy that causes pain in his legs and arms, and severe visual impairment caused by retinopathy. Skilled nursing would be appropriate to administer the injections, since the patient is unable to self-inject.

Documentation Considerations

In this example the patient is physically unable to self-inject. His reasons for being homebound include severe visual impairment and ambulation with assistance of walker only.

In home care, effective clinical documentation paints a picture of the patient, his or her problems and assessed needs, planned and actual interventions and actions, and the evaluation of those actions. For this patient, the documentation would include that the insulin was administered, the time, the amount and specific type of insulin administered, the method (e.g., subcutaneously), the specific site injected, any reaction to the injection or medication, and the teaching or training that was provided. Usually the skilled nursing note may have areas to check off and complete—important parts of the documentation from a reimbursement perspective as it supports coverage, quality, and risk management. Figure 7-1 is an example of a skilled nursing note.

Standards of Practice for Excellence

For all medications, it is important that nurses review what they learned in nursing school about the five rights of medication administration. They are: the right patient, the right drug, the right reason, the right route, and in the right dose for the patient. Home care nurses should have an up-to-date drug text that is used across the organization to standardize care.

Conformance with physician orders related to drugs and other treatments is very important. The home care nurse must check all medicines a patient may be taking to identify possible ineffective drug therapy or adverse reactions, significant side effects, drug allergies, and contraindicated medications and promptly report any problems to the physician.

Medication administration and management are large components of home care nursing practice. There are studies that confirm what all home care nurses think—that patients over age 65 are taking an average of over 10 medications at any given time. In my experience in home care, there are many patients who have twice that many.

The essential skills related to medications are many and include identifying what the patient is currently taking or takes on a daily basis, observation and assessment related to the actual medications and their effects, compliance, knowledge related to drug classifications, and keeping up with myriad new drugs that come on the market. Other skills include venipuncture related to therapeutic versus toxic dosages, possible dietary and drug interactions or drug/drug interactions, and patient teaching considerations. The pharmacist is an important team member in home care and can act as a resource for home care nurses and other team members.

Tube Feedings

Coverage Considerations

- Nasogastric and percutaneous tube feedings (including gastrostomy and jejunostomy tubes).
- Covered services include replacement, adjustment, stabilization and suctioning of the tubes, which are skilled nursing services.
- If the feedings are required to treat the illness or injury, the feedings and replacement or adjustment of the tubes would be covered as skilled nursing services.

Patient Example

A physician has referred a patient to home care who has recently moved in with her daughter. The patient is an 86-year-old woman who had home care nurses in her previous home and has been on tube feedings since she had a resection for cancer some years ago. The daughter and patient provide the actual feedings; home care is responsible for the adjustment and care of the tubes and the daughter's education about the care.

Documentation Considerations

In this example the care related to the tubes would be covered (i.e., observation, assessment, teaching, and training related to the tube). This patient is homebound because she needs assistance to ambulate. The documentation should specify the type or kind of tube, the history of use of the tube, when it was last changed, site care to date, findings on physical assessment related to weight, site of tube, intake and output history, the caregiver's ability and willingness to learn and provide care, and other information related to the feeding tube and the hydration and nutrition status of this new patient.

Standards of Practice for Excellence

Many home care organizations have wound care specialists or enterostomal therapists (ETs) to assist in planning care for patients with wounds or skin sites that are at risk. This patient could be appropriate for such a referral, or the case manager could report the skin site findings to the ET nurse. Besides the tube care, this patient is very appropriate for observation and assessment and should have weight checked every visit. Depending on the findings at the visit, the case manager may also want to case conference with the dietitian about this new patient. Educational materials may also be helpful for the daughter who will need education and support as she learns to care for her elderly mother.

Nasopharyngeal and Tracheostomy Aspiration

Coverage Considerations

- Nasopharyngeal and tracheostomy aspiration (suctioning) are skilled nursing services and, if required to treat the patient's illness or injury, would be covered as skilled nursing services.

Patient Example

A 66-year-old man with lung cancer was admitted to hospice. The home care nurse provides care and support, suctions the patient as necessary, and teaches the family about care. The suctioning would be reasonable and necessary to the treatment of the illness or injury.

Documentation Considerations

In this example the documentation should reflect the suctioning, the patient's response to the treatment, the specific supplies used, and that universal precautions were maintained in technique and care. This patient is homebound because of his debilitating disease and severe shortness of breath.

Standards of Practice for Excellence

Universal precautions are the hallmark of infection control. Effective hand washing is the most important deterrent to the spread of infections. The risk of cross-contamination exists in home care and particularly around respiratory patients and problems; the strictest infection control standards should be maintained when handling supplies, including the catheter, the water, and the suction equipment.

Catheters

Coverage Considerations

- Insertion and sterile irrigation, replacement of catheters, care of a suprapubic catheter, and, in selected patients, urethral catheters, are skilled nursing services.
- Frequency appropriate to the type of catheter used:
    Foley—every 30 days
    Silicone catheters every 60-90 days
- When complications require more frequent visits related to the catheter, this care would be covered, with adequate documentation.
- PRN visits are usually appropriate.

Patient Example

A patient who has a Foley catheter because of loss of bladder control resulting from multiple sclerosis (MS) has a history of frequent plugging of the catheter and urinary tract infections. The physician has ordered skilled nursing visits once a month to change the catheter and has left a PRN order for up to three additional visits per month for skilled observation and evaluation and/or catheter changes if the patient or family reports signs and symptoms of a urinary tract infection or a plugged catheter. During the certification period, the patient's family contacts the HHA because the patient has an elevated temperature, abdominal pain, and scant urine output. The nurse visits the patient and determines that the catheter is plugged and there are symptoms of a urinary tract infection. The nurse changes the catheter and contacts the physician to advise him of her findings and to discuss treatment. The skilled nursing visit to change the catheter and to evaluate the patient would be reasonable and necessary to the treatment of the illness or injury.

Documentation Considerations

In this example the findings reported in the previous paragraph would need to be in the clinical documentation. This patient is homebound because of his MS and because he needs assistance to leave home and/or ambulate. Document the color, appearance of urine, any culture and sensitivity results, and details of sending the specimen to the laboratory.

Standards of Practice for Excellence

The nurse should check with her or his supervisor about the policy, but most home care organizations keep statistics on patients who acquire infections. Urinary infections are usually tracked in home care as a part of ongoing infection control and surveillance activities. Patient and care-giver teaching and training related to maintenance of the catheter, the importance of hygiene, and intake and output observational skills are all important.

Examples of problems that patients in home care with catheters may experience are constipation and resulting pressure on the bladder; uri-nary tract infections; catheter position changes causing leakage or pain, which necessitates an assessment for the possible need for another or different kind of catheter; bladder spasms; and increased sediment in the urine. For these reasons PRN visits should be obtained on catheter patients so that the nurse can visit and assess the patient's needs.

Wound Care

Coverage Considerations

- Thirteen kinds of wounds are listed for which the skills of a nurse are usually reasonable and necessary.
- It is important to remember that there are three covered services re-lated to wound care:
  1. Hands-on care (e.g., dressing change)
  2. Observation and assessment or monitoring of the wound
  3. Skilled teaching and training related to the wound and care. When one of the three covered services is provided, services are covered.

Patient Example

A patient has a second-degree burn with full-thickness skin damage on his back. The wound is cleansed, followed by an application of Sulfamylon. The wound requires skilled monitoring for signs and symptoms of infection or complications, and the dressing change requires skilled nursing services.

Documentation Considerations

In this example two skilled services are provided, hands-on care and skilled monitoring for infection. This patient may be homebound be-cause of medical restrictions relating to the burn or pain caused by the burns, because he needs assistance to ambulate, or for other reasons, based on the patient's unique condition and assessed findings.

For skilled nursing care to be assessed to be reasonable and neces-sary to treat a wound, the size, depth, nature of drainage, (color, odor, consistency and quantity), and condition and appearance of the skin sur-rounding the wound must be documented in the clinical findings. Cov-erage or denial of skilled nursing visits for wound care may be based not solely on the stage classification of the wound, but rather on all of the documented clinical findings. In addition, the POC (HCFA 485) must contain specific instructions for the treatment of the wound.

For each wound care visit, document the skilled care provided, the patient's response to the intervention/care, the patient's homebound status, and the plans for continued care. Observation and assessment include vital signs, including pain; teaching and training include training specific to that visit and the patient's response to the information/teaching. Documentation of the actual hands-on wound care should include the kind of dressing used and other physician orders specified in the plan of care.

Standards of Practice for Excellence

Wound care is a large part of home care practice. There are wide variations in the types of wounds, the kinds of interventions and products, and different staging tools used in practice. As home care and hospice move toward more outcome-focused care, the standardization of care and care processes should contribute to less variation and hopefully will facilitate improved data collection and evaluation of goal achievement. Resources for case managers caring for patients with wounds are the ET nurse and the dietitian.

Infection control plays a big part in wound care home visits. Hand washing, setting up work space, placing a barrier under your nursing bag, correctly disposing of soiled dressings and supplies, and aseptic or clean technique all contribute to quality in wound care (see Chapter 12).

Ostomy Care

Coverage Considerations

- Postoperative care
- Teaching is skilled, regardless of the presence of complications
- PRN visits may be appropriate

Patient Example

A 76-year-old man is sent home after receiving a colostomy as a result of cancer of the colon. His 74-year-old wife is his caregiver. The ostomy site is reddened and sore, and he complains to the nurse about "not being able to eat all the foods I like to eat."

Documentation Considerations

In this example the documentation should consist of the teaching accomplished and the observation and assessment of the patient, the postoperative stoma site and care, and efforts directed toward self-care. This patient is homebound because he is weak status post surgery with new ostomy, medically restricted because of new colostomy, and unable to leave home without assistance.

Standards of Practice for Excellence

Ostomy care requires sensitivity toward the patient. The loss of "regular" bowel function is very difficult for most patients and sometimes complicated by knowing they have or have had cancer and the fear of its recurrence. Monitoring bowel and bladder habits for patients is an important part of all home care, not just for ostomy care. Most impactions are preventable with an effective regimen of diet, stool softeners, and laxatives or suppositories when needed. Physician orders are needed for medications related to bowel maintenance regimens.

As discharge approaches for patients, the nurse should know that support groups can be very helpful for patients with new ostomies in providing both peer support and resources. Many times they have transportation for participants who need this assistance. Usually the support groups are led by an ET nurse who has experience and answers for the participants (see Chapter 12).

Heat Treatments
Coverage Considerations
- This service is rarely used.
- Requires skilled observation and monitoring.
- Consider safety related teaching.

Standards of Practice for Excellence

All heat-related treatments have implications for safety. In home care nurses care for a vulnerable patient population who may have limited sensation to feel heat (or cold) because of neuropathies, diabetes, and other health problems.

Medical Gasses
Coverage Considerations
- Initial phases of a regimen involving the administration of medical gasses that are necessary to the treatment of the patient's illness or injury.
- Requires skilled observation and evaluation of the patient's reaction to the gasses.
- Teaching the patient and family when and how to properly manage the administration of the gasses.

Standards of Practice for Excellence

Oxygen is the most common "gas" seen in home care. Patients and families may have questions about the setup, safety, use, and other informational needs. Some home care programs provide a pamphlet or flyer about the use of oxygen and home safety related to the use of oxygen.

Often home care organizations contract with home medical equipment companies to provide the oxygen and associated supplies. It is important that the home care nurse know where the equipment in the home came from to be able to communicate about any problems related to the patient and patient care related to the oxygen.

Rehabilitation Nursing
Coverage Considerations
Rehabilitative nursing procedures, including the related teaching and adaptive aspects of nursing that are a part of active treatment (e.g., the institution and supervision of bowel and bladder training programs), would constitute skilled nursing services.
Standards of Practice for Excellence
Rehabilitation nursing is a growing field in home care, and standards are starting to emerge from some of the national associations related to this specialty.

Venipuncture
Coverage Considerations
- Physician's orders for laboratory tests should be associated with a specific symptom or disease (e.g., fasting blood sugar—diabetes mellitus)
- Frequency of visits must be reasonable within accepted standards of medical practice for treatment of the illness or injury
- Frequency of testing should be consistent with accepted standards of medical practice for continued monitoring of a diagnosis, medical problem, or treatment regimen.
- Even when the laboratory results are consistently stable, periodic venipuncture may be reasonable and necessary because of the nature of the treatment.
- Documentation is very important in justifying the necessity of venipuncture and particularly in cases in which there is testing more frequently than stated in the Coverage of Service Section of the *HHA Manual—Pub. 11* (HCFA). Examples in the manual of reasonable and necessary venipunctures, the blood tests, and frequencies for stabilized patients include: captopril, dilantin, insulin and fasting blood sugars, and prothrombin times.
Patient Example
A patient with coronary artery disease was hospitalized with atrial fibrillation and was subsequently discharged to home care with orders for anticoagulation therapy. Monthly venipunctures as indicated are necessary to report prothrombin (protime) levels to the physician, notwithstanding that the patients' prothrombin time tests indicate essential stability.

Documentation Considerations

In this example, the documentation should clearly state the continuing need for the venipunctures and that the patient cannot leave without maximum assistance to have them drawn at the physician's office. Even though the patient is essentially stable, the care is still skilled care.

Standards of Practice for Excellence

Most home care organizations have standardized processes for the collection of specimens such as venipunctures. Because of infection control considerations, many use vacutainers and other systems for the actual collection to standardize care among the nurses. The disposal of sharps continues to be a risk in home care as well as other health care settings.

Student Nurse Visits

Coverage Considerations

- Visits made by a student nurse may be covered as skilled nursing care when the agency participates in training programs that use student nurses enrolled in a school of nursing to perform skilled nursing service in a home setting.
- The services must be reasonable, and necessary skilled nursing care must be performed under the general supervision of a registered or licensed nurse. The supervising nurse need not accompany the student nurse on each visit.

Standards of Practice for Excellence

Nursing students need home health experience where they can gain practical experience to become professional nurses. Home care exposure during nursing school introduces the nursing student to home care and the unique nuances of practice in the community. If you have the chance at your home care organization, accept and work with the nursing students; they help all nurses question and rethink our processes, as well as some of our belief systems. They also just may motivate us to go back to school.

Psychiatric Evaluation, Therapy, and Teaching

Coverage Considerations

- Evaluation, psychotherapy, and teaching activities.
- Patient has a diagnosed psychiatric disorder requiring active treatment.
- Must be a psychiatrically trained nurse who has specialized training and/or experience beyond the standard curriculum required for a registered nurse.
- The services of the psychiatric nurse are provided under a POC established and reviewed by a physician.

Patient Example

A patient is homebound for medical conditions, but has a psychiatric condition for which he has been receiving medication. The patient's psychiatric condition has not required a change in medication or hospitalization for over 2 years. During a visit by the nurse, the patient's spouse indicates that the patient is awake and pacing most of the night and has begun ruminating about perceived failures in life. The nurse observes that the patient does not exhibit an appropriate level of hygiene and is dressed inappropriately for the season. The nurse comments to the patient about her observations and tries to solicit information about the patient's general medical condition and mental status. The nurse advises the physician about the patient's general medical condition and the new symptoms and changes in the patient's behavior. The physician orders the nurse to check blood levels of medications used to treat the patient's medical and psychiatric conditions. The physician then orders the psychiatric nursing service to evaluate the patient's mental health and communicate with the physician about whether additional intervention to deal with the patient's symptoms and behaviors is warranted.

Documentation Considerations

In this example the patient's changes in behavior and dress would be documented to show a change that initiates a call to the physician and the plan of care for a psychiatric nurse evaluation. The patient in the example is homebound for medical problems. However, sometimes patients receiving psychiatric services may be homebound for psychiatric reasons, including depression, agoraphobia, psychotic thinking processes, and severe anxiety.

Standards of Practice for Excellence

Medicare has special criteria for nurses who provide psychiatric home care. Each RHHI reviews the resumés of the nurses for their geographic regions and initiates a process for approval (see Chapter 10).

Physician-Approved Plan of Care

The services provided must fall under a POC established and approved by a physician. The POC content must include pertinent diagnoses; patient's mental status; types of services, supplies, and equipment required; frequency of visits; patient prognosis; rehabilitation potential; functional limitations; activities permitted; nutritional requirements; all medications and treatments; safety measures to protect against injury; instructions for timely discharge or referral; and any additional items the organization or physician chooses to include.

The POC or 485 form must be completed for every Medicare patient on admission and every 62 days thereafter. These 62-day periods of care are called certifications for the initial period and recertification for subsequent certifications. The physician certification then may cover a period less than but not greater than 62 days.

By signing the 485, the physician certifies the following:

1. The home health services are or were needed because the patient is or was confined to the home as defined in the Home Health Agency Manual per "homebound."
2. The patient needs or needed skilled nursing services on an intermittent basis, physical therapy, or speech-language pathology services or continued or continues to need occupational therapy after the need for skilled nursing care, physical therapy, or speech-language pathology services has ceased.
3. A POC has been established and is periodically reviewed by a physician.
4. The services are or were furnished while the patient is or was under the care of a physician.

Documentation Supports Care Covered

The clinical documentation must support the coverage of covered care. *Reimbursement in home care hinges solely on documentation.* The home care nurse has a pivotal role in creating documentation that supports coverage for patients who meet the criteria and have Medicare. Documentation then must be valued and as important as the care provided. Chapter 7 addresses the complexities and requirements related to home care documentation. The nurse as case manager, team leader, or care coordinator is responsible for providing this support and evidence in the clinical documentation.

SUMMARY

Medicare home care has set many of the standards for home care. Nurses in home care must integrate the Medicare rules into daily practice and operations to be able to explain it to patients.

The role, scope, and complexity of home care nursing will only be more valued in the years to come. The COPs and the Medicare coverage guidelines must be operationalized for the home care nurse to meet requirements while maintaining professional standards of practice. Medicare skilled nursing services may be covered when the beneficiary meets the qualifying requirements, when the patient is homebound, when the services are medically reasonable and necessary based on the patient's unique medical condition, and when the clinical documentation supports coverage of covered services.

REVIEW EXERCISES

1. What requirement listed below is not one of the main coverage criteria for Medicare home care?
   a. Skilled care
   b. Under a physician plan of care
   c. Homebound
   d. Patient needs daily and full-time care
2. Describe homebound with patient examples.
3. List the services covered under Medicare Part A.
4. Define five of the 15 Medicare covered skilled nursing services.
5. Medicare is a medical insurance program and as such is like any other insurer, i.e., there is covered care as well as exclusions to coverage. True or False?
6. It is the home care team member's clinical documentation that ultimately either supports (or does not support) coverage. True or False?

FOR FURTHER READING

HCFA: *Your Medicare handbook,* Baltimore, 1996, Health Care Financing Administration. This handbook is also available on audiotape for the visually impaired and on the Internet. HCFA's WEB site address is: http:www.hcfa.gov. To obtain the handbook, write to: Health Care Financing Administration, Office of Beneficiary Relations, N-1005, 7500 Security Blvd., Baltimore, MD 21244-1850.

Marrelli TM: *Handbook of home health standards and documentation guidelines for reimbursement,* ed 3, St. Louis, 1998, Mosby.

6
INTAKE REFERRAL PROCESS

Tina M. Marrelli, MSN, MA, RNC

"If you always do what you've always done, you'll always get what you've always gotten."

Jay Katz

In health care and home care, we must try to improve the way we do things; without improvement or change, outcomes will remain the same. This is particularly important to remember about the intake or referral process.

The entire patient process, beginning with intake and admission, through care and planning, and ending with discharge, is a key component of an effective orientation. The intake or referral process is the data collection point of entry for new home care patients; it is how referral sources such as case managers, discharge planners, physicians, or patients initially contact home care. In some home care organizations, this area may also be called the admission department. Once the patient is into the home care system, the intake process consists of a series of questions and initial data collection for determining how best to meet the patient's home care needs. Larger home care organizations have intake offices staffed by nurses and coordinators, support team members who collect the data before passing the information on to a nurse for review and distributing it to a manager for assignment. No matter what titles and individual processes or referral/intake forms are used, the functions in this areas must occur as accurately and timely as possible. Skills for home care nurses who work in the intake area include active listening, home care experience, a broad knowledge of insurance reimbursement, impeccable customer service and phone skills, and up-to-date information about resources in the community. The new nurse in home care may spend time with the admissions area manager to better understand the organization and work flow that are initiated in the intake referral area.

BOX 6-1	**REFERRAL SOURCES IN HOME CARE**
Social workers	Nurses from inpatient areas
Case managers	Community services
Physicians	Family members or friends of
Ambulatory care sites	patients
Hospital discharge planners	Clergy or community leaders
Liaison coordinators	Legal guardians or trustees
Physician office staff	Others

Intake nurses must use their professional judgment to determine whether a prospective referral is appropriate for home care. This analysis is based on the demographic information (e.g., is the patient in the defined geographic catchment area of the home health agency (HHA)), the patient's diagnoses, and medications and associated health care problems that contribute to the determination of meeting patient needs safely and effectively. Your home care organization has policies related to guidelines for referrals and the timeline during which patients must be seen. An example is "that patients are visited and assessed for home care within 24 (or 48) hours of discharge from the hospital or of the referral." As home care patients are sent home sooner because of the decreasing length of hospitals stays, more and more often they will be seen the same day (e.g., the infusion patient who is discharged and needs a dose of intravenous medication later that evening or the wound care patient who needs the second of the BID dressing changes later in the day of discharge). When these visits occur on the same day as the hospital discharge, it is very important that the nurse's documentation explain the reason for that visit so that insurers do not see the service as a duplication of the service provided in the hospital the same day. For all these reasons, many organizations are increasing the hours and flexibility of the intake or admissions areas to cover evenings, weekends, and other traditional after-office hours to more effectively meet patient and referral source needs (Box 6-1).

Referrals to home care can occur in a variety of ways. They commonly occur by telephone, but they are also faxed, e-mailed, and downloaded as technology becomes more able to support health care systems. Regardless of how the referral is initiated, the data collected at the onset must be correct. Intake team members or anyone who takes referrals must have multifaceted listening skills to elicit needed information. One of the roles is to assist the patient "through the system." Nurses have

---

BOX 6-2   **LIST OF NEEDED INTAKE
              REFERRAL INFORMATION**

Date referral obtained
Referral source (name and
    phone number, setting)

Patient Information
Patient's name
Address
Phone number
Date of birth
Emergency contact (next of kin)
    name and phone number
Anticipated date of discharge
    from hospital
Directions to home
Referring physician
Unique physician identification
    number (UPIN)

Has this patient been a home
    care patient before here?
If yes, when? Nurse? (internal use)
Allergies
Reason for home care referral,
    including MD orders
Other

Insurance Information
HIC Number
Primary insurer
Name of contact at insurer and
    phone number
Need for prior authorization?
If Medicare, does patient belong
    to a Senior Plan?
Other

---

all had encounters with patients and their families who were just told to
call but who can't tell them why.

From the intake process, the patient or referral information is then
directed to the appropriate manager and team. The data gleaned from
the steps in the intake information/referral process are very important.
Box 6-2 lists the needed intake referral information for admission, care,
and billing.

FROM INTAKE TO BILLING
From Intake to Team Assignment

Home care organizations are usually comprised of teams. There are different models or configurations for care delivery in home care. These
teams may be organized geographically, by clinical specialty, or by a combination of these two. For example, a new referral of a patient pending
hospital discharge with a pressure ulcer may be referred to the team with
a wound care specialist as a manager, or a new postpartum patient would
be referred to the manager of the maternal-child program. For quality and
safety reasons, most home care organizations try to match new patients
with the skills of the nurse to be assigned as the care manager.

The need for information to be accurate at the front end of the process becomes very clear with a review of the model in Figure 6-1 that shows how patients (the clinical side of home care practice) and the administration (the billing and regulatory side of home care operations) must fit together for effectiveness and efficiency. As shown in this model, the two side pieces must fit together to make the whole organization work to provide patient care and be reimbursed appropriately for care provided.

Reimbursement Considerations

Like the clinical data initially collected during the intake process, the billing information must be accurate and, when possible, obtained even before the patient's admission. Nurses in hospitals traditionally left "billing functions" to the business office. In home care the two are intertwined from patient admission through discharge.

Much preplanning goes into the setup of the billing and business operations in home care programs. As the nurse manager reviews the intake information to determine the clinician who will care for the patient, simultaneously the billing clerk is identifying or validating the insurance information and may be data entering the information about this pending patient.

About now you may be saying, "I'm a nurse, what does this have to do with me?" Nurses in home care are pivotal to claims (or bill) payment or denial of payment based on their clinical documentation. Home care documentation will be discussed in depth in Chapter 7, but suffice it to say that the nurse's performance related to care and the documentation of that care can impact on the financial health of the home care organization where she or he works.

Home Care Nursing and Reimbursement: Important Interface

Determinations concerning home care coverage by Medicare are made well after the care has been provided by the nurse. Congress has provided the regional home health intermediaries (RHHIs) with a very limited medical review budget to look at claims. What this means is that they process and pay millions of home care and hospice claims and clearly cannot review each one to see that organizations and individual team members follow the admission criteria and coverage guidelines.

Thus a paid claim is not necessarily a covered claim, and the RHHI may come back many months later with denials or requesting money back from the organization because of an "overpayment." The RHHIs by law, as Medicare contractors, can only pay for covered care. They have front-end

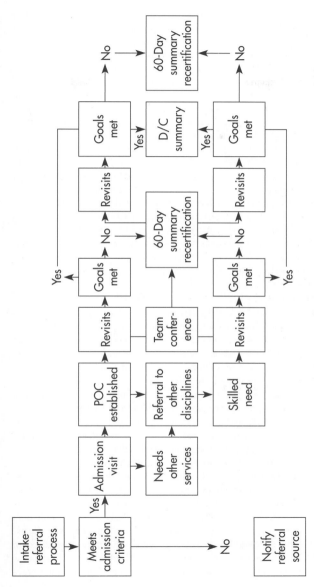

FIGURE 6-1 Workflow model.

edits or screens that assist in identifying claims that stand out or appear to be problematic (e.g., an organization provides many more visits than its peers in the same city or state, or the organization provides fewer home health aide services than "like" peers, or other aberrant practice patterns).

Once a problem is identified, the nurse reviewers at the RHHI may request additional records, perform a "coverage compliance review," or otherwise more closely review the home care documentation. The intermediary may pay or deny visits/services based on information provided on the Health Care Financing Administration (HCFA) 485 series forms (485,486,487). When the information on these forms is not sufficient to make a coverage decision, the HCFA form 488 is used to request additional information and/or the medical record. Routine submission of additional information is requested by the intermediary only when absolutely necessary. As a home care nurse then, your documentation must support covered care, and the form 485 must contain the information needed for a coverage determination. In "The Admission Process" section, a form 485 (HCFA Form 485—Home Health Certification and Plan of Care) is completed on the patient, Mr. Smith. This example shows how important all the details on the form 485 are to all involved in the patient's care and planning.

Working with Case Managers from Managed Care Companies

Managed care companies have nurse case managers who authorize any care for their patients. Usually these referrals come directly from the managed care nurse to the home care or hospice organization that has the contract to provide care to a defined group of their patients. In these instances the home care or hospice nurse must receive prior or preauthorization for any visits after the initial (and authorized) assessment visit. The case managers are paying the home care or hospice organization not so much for the task or activity, but for higher-level nursing skills such as observation and assessment, teaching and training directed toward caregivers or the patient for self-care, care coordination, and medication management.

Historically, and perhaps because of the Medicare model and the "15 covered skills," some see home care as task-oriented. This is a concern. The following example illustrates a patient case in which tasks are important, but the higher-level skills must also be valued. The nurse can teach Mrs. Jones to pack Mr. Jones's wound. However, she or he cannot teach Mrs. Jones the baseline knowledge that compares Mr. Jones' wound with the other hundreds the nurse has seen or the other facets of professional practice related to infection control, asepsis, observation and assessment of the wound, and integration and analysis of the entire picture toward projection of healing or dehiscence. This role of communicating to the nurse case managers the care provided to the patient is a very important aspect of the home care nurse's activities. The nurse must keep in mind that it is the framework encompassing the group of activities, within the state nurse practice act, that defines home care practice.

For all these reasons it is imperative that the operations that support the organization, such as the effectiveness, accuracy, and timeliness of the clinical documentation, be seen as equal to the care provided to patients; from a business survival focus, they must be. This information all comes together as nurses admit, care for, and discharge the patient in the following chapters. Refer to the Model of Work Flow (see Figure 6-1) for a visual review of the nurse's role in the process and to help see the "bigger picture" of home care.

THE ADMISSION PROCESS

The admission process is initiated by the decision of the nurse manager to accept the referral and scheduling the home care nurse to perform the admission evaluation visit. The admission process is the review and analysis of all the information, including the patient and the patient's environment, to make a determination for care and care planning. The knowledge needed for effective admissions and the sharing of complex information from multiple sources with patients includes a knowledge of the admission process, the admission criteria per the organizational policy, nursing and organizational standards of care, and the organization's mission and philosophy. At the same time, the patient may be in personal crisis, depressed, in pain, worried about his or her family, or otherwise preoccupied with appropriate health concerns. It is easy to see why an effective admission and assessment visit may take more time than anticipated.

In your orientation one of the policies that may have been provided to you for review is the "Admission Policy (or) Admission Criteria." Box 6-3 contains sample admission criteria; it is very important that you learn your organization's admission policies and, when you have questions, call your supervisor for direction.

Because team members of the home care organization must uphold the policies, if there is not compliance with the stated policy, the patient is not admitted. Simply put, admission criteria are the realistic plans for care, given the patient's home environment, care needs, the availability of specialty or other staff or resources, and other factors. At the completion of the admission visit, the home care nurse makes a determination for admission to home care based on the organization's admission criteria and speaks with the supervisor for direction and possible referral to other community resources.

BOX 6-3   **SAMPLE ADMISSION CRITERIA**

1. An initial assessment visit is made to determine that the patient is homebound (if Medicare), the patient's care needs, and that these needs can be met safely and adequately in their home environment.
2. Services are provided on an intermittent or part-time basis and are available to patients in their homes 7 days a week, 24 hours a day.
3. The patient must live in the geographic catchment area (defined counties, towns, areas).
4. The referring physician and the patient and patient's caregiver must be active participants in care and care planning.
5. Eligibility for participation is open to all, without regard for the patient's race, creed, color, sex, age, handicap, or other factors.
6. The patient meets the specific criteria for the insurance company related to skilled care and other criteria.
7. Other criteria, based on the organization's policy.

Initial Care Coordination and Communications

The supervisor provides the nurse with information about the patient needing the evaluation (also called an assessment or initial) home visit. Usually the manager provides all the information that is known about the patient and the patient's projected care needs as communicated by the referral source. Before the visit, physician orders are needed to initiate the care (i.e., the initial home visit). Usually this is done by telephone and noted in the documentation, followed up in writing with a verbal order form that is then signed by the physician. Services and care may be provided before obtaining the physician's plan of care (POC) (form 485) *based on documented verbal orders.* The intake/referral information and this verbal MD order, taken by the nurse, begin the patients' clinical record and care process.

For example, a patient named Mr. Smith will be followed from admission through care to discharge from home care services. Mr. Smith is a 74-year-old patient who was referred from St. Elsewhere Medical Center on discharge after a recent exacerbation of congestive heart failure (CHF) and chronic obstructive pulmonary disease (COPD) complicated by bronchitis. He was reported to be dehydrated on admission to the hospital and had a poor nutritional status, as evidenced by weight loss and weakness. Mr. Smith is married, and the social worker at the hospital called to say that Mrs. Smith could not visit him in the hospital due to her own health problems.

Planning the Admission Visit

The nurse then contacts the patient or designated caregiver contact and schedules the initial home visit. At this time the home care nurse introduces herself or himself, verifies that the patient is home (if an inpatient setting referral), verifies the address and directions to the home (sometimes at the last minute patients choose to go to a family member's), and briefly explains the reason for the visit. The following is an example of this interaction:

Nurse: Mr. Smith, this is Sarah James from XYZ Home Health in Anytown. I am a registered nurse, and your doctor, Doctor Kildare, asked that I come out and see how you are doing after your hospitalization.

Mr. Smith: Hang on, speak louder, I'm hard of hearing—I'll get my wife.

Mrs. Smith: He can't hear good anymore.

Nurse: Mrs. Smith, it's the nurse. I was calling to say I'd like to come out this morning at 11 AM and visit you and Mr. Smith and see how he is doing after the hospitalization.

Mrs. Smith: That would be fine.

This example points out a patient problem that was not communicated—the referral did not mention that Mr. Smith was hard of hearing. Including these kinds of details creates a culture in which individual patient needs and problems are valued and patients feel cared for by the home care team. This is the kind of information (i.e., that Mr. Smith is hard of hearing) that needs to be communicated to all team members who work with him and his family and the coordinator who schedules the home health aides, noted in the on-call book for the on-call nurses, and so on. Some agencies put details such as this on the front of the patient's chart so that, when the nurse is speaking with a home medical equipment vendor about a supply need for Mr. Smith, the vendor knows and can tell his team. All of these details contribute to satisfied customers for whom care is provided the right way and the first time.

The actual assessment or initial visit is a lengthy process and may take up to 2 hours, depending on the patient's problems and care needs. During your orientation you may have observed your preceptor or another experienced home care nurse making admission visits. In this observation role you may have noticed that there is a standard format for the organization of the work surrounding the admission process. The completion of forms, the health history, the explanation of the patient bill of rights and responsibilities, as well as information about advance directives and safety, may be provided in a certain order and in a standardized manner in the organization. This is another way that organizations standardize care processes so that whomever the caregiver is, the patient gets the same level and kind of care. Box 6-4 contains a list of

BOX 6-4   ADMISSION CHECKLIST

Regulatory Items

✔ Initial MD orders for patient to be seen

✔ Patient rights and responsibilities

✔ Consent for care and services

✔ Brochure

✔ Advance directive information

✔ Assignment of benefits (if insurance care)

✔ Notice on noncoverage (Medicare only)

✔ Medicare secondary payor (Medicare only)

✔ Financial responsibility

✔ Emergency checklist/plan

✔ Home safety assessment/information

✔ Clinical care items:

   ✔ Nurse bag:

     (Clean side) universal precaution supplies, personal protective equipment, alcohol swabs, newspapers, paper towels or plastic barrier, disposable supplies, laboratory specimen tubes and/or containers, venipuncture supplies, others. Some organizations also bring out a new thermometer and a mediset with the home care organization's name and number on it for each new patient.

     (Dirty side) tape measure, pen light, sharps box, blood pressure cuff and stethoscope, thermometer, glucometer, germicide or cleaning foam, others.

✔ Others: Laboratory supplies and forms, scale, map and directions.

Care

✔ Environment and safety assessment

✔ Entire systems review

✔ Comprehensive health history

✔ Physical and other assessments

✔ Initial ordered care (e.g., medication management and teaching, observations and assessment)

The Admission Forms Packet

✔ Initial assessment form (sometimes these are specific to patient and or home care program (e.g., pediatric, hospice, infusion care, psychiatric)

✔ Visit note (if not on the initial assessment tool)

✔ Medication profile

✔ Physician's orders (HCFA Form 485)

✔ Interdisciplinary care plan

✔ The OASIS form

Others

✔ Teaching guides

✔ Home safety information

✔ Calendar for the patient and team to track visits and schedule

✔ Others, per organizational policy

supplies and forms that may be needed for the initial assessment visit categorized for review. Other items may be needed, based on the patient and the home care organization.

The Admission/Evaluation Visit

Your supervisor reported that Mr. Smith needed to be seen and admitted for observation and assessment, follow up of his lengthy hospitalization, and multiple medication management and may be candidate for management and evaluation of the care plan.

As you drive to the home and walk up the stairs and into the home, you began the assessment related to the environmental safety and stability.

On the admission visit, when you arrive, you reintroduce yourself to Mr. Smith, who answers the door, and ask to come in. Mr. Smith explains that he can read lips and can hear you if you look at him when you speak. You tell him why you are there, explain the home care program, and encourage him to talk about himself. This is when you can "hear" what the *patient* wants from the home care nurse, which sometimes can be (very) different from *your* reason for being there. In the interest of customer service, it is important that you work to the meet patient needs.

Infection Control and the Home Visit

Mr. Smith walks you back to the kitchen where you both sit down; he explains that Mrs. Smith is now taking a nap. You ask if you can wash your hands and note that Mr. Smith has paper towels and liquid soap at the sink, which you use, turning off the handles with the paper towel.

You note that Mr. Smith is very tall and thin, is short of breath, and has cigarette burn holes in his shirt ("I'll probably never be able to quit," he says when you obtain the history about smoking), and reports that he usually cooks for himself and his wife. His wife is 8 years older and has periods of confusion, so she can no longer use the stove ("She about burned the house down").

When you ask to see his medications, Mr. Smith brings out a large shoebox packed with pill bottles and inhalers. He says that during this hospitalization they started him on two new asthma medications because he had trouble keeping track of all the other medications he was taking—he had been on nine medications, and the doctor said they made him lose too much fluid, and sometimes he ran out of them because they "cost too much" (in the back of your mind consider the need for social work, since lack of money to buy the needed medications would be an impediment to the POC being effectively implemented). The medications listed on the referral information are validated with the internist by calling from Mr. Smith's home. The medication regimen is: theophylline

PO, proventil inhaler, prednisone, digoxin, ampicillin, and aceta-
minophen (Tylenol) for his pain on coughing. The only allergies reported are paper tape, betadine, and pineapple.

Using All Your Assessment Skills: Initial Assessment

Home care nursing uses all your skills and, with experience, makes you
a very perceptive person. The initial assessment uses all your senses to
see the environment and patient, identify possible safety or other problems, begin the assessment of family dynamics, see the patient functioning in his or her own space, and collect data for the plan. If there is
a caregiver in the home, the nurse evaluates the caregiver's ability,
availability, and willingness to assume the care and support role. In this
case, Mrs. Smith may or may not be able to assist Mr. Smith; in fact, it
sounds as if he is the caregiver for both of them. This is also the time to
consider resource needs and availability. Consider the niece as a support
or backup caregiver for the Smiths, should he need assistance with shopping, house cleaning, errands, and other activities.

During the home assessment, you notice and hear the following:

- Mr. Smith is unshaven but dressed in shorts and a gold shirt that
  match.
- He states that "it takes me all morning to get bathed, and I can't
  reach my feet anymore—I want help with that; I used to have diabetes until I lost all this weight."
- The oxygen is in the corner, shut off, and you notice dust on the
  oxygen unit's housing.
- You notice that the dials for the electric stove have all been removed from the oven.
- There are no audible wheezes or coughing, but Mr. Smith uses upper accessory muscles to breathe at rest.
- He has clubbing of his fingers.
- There is an ashtray full of cigarette ashes and butts.
- He cannot bend over without increasing shortness of breath, and
  he has shiny ankles and edema.
- Mr. Smith appears happy to be home and back with Mrs. Smith
  (he explains that his niece came every night and stayed over with
  her while he was in the hospital and the neighbors checked in on
  her during the day and brought meals).
- Other observations

A comprehensive history and physical assessment follows. During
this time consider any medical equipment or supplies to support safe

care in the home. Paperwork, including clinical forms, findings, and nurse recommendations should be completed at the patient's home (unless there is safety concern). The initial assessment documentation includes the home visit and findings, the completion of the assessment tools and forms, the interactions with the patient and family, the care provided during the visit, the patient's response to the care, and the plan for continued care.

The first visit is the time to tell the patient that, since Medicare or another insurer is the payor, there is paperwork that must be completed; the patients all understand. Make it a standard practice to spend the last 5 to 10 minutes of every visit completing visit notes, updating the medication lists, completing the calendar, and performing other written or automated data entry patient-related tasks. Invariably, when the nurse leaves, the patient may have questions that he or she did not think of during the visit. This quiet time at the end of the visit saves many phone calls.

Complete the witness spaces and the dates on the regulatory items (listed in Box 6-4) and write the physical assessment findings directly on the nursing assessment form. Integrated into the information on the assessment tool are questions related to nutritional assessment (for which Mr. Smith is high risk, given his history, weight, and height) and screening for abuse and neglect. If you are automated and have computer data entry, this information would be directly keyed as obtained or as instructed by the organization's policies.

The following paragraphs address the nursing process used to create the POC for Mr. Smith. All data that are collected from the history; the assessment of the physical environment; and the physical findings from auscultation, weight, blood pressures (sitting and standing due to history of dehydration), and other vital signs (including pain) are analyzed to create the individualized POC for Mr. Smith. At the onset, and especially after explaining or reading to Mr. Smith the patient rights and responsibility forms, it is important that Mr. Smith know he is an equal partner in care and care planning.

When you ask what his immediate health problem is that requires your help, he explains that he is very constipated from the hospitalization and his hemorrhoids are, as he reports, "torqued up." He says he had the neighborhood pharmacist deliver something, but it has not helped. He also says he believes he is more short of breath than usual because, since he's been home, his wife has been up at night; thus he can't sleep through the night (like the hospital, he says) and feels very tired. During the review of current problems, this is a good time for the nurse to assess the need for other disciplines or services. With Mr. Smith the occupational therapist (OT) may be very appropriate for breathing exercises and conservation of energy techniques and teaching. In addition the OT may recommend assistive or adaptive devices and identify ways for Mr. Smith to more safely perform cooking and other activities of daily living (ADLs).

You complete all of the forms on the Admission Checklist per agency policy and give Mr. Smith a copy of all the papers that he signed. You also give him a "Home Safety Guide" that addresses issues related to bathroom safety; medication safety; and electrical, environmental, and fire safety. He says that he will read it and that he is very aware of safety because of his wife. In fact, he refrigerates all his medications except the inhaler because she doesn't go near the stove or the refrigerator anymore. "I am chief cook and bottlewasher," he says with a grin. You also give Mr. Smith an education booklet about "You and COPD," a magnet for the refrigerator, and a home care brochure. You again tell him how to reach the nurse or the on-call system after office hours.

Nursing Interventions and Actions

During the initial visit you provided the following skilled nursing services:

- Skilled observation and assessment of patient following hospitalization who has bronchitis and CHF and is at high risk for recurrent lung process because of smoking
- Assessment of nutrition and hydration status
- Management and evaluation of the patient POC
- Monitoring of cardiac, respiratory, integumentary, and other systems
- Teaching and assessment of signs and symptoms of digoxin toxicity
- Referral of patient to home health aide services for personal care and ADL assistance
- Other interventions, based on teaching and care provided

The Plan

You explain that you will be back to visit in 3 days, tell Mr. Smith the day and date, and write this information on the calendar you brought for him so he would know what team members would come when. You explain that you will call the physician and get orders for a bowel regimen and have this called into his local pharmacy for delivery. You explain that you will call him tomorrow about home health aide services who will help him with his bathing and grooming and that the OT will call to set up an appointment (he knew about OT because of the hospitalization).

You also explain that you'd do your best to be there for the home health aide's installation visit. You thank him for his time and the visit and leave. The following nursing diagnoses may apply to Mr. Smith:

- Activity intolerance, risk for
- Altered nutrition, less than body requirements
- Breathing pattern, ineffective
- Cardiac output, decreased
- Caregiver role strain, risk for
- Constipation
- Fatigue
- Fluid volume excess, risk for
- Gas exchange, impaired
- Infection, risk for
- Knowledge deficit (medications, self-care regimens)
- Management of therapeutic regimen, ineffective
- Mobility, impaired physical
- Nutrition, altered
- Self-care deficit (bathing, grooming)
- Sleep pattern disturbance
- Others

The nursing diagnoses are identified to integrate into Mr. Smith's POC. The creation of the plan is a thoughtful process that integrates all the data from all sources into a comprehensive tool that becomes the basis for initial care planning and care coordination among team members. Many times in the initial assessment visit all the facets of assessment may not be completed, particularly in relation to caregivers. In this case, the nurse's meeting of Mrs. Smith would be helpful in providing her with information about the stability of the situation. For example, if Mrs. Smith is very confused, the social worker would be called in sooner (as she will also address the medication and financial concerns) to help Mr. Smith with future planning and community resources where he may get respite on certain days. The multifaceted roles of the home care nurse come to the foreground during any patient admission visit. Roles of assessor, planner, coordinator, and advocate all come together and are prioritized based on the patient's needs.

When Evaluations do not Become Admissions

It is important to note that not all patients are admitted to care after the initial visit by the home care nurse. When a patient is not admitted after the initial visit, it usually means that the patient did not meet the home care organization's admission criteria. This may occur when the patient has extensive care needs, such as 24-hour care, and needs inpatient hospital– or skilled nursing facility–level care and the safety of the patient would be compromised with only intermittent or part-time visits. Another example is when the patient has specialty care needs that cannot be safely provided at home (e.g., the sick and high-risk infusion patient who lives alone on an island and has no refrigerator for storage of the drugs and fluids nor a telephone for communications). These situations could place both the patient and the organization at risk because of the identified safety concerns for the patient. When these circumstances occur, the manager usually calls the referral source and physician to communicate the problem and the reason the patient was not admitted to care. Alternatives are discussed, and the patient is not admitted. The records of these patients, which are comprised of the referral intake information and the admitting documentation, are usually filed by the organization as "patients assessed but not admitted."

ORIENTATION ASSIGNMENT

Ask your supervisor/preceptor for your organization's clinical forms, including comprehensive nursing assessment tool, medications/drug regimen sheet, visit note, and home environment safety checklist. These forms may be completed for a given patient from your organization, as assigned by your supervisor/preceptor or according to the Mr. Smith example.

Completing a HCFA Form 485

The HCFA form 485, Home Health Certification and Plan of Care, contains the data necessary to meet regulatory and certification requirements for the physician's POC and certification.

The first form 485 completed for your patients will be the "initial certification." Subsequent form 485s will be known as "recertifications" or "recertification periods" and are used when care continues beyond the certification period.

The form 485 is the basis of the care ordered and provided in home care. *The form 485 is the POC.* Because of this, the correct completion of the form 485 cannot be overstated. For Medicare and some other payors, it is the document that determines payment or denial for patient services. Because the form 485 serves as the physician orders and source of certification, it is the cornerstone on which all interventions, clinical forms, and documentation are based. HCFA requires that the nurse obtain a signed physician certification as soon as practical after the start of care (SOC) and before submission of the claim for payment to the Medicare RHHI. The physician-signed form 485s are retained in the home care clinical record. Many organizations use the 485 form for all patients, regardless of payor source.

For example, Mr. Smith's SOC date is 06/14/--, the date of the initial nursing assessment when he was admitted to home care and received covered skilled services. The completed form 485 for Mr. Smith may be found in Figure 6-2.

The following information provides the rationale for how this information is formulated and completed. The overall goal for the completion of the form 485 is that all data elements are completed and the information is accurate. This is the "detail-oriented" part of home care that leads to both clinical and operational excellence. The home care nurse usually completes elements 1 to 23.

1. *Patient's HI Claim Number (HICN).* Write the patient's HICN here. It contains numeric plus alpha indicators. This information is on the patient's Medicare card. For example, Mr. Smith's Medicare HICN is 123-45-6789A.

2. *Start of Care Date.* This is one of the most important entries on this form. The form 485 is tied to billing and clinical operations, and the SOC date is the pivotal point that initiates the activities for certification, recertification, and any mechanisms to prevent gaps in the POC certification periods. In addition, from a Medicare payor perspective, all entries related to the patient use the SOC as a key date for tracking and identification. As noted in Mr. Smith's example, the date must be a 6-digit month, day, and year. This date is the date of the first Medicare billable visit. "Billable" means that the patient meets the coverage criteria and was provided covered, skilled nursing care in the 15 skilled nursing services as defined in the *HHA Manual—Pub. 11* (HCFA). In Mr. Smith's case, because of the medication teaching, observation, and assessment provided, he had covered, billable care. Of course, the clinical documentation of that care would support this information, using the language, where possible, from the *HHA Manual—Pub. 11* (HCFA).

   This date remains the same on subsequent plans of treatment (recertifications) until the patient is discharged. Home health care may be suspended and later resumed under the same SOC date in accordance with the internal operations of the nurse's organization.

3. *Certification Period.* The certification period identifies the period covered by the physician's POC. The dates span from the SOC

Department of Health and Human Services
Health Care Financing Administration

Form Approved
OMB No. 0938-0357

HOME HEALTH CERTIFICATION AND PLAN OF CARE

1. Patient's HI Claim No.	2. Start Of Care Date	3. Certification Period	4. Medical Record No.	5. Provider No.
123-45-6789A	06-14-	From: 06-14- To: 08-14-	01-23	12-3456

6. Patient's Name and Address
Mr. Harry Smith
123 St. Mary's Road
Anytown, CA 12345

7. Provider's Name, Address and Telephone Number
XYZ Home Care Organization
12 Main Street
Pleasonton, CA 56789

8. Date of Birth 02-23-26 **9. Sex** [x] M [ ] F

10. Medications: Dose/Frequency/Route (N)ew (C)hanged Theophylline 200 mg qid po, (N), O_2 2-3 l per nasal cannula prn, proventil inhaler–3 puffs q8h as directed (C) prednisone 5 mg x 6 days bid; then call physician for adjustment (N), digoxin .125 mg po q am, lasix 20 mg po q am/(C), ampicillin 250 mg qid po x 1 week only (N), KDur 20 mEq 1 po q am (N), tylenol 2 tabs prn q4h pain (N), metamucil 1 T qod am prn po (N), anusol HC suppositories pr prn for hemorrhoidal pain (C)

ICD-9-CM	Diagnosis	Date
11. ICD-9-CM: 466.0	Principal Diagnosis: Bronchitis	6-14
12. ICD-9-CM	Surgical Procedure: N/A	6-14
13. ICD-9-CM: 496	Other Pertinent Diagnoses: COPD	
428.0	CHF	Unk.

14. DME and Supplies Oxygen concentrator and cannula, walker, and venipuncture supplies.

15. Safety Measures: Infection control, remove scatter rugs, oxygen safety instructions

16. Nutritional Req. low sodium diet

17. Allergies: allergies — paper tape, betadine, pineapple

18.A. Functional Limitations
1 [ ] Amputation 2 [ ] Bowel/Bladder (Incontinence) 3 [ ] Contracture 4 [x] Hearing 5 [ ] Paralysis 6 [x] Endurance 7 [x] Ambulation 8 [ ] Speech 9 [ ] Legally Blind A [x] Dyspnea With Minimal Exertion B [ ] Other (Specify)

18.B. Activities Permitted
1 [ ] Complete Bedrest 2 [ ] Bedrest BRP 3 [x] Up As Tolerated 4 [ ] Transfer Bed/Chair 5 [x] Exercises Prescribed 6 [ ] Partial Weight Bearing 7 [ ] Independent At Home 8 [ ] Crutches 9 [ ] Cane A [ ] Wheelchair B [ ] Walker C [ ] No Restrictions D [x] Other (Specify) SOB

19. Mental Status: 1 [x] Oriented 2 [ ] Comatose 3 [ ] Forgetful 4 [ ] Depressed 5 [ ] Disoriented 6 [ ] Lethargic 7 [ ] Agitated 8 [ ] Other

20. Prognosis: 1 [ ] Poor 2 [ ] Guarded 3 [x] Fair 4 [ ] Good 5 [ ] Excellent

21. Orders for Discipline and Treatments (Specify Amount/Frequency/Duration)

SN (NSG)	3 x week x 3 weeks	observation and assessment
	2 x week x 2 weeks	venipuncture for blood levels
	1 x week x 4 weeks	medication and self-care teaching
H/Aide	3 x week x 9 weeks	personal care, ADL assistance
OT	2 x week x 4 weeks	evaluation, conservation of energy techniques, home eval related to above, eval and teach re: assistive adaptive devices
MSS	2 x week x 1	evaluation related to financial concerns impacting ability to obtain medications, home safety concerns

22. Goals/Rehabilitation Potential/Discharge Plans Goals: (SN) verbalizes and adheres to care regimen related to meds, bowel regimen, smoking and diet. Venipunctures results reflect therapeutic dosages of theophylline and digoxin. (H/Aide) Patient clean and comfortable. (OT) Patient uses conservation of energy techniques and assistive/adaptive devices. (MSS) Patient provided with community linkage, able to obtain medications per plan of care.

Rehab potential: Good for returning to previous self-care status with assistance related to above problems. Projected time frame – less than 60 days.

Discharge plans: Mr. Smith will be discharged back to self-care status in his home with support of community elder services and followed by his physician.

23. Nurse's Signature and Date of Verbal SOC Where Applicable: 06-13-, T. Marrelli, RN

25. Date HHA Received Signed POT

24. Physician's Name and Address
J. Heal, M.D.
111 Carrick Road
Everytown, CA

26. I certify/recertify that this patient is confined to his/her home and needs intermittent skilled nursing care, physical therapy and/or speech therapy or continues to need occupational therapy. The patient is under my care, and I have authorized the services on this plan of care and will periodically review the plan.

27. Attending Physician's Signature and Date Signed

28. Anyone who misrepresents, falsifies, or conceals essential information required for payment of Federal funds may be subject to fine, imprisonment, or civil penalty under applicable Federal laws.

Form 1488LR BRIGGS, Des Moines, IA 50306 (800) 247-2343 PRINTED IN U.S.A. Form HCFA-485 (C-4) (02-94) (Print Aligned)

FIGURE 6-2 Completed form 485 for Mr. Smith. *(Form reprinted with permission of Briggs Health Care Products, Des Moines, Iowa.)*

date up to, but never exceeding, 2 calendar months and mathematically never exceeds 62 days. In this example, the certification period is 06/14/-- to 08/14/--. Always repeat the "To" date on a subsequent recertification as the next sequential "From" date. *Services delivered on the "To" date are covered under the next certification period.* This is because the "To" date is not a "Through" date and the certification ends on the "To" date if not extended to a recertification.

Example: Initial Certification   "From" date   06/14/--
           Initial Certification   "To" date   08/14/--
           Recertification "From" date   08/14/--
           Recertification "To" date   10/14/--

4. *Medical Record Number.* Enter the patient's medical record number that your home care organization assigns. From a Medicare perspective, this is an optional field, but most organizations assign medical record numbers for record reviews and other quality initiatives when the patient name may not be used. For this example use only the number 123-456.

5. *Provider Number.* Every home care organization that is Medicare participating receives a provider number from HCFA. This is the 6-digit number given by Medicare to the home care organization after achieving certification. For our example only, it is 12-3456. Sometimes home care organizations may have forms or computer screens that complete this information for the nurse.

6. *Patient's Name and Address.* This is the patient's last name, first name, and middle initial as shown on the health insurance card, followed by the street address, city, state, and zip code. For this example only, this is completed as Smith, Harry, 123 St. Mary's Road, Anytown, CA 12345.

7. *Provider's Name, Address, and Telephone Number.* This is the name of the home care organization and/or branch office (if applicable), street address (or other legal address), city, state, and zip code and telephone number. For our example, this is XYZ Home Care Organization, 12 Main Street, Pleasonton, CA 56789, (123) 456-7890.

8. *Date of Birth.* This is the patient's date of birth and has 6 digits (month, day, year) in numbers. For this example, Mr. Smith's date of birth is 02/23/26.

9. *Sex.* Just check the appropriate box; in this case, M.

10. *Medications: Dose/Frequency/Route.* This section begins the clinical components of the form 485 completion. This is the section in which physician orders for all medications are listed, including the dosage, frequency, and route of administration for each.

- When patients have more medications than can be listed in this space on the form 485, use the addendum HCFA-487 to list the rest.
- Place the letter (N) after medications that are "new" orders. "New" orders refer to medications that the patient has not taken recently (i.e., within the last 30 days).
- Place the letter (C) after medications that are "changed" orders. Changes include dosage, frequency, or route of administration changes. "Change" orders for medications include dosage, frequency, or route of administration changes within the last 60 days.

In our example, Mr. Smith's entire medication regimen, except for the digoxin, was changed, and this is noted on the sample 485 form.

11. *Principal Diagnosis.* The principal diagnosis is entered here. This diagnosis code is the diagnosis *most related to* the current treatment plan. It may or may not be related to the patient's most recent hospitalization, but it must relate to the service the home care organization is providing. If more than one diagnosis is treated concurrently, determine and use the diagnosis that represents the most acute condition and requires the most intensive services.

For example, even though Mr. Smith has both COPD and CHF, his COPD is the primary or principal diagnosis because the bronchitis and the CHF are problems related to but different from his COPD, and the services provided (e.g., new medication regimen and management, antibiotic therapy for the bronchitis, OT for conservation of energy) all relate more to the lung processes associated with COPD.

Here you enter the ICD-9-CM code in the space provided. The code must be the full ICD-9-CM diagnosis code, including all digits. V codes are acceptable as both primary and secondary diagnoses. In many instances, the V code more accurately reflects the care provided. However, do not use the V code when the acute diagnosis code is more specific to the exact nature of the patient's condition. The acceptable V codes, according to the *HHA Manual—Pub. 11* (HCFA), are contained in Box 6-5. List the actual *medical* diagnostic term next to the ICD-9-CM code. Do not use surgical procedure codes here. The date should be represented by six digits (MMD-DYY); if the exact day is not known, use 00. The date of onset is specific to the medical reason for the home care services. When the condition is chronic or long-term in nature, use the date of the exacerbation. Always use the latest date and complete all dates as close as possible to the actual date, to the best of your knowledge. For our example, the date listed is the date that Mr. Smith went to the physician's office and was admitted to the hospital for severe respiratory

BOX 6-5	**ACCEPTABLE V CODES**		
V45.6	Status following surgery of eye and adnexa	V54.8	Orthopedic aftercare, Kirschner wire, plaster cast, external splint, external fixation device, or traction device
v45.81	Postsurgical status, aortocoronary bypass status		
V45.89	Postsurgical status, presence of neuropacemaker or other electronic device	V54.9	Unspecified orthopedic aftercare
V46.0	Dependence on aspirator	V55.0	Attention to tracheostomy
V46.1	Dependence on respirator	V55.1	Attention to gastrostomy
V52.0	Fitting and adjustment of artificial arm	V55.2	Attention to ileostomy
		V55.3	Attention to colostomy
V52.1	Fitting and adjustment of artificial leg	V55.4	Attention to other artificial opening of digestive tract
V53-5	Fitting and adjustment, ileostomy or other intestinal appliance	V55.5	Attention to cystostomy
		V55.6	Attention to other artificial opening of urinary tract
V53.6	Fitting and adjustment, other urinary devices		
V54.0	Orthopedic aftercare involving removal of internal fixation device	V58.3	Attention to surgical dressing and sutures
		V58.4	Other aftercare following surgery

From HCFA: *HHA Manual—Pub. 11* (HCFA).

distress and wheezing. This is the date of the exacerbation of the COPD that facilitated the need for home care.

Other examples include the following:

- A patient is surgically treated for a subtrochanteric fracture (code 820.22). Admission to home care is for rehabilitation services (V57.1). Use 820.22 as the primary or principal diagnosis, since V57.1 does not specify the type or location of the fracture.
- A patient is surgically treated for a malignant neoplasm of the colon (code 153.2) with exteriorization of the colon. Admission to home care is for instruction in care of the patient's colostomy (V55.3). Use V55.3 as the primary or principal diagnoses, since it is more specific to the nature of the service provided.

The principal diagnosis may change on subsequent form 485s only if the patient develops an acute condition or an exacerbation of a secondary diagnosis requiring services different from those on the established POC.

12. *Surgical Code.* Enter the surgical code relevant to the care rendered (e.g., a patient with a below-knee amputation (BKA) who would have both a medical and a surgical code; thus both 11 and 12 would be completed with codes). Do not leave blank; either complete when the patient has a related, relevant surgical intervention or put N/A (not applicable). For Mr. Smith this is N/A. If the exact date of the surgery is unknown, put "00" as the day, but complete the month and year.

13. *Other Pertinent Diagnoses.* Other pertinent diagnoses are listed here. For Mr. Smith CHF would be listed. All diagnoses that coexisted at the time the POC was established or that developed later are listed. Excluded are diagnoses that may have occurred earlier but that have no bearing on the POC. These diagnoses can be changed by the home care nurse to reflect changes in the patient's condition. Place them in the order that best reflects the seriousness of the patient's condition and justifies the disciplines and services provided. If there are more than four pertinent diagnoses, use HCFA-487, the addendum, to list them. Enter N/A if there are no additional pertinent diagnoses.

   Effective documentation helps paint a picture of the patient to any reviewer. This information assists in communicating to the reviewer the severity or complexity of the patient's condition.

ORIENTATION ASSIGNMENT

Either complete a form 485 for a given patient from your organization, as assigned by your supervisor/preceptor, or according to the Mr. Smith example.

The source for codes is the current edition of the ICD-9-CM. The ICD-9-CM system contains more than 10,000 diagnosis code categories and more than 40,000 cross-referenced diagnosis terms. Specific ICD-9-CM and V codes for the most common diagnoses in home care are alphabetically listed for easy identification, by patient problem, in the *Handbook of Home Health Standards and Documentation Guidelines for Reimbursement* (Marrelli, 1998). The ICD-9-CM system sometimes requires secondary codes for complete description of the diagnostic entity. For example, pneumonia in the presence of acquired immune deficiency syndrome (AIDS) is coded as both 486 (pneumonia) and 042 (AIDS). It is important in such instances to use all codes given in the order given. In instances in which the RHHI has preferred or recommended codes, those codes should be used when appropriate for your patient. These codes may be communicated through the RHHI's newsletters. Medical diagnosis codes have three digits before the decimal point and in some cases have no decimal at all. Operative or surgical codes have only two digits before the decimal and are always followed by one or two digits following the decimal. An example follows:

Diagnosis (medical) osteomyelitis, lower leg 715.96

Surgical/operative procedure status/post (s/p) BKA 84.15

Remember that modifiers to diagnosis codes may be important. Modifiers such as acute/chronic, unilateral/bilateral, upper/lower, adult/juvenile, insulin-dependent/noninsulin dependent, or diabetes with complications/diabetes without complications frequently require differentiation in the ICD-9-CM codes.

14. *DME and Supplies.* List DME ordered by the physician that will be billed to Medicare. Listing the DME supplies such as a hospital bed or wheelchair also helps to show that the patient is homebound. Supplies need to be on the POC because they must be ordered by the physician. Supplies to be listed vary among organizations, so ask your manager about which supplies should be listed and in what specificity. Again, the supplies listed can help show the patient's problems and need for care. Examples include venipuncture and Foley catheter supplies. For Mr. Smith the home medical equipment noted is the oxygen and a walker in the corner of the kitchen. In the example supplies are venipuncture supplies for obtaining digoxin and theophylline levels.

15. *Safety Measures.* These are the "physician's instructions for safety measures" according to the *HHA Manual—Pub. 11* (HCFA). More realistically, they are what the nurse notes and communicates to the physician or recommends for the patient's safety in his or her home environment. This can include "patient has personal emergency response system (PERS)," remove scatter rugs, and others.

16. *Nutritional Requirements.* Complete the physician's order for the patient's diet. This includes specific therapeutic diets and/or any specific requirements such as supplements, as well as fluid restrictions or additional fluid needs. Total parenteral nutrition can be listed here also and/or under medications and continued on the HCFA-487 Addendum.

17. *Allergies.* List here the patient's allergies. This should include all known allergies (e.g., to medications, foods, adhesive or other tapes, or iodine). If the patient reports no known allergies, enter this response.

18A. *Functional Limitations.* This is another area that can help paint a
picture of your patient. All the boxed areas that describe the patient's
current limitations as assessed by the physician and nurse should be
completed. This box and 18B assist in supporting the patient's homebound status. Use "other" when needed. Remember that pain can be
a limitation, as can oxygen, severe shortness of breath, immunosup-
pression, incontinence, pitting edema, and other clinical findings that
impact what your patient can and cannot do.

18B. *Activities Permitted.* Check here the activities that the physician
allows and/or for which physician orders are present. Again, this box
supports the patient's homebound status. Do not mark "Up as tolerated" or "Independent at home" or "No restrictions" without explaining clearly how he or she is still homebound. Otherwise, it can look as
if the patient is not homebound. If the patient is not homebound, he or
she is not covered by the Medicare home care program and should
not be admitted to home care as a Medicare patient.

19. *Mental Status.* Check all the boxes that apply to your patient.
"Other" can be marked and explained. An example is "occasional
confusion in the evenings." Again, the nurse is providing more information to paint a picture of the patient.

20. *Prognosis.* Check the box that best describes the most appropriate
prognosis for your patient. This is realistically how he or she will
do, given his or her unique condition.

21. *Orders for Discipline and Treatments (Specify Amount/Fre-
quency/Duration).* These are all the services to be provided to the
patient and include all the services ordered (e.g, SN, PT, SLP, OT,
MSW, HHA). These usually also include other services, even those
that are not covered by Medicare and may be billed to other payors.
Frequency means the number of projected visits to be provided, by
discipline, and is written in days, weeks, or months. Duration refers
to the length of time the services will span. An example for Mr.
Smith is:

DISCIPLINE		TREATMENTS/SPECIFIC ORDERS
SN	3 × week × 3 weeks	Observation and assessment
	2 × week × 2 weeks	Venipunctures for blood levels
	1 × week × 4 weeks	Teaching related to medications
HHA	3 × week × 9 weeks	Personal care, ADL assistance
OT	3 × week × 4 weeks	Evaluation, conservation of energy, home eval related to above, ADL retraining, eval for assistive/adaptive devices

Usually, if the patient is admitted and the patient and the nurse believe the patient will need the certification period of 62 days, it is better to project and have orders certifying (signed) the entire certification period. Home care organizations usually use 9 weeks as the term to cover the 62-day span, since some months have 5 weeks and, without the extra week, the nurse could provide care that is not certified (and therefore not under a POC and not covered). Project for a 9-week period when completing this area or as directed by your manager.

Because patients often have a higher acuity when initially admitted to home care, the visits are usually more frequent and then taper or decrease toward stability. The following section, Frequency and Length of Stay Considerations, addresses the judgments related to projecting the patient's needs and the many factors that are a part of this decision.

The nurse should always count visits as they are made to ensure that she or he is staying within physician orders per the POC. If the patient needs additional visits, the nurse must obtain a verbal order from the physician explaining the need for the additional visits, document this information, and follow up with a signed physician order. An example of a calendar that may be used for each patient is found in Figure 6-3.

22. *Goals/Rehabilitation Potential/Discharge Plans.* Three different pieces of information need to be completed in this section. They should be thorough, descriptive, and based on the nurse's judgment after assessing and caring for the patient. They can be numbered as follows: (a) goals, (b) rehabilitation potential, and (c) discharge plans. These three areas communicate the plans for the patient through their home care stay.

   a. The goals need to be realistic and quantifiable or measurable. One definition of outcomes is that they are quantifiable or measurable goals for care. Examples are:
      • Patient verbalizes and adheres to medication regimen (i.e., patient verbalizes this, lung processes are stabilizing, and laboratory value results show therapeutic doses of theophylline and digoxin)
      • Healing of leg ulcers (objective vision and wound measurement)
      • Maintain patency of Foley catheter and patient remains infection free (urinary C&S, catheter draining without problems)
      • Ability to demonstrate correct insulin preparation and administration
   b. Rehabilitation potential: The rehabilitation potential realistically addresses (1) the patient's ability to attain the above goals, and

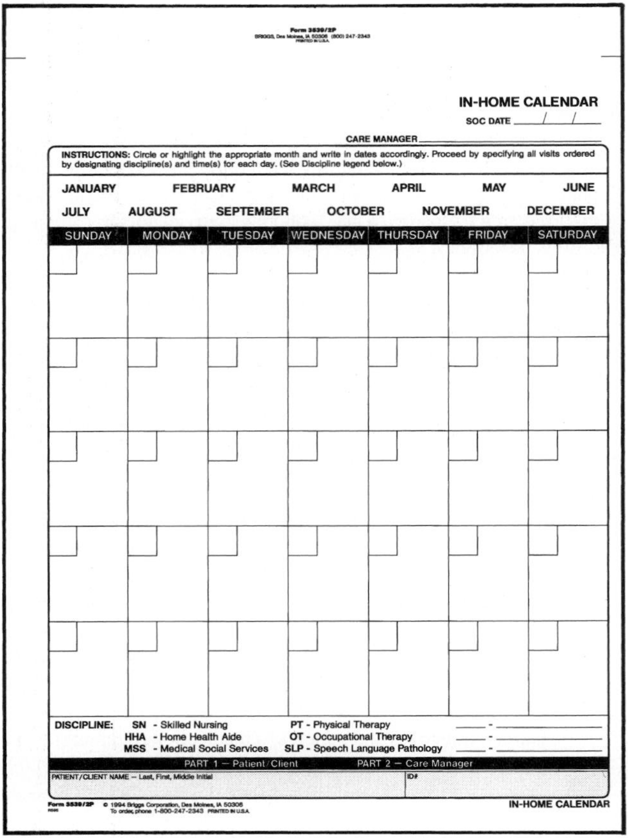

Form 3539/2P
BRIGGS, Des Moines, IA 50306 (800) 247-2343
PRINTED IN U.S.A.

IN-HOME CALENDAR

SOC DATE ____/____/____

CARE MANAGER ______________________

INSTRUCTIONS: Circle or highlight the appropriate month and write in dates accordingly. Proceed by specifying all visits ordered by designating discipline(s) and time(s) for each day. (See Discipline legend below.)

JANUARY FEBRUARY MARCH APRIL MAY JUNE
JULY AUGUST SEPTEMBER OCTOBER NOVEMBER DECEMBER

SUNDAY	MONDAY	TUESDAY	WEDNESDAY	THURSDAY	FRIDAY	SATURDAY

DISCIPLINE:
SN - Skilled Nursing
HHA - Home Health Aide
MSS - Medical Social Services
PT - Physical Therapy
OT - Occupational Therapy
SLP - Speech Language Pathology
____ - ________
____ - ________
____ - ________

PART 1 — Patient/Client PART 2 — Care Manager

PATIENT/CLIENT NAME — Last, First, Middle Initial	ID#

Form 3539/2P © 1994 Briggs Corporation, Des Moines, IA 50306
To order, phone 1-800-247-2343 PRINTED IN U.S.A.

IN-HOME CALENDAR

2428 p1 f1 hh

FIGURE 6-3 Example of an in-home calendar. *(Reprinted with permission of Briggs Health Care Products, Des Moines, Iowa.)*

(2) an estimate of the time frame needed for achievement of the goals. Remember that terms such as "fair" or "good" are not a description and as such are not acceptable. For example, Mr. Smith's rehabilitation is good for returning to previous self-care status with assistance related to documented problems. Projected time frame: less than 60 days (if realistic from your perspective, taking into account all the factors related to the patient's environment and care needs).

Note: When patients have daily nursing care (daily defined by Medicare as 5, 6, or 7 days a week), there must be a finite and projected end point. If a patient has had a wound for 2 years and is evaluated for admission to home care, this patient may not be appropriate for home care under Medicare. Medicare does not pay for long-term or full-time care; daily visits need a projected and predictable date for ending that is realistic to the patient and the patient's history. (Insulin is the only exception to daily, although it is recommended that the nurse ultimately work toward patient self-teaching and discharge.)

c. Discharge plans: This area includes a statement about how and/or where the patient will be cared for once home care is no longer provided. For example, Mr. Smith will be discharged back to self-care status in his home with support of community elder services and followed by his physician.

23. *Nurse's Signature and Date of Verbal Start of Care.* This section verifies that a nurse spoke with a physician and received verbal orders to authorize the initiation of home care services. Rubber stamps are not acceptable—a handwritten signature is required. This helps to ensure that the care was provided under a plan and verifies for state or other surveyors, intermediaries, and reviewers that a nurse spoke with the physician and coordinated care orders. This date *may precede* the SOC date in Item 2 and the "from" date in Item 3. This field may be used to document verbal orders to begin, modify, or continue care. It is most frequently used to initiate care and demonstrate the presence of verbal orders. As always, initial and ongoing communications with the physician are to be documented with the physician. Use N/A if the physician has dated and signed the form 485 on or before the SOC or recertification date or if he or she has submitted a written order to start, modify, or continue care on another document.

24. *Physician's Name and Address.* Complete this area by printing the physician's name and address. Some agencies include the phone number for easy retrieval of that information. This is the physician

who established the POC and certifies and recertifies the need for (medical necessity) home health services.

25. *Date HHA Received Signed POC.* This is the date that the HHA received the signed POC back from the physician. In many organizations, the POC is dated when the mail is opened and distributed. The nurse should ask his or her supervisor about the procedure at the organization; regardless of the process, this needs to be completed. Many times state licensing laws define timelines when MD orders must be signed. To remain in compliance, the date must be within the stated time frame.

26. *Physician Certification.* This statement verifies that the physician has reviewed the POC and certifies the need for the services, including that the patient is homebound and requires the skilled care per Medicare or other regulation, the POC has been established and is or will be periodically reviewed, and the services are authorized by and furnished while under the care of the attending physician.

27. *Attending Physician's Signature and Date Signed.* The physician signs and dates the POC/certification prior to claim submission. The form may be signed by another physician who is authorized by the attending physician to care for his or her patient in his or her absence. Usually if this area is sent back and the physician did not date it, the organization or nurse completes the date.

This signed POC is kept at the HHA in the medical records and may be used for verification of certification in audits.

28. *Penalty Statement.* This statement specifies the penalties imposed for misrepresentation, falsification, or concealment of essential information on the form 485.

FREQUENCY AND LENGTH OF SERVICE CONSIDERATIONS

The frequency of visits and the length of service are usually based on the professional nurse's assessment and ongoing evaluation of the patient's clinical status, as well as on the patient's biopsychosocial and unique family system needs. The current health care environment and the increasing emphasis on quality initiatives demonstrated by positive patient outcomes identify the need for research and evaluation regarding the determination of how frequently and for how long the patient needs to be under care. A discussion follows of the process and the knowledge that may assist in making the best determination of frequency and duration of care needed. Throughout this discussion, remember that all visits require orders by the physician and that the nurse must maintain compliance with the Medicare conditions of participation, state licensing, surveyor directives, and other regulations or laws.

A number of considerations help to determine the appropriate frequency of home care visits. *This discussion does not take the place of ongoing meetings with the home health care manager to determine patients' unique frequency and duration needs.* Rather, it provides a framework to help the nurse be aware of the many factors that go into making this determination and to help her or him make the determination appropriately.

The introduction of diagnosis-related groups and other prospective payment systems (PPSs) in inpatient settings has increased the scrutiny of admission, frequency, and duration of home health services. Nurses practicing in the community are acutely aware of the decreased lengths of stay in hospitals and the increased patient acuity in both the hospital and the home care setting. The increasing complexity of patient needs is demonstrated in the changing case mix of the home health nurse's case load. Early discharge and shorter lengths of stay in acute care facilities result in a greater number of high-acuity home care patients who require services necessitating expanded skills and improved knowledge of the home health nursing staff (Twardon and Gartner, 1992).

In addition, most health care analysts, payors, and consumers of health care realize that forms of PPSs such as the Medicare hospice benefit will continue to expand to other areas of health care, including home health care. The Medicare Home Care Prospective Payment Demonstration is continuing to collate needed information on this significant change in payment to home care programs, which is expected to occur in the near future.

Experienced home care, hospice, and community health nurses know that they are in an important position to identify the patient's specific service and visit frequency needs. The objective findings, as found through the nursing assessment, are the basis for these recommendations that are made by the nurse and communicated to the physician. It is also important to note that some patients may be seen infrequently by their physician after discharge—the patient may lack adequate transportation to the physician's office, or the patient may be considered "homebound," but the physician does not or will not make needed home visits. The professional nurse's judgment skills can help in making these important visit frequency decisions.

Some frequency determinations are easy; for example, when there are generally recognized medical or nursing practice standards, such as the elderly, homebound patient needing monthly B_{12} injections. Usually these injections are given once a month; thus the nurse creates the plan with skilled nursing visits scheduled for once a month for the injection.

The *HHA Manual—Pub. 11* (HCFA) states the following about frequency in the text addressing the completion of element 21 on the form 485: "Frequency denotes the number of visits per discipline to be rendered, stated in days, weeks, or months. Duration identifies the length of time the services are to be rendered and may be expressed in days, weeks, or months." Realistically and operationally, other factors besides recognized medical or nursing practice standards are important to scheduling and frequency decisions. They include staffing trends, standards of practice, geographic location of patients, family and referral support systems, and the availability of qualified staff for patients with particular conditions or problems. When conflict occurs between patient needs and the agency's ability to meet those needs, other courses of action should be implemented (e.g., transferring the patient to another agency or program in which the patient's needs can be safely and adequately met).

Box 6-6 outlines some of the factors that are considered in the process of determining frequency and duration of care. For this discussion, duration, usually referred to as 60 to 62 days, is the length of stay (LOS) for which the patient is projected to need home care services to safely and effectively meet the patient's unique medical and other needs.

A review of form 485, Section 18, A and B, "Functional Limitations" and "Activities Permitted," may also assist the nurse in the determination of frequency and duration of home care services. The nurse's rationale, experience, and, sometimes, intuition contribute to the decision-making process related to frequency and length of stay. According to Benner, "Intuitive judgment is what distinguishes expert human judgment from the decisions that might be made by a beginner or by a machine" (Benner and Tanner, 1987). Home health and hospice are settings in which experienced professional nurses use their broad knowledge base to make effective patient care decisions, such as those determining frequency and LOS, that can have a direct impact on patient outcomes. The nurse can look to the manager for specific information, feedback, and standards of the agency or program.

Health care reform is primarily addressing three of the largest problems within the U.S. health care system—access, cost, and quality. Cost is the issue that home care and hospice programs address daily when a case management company questions or limits needed visits. As home care experts, nurses, managers, and administrators must articulate to a case manager or third-party payor the objective rationale and plan for projected visits. For example, simply because a patient can perform the

BOX 6-6 LIST OF PATIENT-RELATED CONSIDERATIONS

The following is a list of the most common patient-related considerations that are evaluated by the nurse as plans are formulated and care is begun. This alphabetical list is not all-inclusive, and other considerations may be as varied as the individual nurse's patient caseload. In addition, many of these factors are interrelated.

- Absence of caregiver
- ADL limitations
- Adaptive or assistive devices
- Affect (e.g., depression)
- Behavioral or mental disorders
- Caregiver support
- Chemical or drug problems (e.g., alcoholism)
- Cognitive function
- Communication
- Compliance/noncompliance
- Disabilities
- Discharge plan
- Drug interaction
- Educational level/barriers
- Environment
- Fatigue
- Fire safety
- Functional limitations
- Goals/expected outcomes
- Handicaps
- History
- Home medical equipment
- Home setting
- Independence
- Instrumental ADLs
- Knowledge of emergency procedures
- Language
- Loneliness
- Loss of significant other(s)
- Medical equipment or supply needs
- Medications
- Mobility
- Motivation
- Nursing assessment and reassessment findings
- Nursing diagnosis
- Nutritional status
- Orthotic needs
- Other considerations, based on patient's/family's unique needs
- Pain
- Parenting
- Pathology
- Physical assessment findings
- Polypharmacy
- Probability of further complications
- Prognosis
- Psychopathology
- Reason for prior hospitalization, for referral to home care/hospice
- Rehabilitation needs
- Resources (e.g., financial, human
- Risk factors
- Safety
- Self-care status
- Skin integrity
- Social factors
- Social supports
- Socioeconomic condition
- Stability
- Swallowing
- Voice

Reprinted with permission from Marrelli T: *Handbook of Home Health Standards and Documentation Guidelines for Reimbursement*, St. Louis, 1998, Mosby dressing or administer the injections, the care is not automatically no longer a skilled service. In fact, continuing visits for observation and assessment, teaching, and training are very often appropriate, based on the patient's unique needs. The patient may still require thorough observation and assessment of the wound, teaching about site care, monitoring of the effects of medications, venipunctures to monitor drug levels, and infection control and safety training for a period of time.

PAYORS PAY FOR THE "HIGHER-LEVEL" SKILLS

Unfortunately, when a nurse says "the patient can do her own dressing," the payor, who is interested in containing costs, may construe that to mean that the patient is ready for discharge. Based on the patients' individual needs, however, this may or may not be true. Nurses must be able to communicate objectively the skills used during every visit and explain why those visits may vary, even though patients may have the same general diagnoses or problems.

Payment is made on the basis of the professional nurse's judgment and observational and other skills. Only nurses can compare that wound to the others seen in their practice experience, make a judgment regarding healing or infection, identify dehiscence, evaluate the wound in relation to other pathology, obtain a baseline assessment and teach the patient and caregivers, and myriad other skills that are provided daily in home to patients. The role and responsibility of home care and hospice professionals is to educate others, including case managers, payors, consumers, and their families about the cost-effectiveness, quality, and demonstrated positive outcomes experienced by patients in home care. An emphasis on continuous quality improvement (CQI) and the need to define home care roles, care, and nuances of individual patient care is appropriate use of limited resources. As CQI initiatives focus on the consumer of services, the industry must move toward standardizing the process, continually looking at methods to improve results (positive patient outcomes) and objectively measuring performance and demonstrated outcomes.

Research-based practice guidelines, outcome measures, and standards of care are important because of the increased emphasis on cost-effective, high-quality care. These practice parameters help home care nurses in determining patient frequency and length of service.

Some HHAs have developed their own standardized care plans based on North American Nursing Diagnosis Association (NANDA) nursing diagnoses and the nurses' experience with particular patient problems. Other home health agencies have developed or purchased automated systems that help them track and define objective findings, demonstrate goal achievement, and discharge based on outcome criteria. Nurses in practice are aware of this ongoing concern regarding provision of adequate patient care in a climate of tighter reimbursement, more limited resources, and frequent ethical dilemmas, along with an emphasis on both quality and effectiveness. This cost/quality equation must balance to maintain patient satisfaction and success, productivity, and viability of health care organizations, as well as the nurses' satisfaction in the ability to meet patient need.

Home care agency managers and nurses need to be adept in articulating and quantifying patient care needs based on objective evidence and supporting documentation. The Omaha Classification System (OCS) was developed by the Visiting Nurse Association of Omaha, Nebraska. The OCS is an orderly nursing diagnosis taxonomy listing of client problems nurses may encounter in community health settings. There are four categories, termed domains, in which each of these problems fall: environmental, psychosocial, physiologic, and health behaviors (Weidmann and North, 1987). Hallmarks of this system include the following:

1. Expected outcomes
2. Standard terminology
3. Integration of the components of quality assurance initiatives into an agency's operations
4. Assigned end dates to patient's outcomes
5. Clearly identifiable resolutions of patient problems demonstrated in the nursing documentation

As nurses identify the need to streamline and more effectively provide and demonstrate care, use of such systems will help in creating and maintaining cost- and time-effective operations and quality improvement. The use of standardized POCs as the basis for individualizing patient care helps to prioritize needs for nurses teaching patients with new or multiple health problems.

SUMMARY

The importance of the nurse's role in admitting a patient to a home care or hospice program cannot be overstated. The admission information assists in the creation of a realistic and outcome-oriented POC. The patient has input into this POC, and feedback (evaluation) is obtained on an ongoing basis. The nurse performs many functions, but her or his roles as case manager, coordinator, and educator stand out. Insurance verification, admissions processing, and initial data identification point make this visit very important because this information becomes the basis for operations across the patient's stay in home care. In this capacity, the nurse integrates the complex information from multiple sources and shares it, in an understandable manner, with patients, families, and caregivers.

Nurses working in home care, hospice, or other community settings must be flexible and able to explain objective reasons for frequency, LOS, or discharge decisions. These decisions and underlying rationale need to be communicated clearly to the nurse's manager or third-party payor representatives who are responsible for tracking, approving, or denying visits. As payors try to decrease the number of patient visits, nurses must be able to articulate the clinical and other needs of the patients. This advocacy role will ensure high-quality care while the patient remains at home. This is more important now as the technology explosion continues and nurses care for patients such as those receiving dobutamine therapy or needing management of infusion care or ventilators in the community. Those who can explain needs based on objective information and patient findings to numerous reimbursement gatekeepers will continue to be successful in home care. The increasing complexity of patients sent home with limited resource and coverage demands these skills for safe, effective patient care.

REVIEW EXERCISES

1. Apply concepts for effective care planning.
2. Describe the use of the nursing process in home care.
3. Complete a HCFA Form 485.
4. List the actions that comprise a home care evaluation visit.
5. Describe the intake and referral process in home health care.
6. Identify the information needed to safely care for a new home care patient.
7. Describe the interface between reimbursement and clinical care in home health care.
8. Identify your RHHI and the role of clinical documentation in the medical review process.
9. Describe and/or demonstrate correct bag technique per your organization's policy.
10. Identify the role of the nurse in the home safety assessment.

RESOURCES

Occupational Safety and Health Administration (OSHA) Helpline is staffed by registered nurses to answer questions about OSHA standards related to bloodborne pathogens and provide updated information regarding the airborne transmission of tuberculosis (TB). Established by Kimberly-Clark, the number is (800)524-3577.

"Lung-Line" is a resource for clinicians who have patients with difficult TB or have questions related to TB, asthma, COPD, or other respiratory problems. Established by the National Jewish Center for Immunology and Respiratory Medicine to discuss treatment and care, their number is (800)222-LUNG or (800)552-LUNG. They also have patient education materials related to these respiratory problems.

Home Care Nurse News is a clinically focused newsletter that has a patient case conference every month that plans care, lists interventions, and projects outcomes for a patient in home care or hospice. To review a copy, call (800)993-NEWS.

REFERENCES

Benner P, Tanner C: Clinical judgment: how expert nurses use intuition, *Am J Nurs* January:23, 1987.

Health Care Financing Administration: *Home health agency manual—Publication 11,* Washington, DC, 1989, Health and Human Services, p.24m4f, Revision, 228.

Twardon C, Gartner MA: Strategy for growth in home care, *J Nurs Admin* 22(10):49, 1992.

Weidmann J, North H: Implementing the Omaha Classification System in a public health agency, *Nurs Clin North Am* 22(4):973, 1987.

FOR FURTHER READING

Bradley P, Alpers R: Home healthcare nurses should regain their family focus, *Home Healthcare Nurse* 14(4):281-288, 1996.

Harris M, Yuan J: "Oh, no, not another hand-washing in-service!" *Gastroenterol Nurs* 16(6):269-272, 1994.

Jaffe M, Skidmore-Roth L: *Home health nursing care plans,* St. Louis, 1996, Mosby.

Marrelli T: *Handbook of home health standards and documentation guidelines for reimbursement,* ed 3, St. Louis, 1998, Mosby.

Marrelli T, Hilliard L: *Home care and clinical paths: effective care planning across the continuum,* St. Louis, 1996, Mosby.

Wendt D: Building trust during the initial home visit, *Home Healthcare Nurse* 14(2):92-98, 1996.

White M, Smith W: Infection control in home health agencies, *Am J Infect Control* 21(3):146-150, 1993.

OVERVIEW OF DOCUMENTATION

Tina M. Marrelli, MSN, MA, RNC

"In God we trust, all others must have data."

Dr. W. E. Deming

This chapter seeks to help both new and experienced home care and hospice nurses in meeting various requirements while assisting clinicians create the specific documentation required by any payor by factually illustrating the patient's condition and responses to teaching or other interventions.

Nurses and nursing practice in home care are described every day to surveyors, peers, and managers through the review of clinical home care records. Nursing visit records, notes, and other information that appear in the home health agency (HHA) record reflect the standard of nursing care, as well as the particular care provided to a specific patient. Home care and hospice nurses must be able to integrate knowledge of regulatory criteria, care coordination, and practice into effective documentation that supports coverage while demonstrating quality to any reviewer. Today, numerous third-party payors make quality and reimbursement decisions based on the care the patient received as evidenced in the clinical record.

The professional home care and hospice nurse's entries in a patient's clinical record are recognized as a significant contribution to the documentation of the standard of care provided to a patient. As the practice of nursing has become more complex, so too have the factors that influence documentation. These factors include requirements of regulatory agencies (e.g., Joint Commission on Accreditation of Healthcare Organizations, Community Health Accreditation Program, state licensure departments), consumers of health care, and legal entities. The home care nurse must try to satisfy these various requirements all at once, often with little time in which to accomplish the important task of documentation. Fortunately, many home care programs have integrated many of these requirements into the HHA's policy and/or procedure manuals. In addition, it is important to note that the written clinical record is also the nurse's best defense against malpractice or negligence litigation. For an in-depth discussion of documentation, the reader is referred to the *Handbook of Home Health Standards and Documentation Guidelines for Reimbursement* (Marrelli, 1998).

The increased specialization of practice, the complexity of patient problems, and the new technology associated with these problems have contributed to multiple and varied services being provided to patients. The clinical record is the only source of written communication, and sometimes the only source of any communication, for all team members. The team members not only contribute their unique and individual assessments of interventions and outcomes, but may also actually base their subsequent actions on the events documented by another team member.

REASONS FOR THE IMPORTANCE OF THE HOME CARE CLINICAL RECORD

The clinical HHA record is the only document that chronicles a patient's stay from start of care through discharge. As such, the actual documentation should be completed as soon as possible. This includes beginning and completing the Health Care Financing Administration (HCFA) form 485 (or other required forms) and the daily visit record or nursing notes as soon as possible. It is recommended that the documentation be completed at the time the care is provided. Many nurses remember performing rounds with the physician in the inpatient setting—it would have been unheard of to not document as care and plans for care were developed for the patients. Documentation may include a change in the patient's plan as discussed with the patient and team members. Important facets of the documentation include the patient's condition, the environment of care, a description of the specific care provided, communications with the physician or other team members, and the observed or verbal patient response(s) to interventions.

The following factors have contributed to the additional emphasis being placed on nursing documentation and have increased the importance of such documentation:

1. Economics of the health care system and emphasis on utilization management
2. Emphasis on continuous quality improvement or performance improvement

   3. Emphasis on standardization of care, policies, and procedures
   4. Increased recognition and empowerment of the nursing profession
   5. Emphasis on effectiveness and efficiency in all health care settings

Economics of the Health Care System and Emphasis on Utilization Management

Patients continue to be discharged from the hospital sooner or stay home while they are very ill. In response to spiraling health care costs, third-party payors (e.g., government, commercial, and business self-insurers) have increased their scrutiny and control of limited resources. Initially these programs, called *utilization review or utilization management,* were influential in decreasing hospital lengths of stay. This review of care then moved into the outpatient and home care arenas. In addition, today many surgeries and other procedures are provided on an outpatient-only basis. As experienced home care nurses know, the same elderly patient who would have required an extensive inpatient hospital stay only 5 years ago may now have a very limited stay, if any, and may need extensive, skilled home care services.

The phrase often heard to describe this phenomenon is "quicker and sicker." In general, these decreased length of hospital stays have increased home care patients' acuity levels. This often translates into increased nursing care and other needs and is evidenced by the increase in the number of visits or hours patients are seen. In addition, some managed care programs are decreasing their home visits while also limiting the patient's inpatient stay, which places stress on the HHA nurse to continue to provide needed care and many times negotiate for the patient so that the appropriate level of safe, effective nursing care is provided. Third-party payors often need substantiating evidence (i.e., documentation) that clearly shows that skilled care was provided; Medicare by law can only pay for covered care. The information in the clinical record is the source third-party payors use to make payment or denial decisions. Documentation then is the objective basis for payment determinations because these notes reflect the care provided to a home care patient.

Emphasis on Continuous Quality Improvement or Performance Improvement

As quality initiatives in all health care settings have evolved, patient outcomes are being recognized as valid indicators of care. Clinical documentation is the written record demonstrating the nursing process based on the plan of care (POC) and movement toward achieving patient-centered, quantifiable goals for care.

The interdisciplinary focus on quality efforts creates an incentive for the entire health team to work together to achieve patient outcomes. The clinical documentation in the written HHA record demonstrates care coordination in the format of team meetings, conferences, or other team activities and communications.

Emphasis on Standardization of Care, Policies, and Procedures

All patients are entitled to a certain level or standard of nursing care. Operationally this means that every nurse provides the same care and many times in the same order that is designated by the organizations and managers. This is a way to ensure standardization of care and care processes. In fact, use of a text such as this by all nurses in a given organization contributes to standardization of patient care.

As patients become more proactive consumers in their purchase of health services, patient satisfaction with the care provided is key to any HHA's reputation and ultimate survival. As patients and their families become more active consumers of health care, more are demanding to receive care in their own homes. Home care nurses, because of their healing skills and other areas of professional proficiency, are pivotal in fostering patient satisfaction. Further, the role of the home care nurse as patient advocate, listener, and teacher has become widely accepted in recent years. In general, it is also known that satisfied patients are less likely to sue.

Although there are more nurses in the work force than ever before, there continues to be a need for qualified professional home care and hospice nurses.

The nurse's notes can become the factor by which documented quality becomes demonstrated quality. All health care professions, including nursing, have recognized standards of care. As society has become litigious, the home care nurse must be aware of state practice and other accepted standards of care. These standards of care are the minimum level that any patient can expect in similar circumstances. Other standards include policies and procedures, state or federal regulations, and the published standards of professional nursing organizations (Guide, 1985). These standards necessitate keeping current and informed of the standards of professional nursing practice through affiliation with nursing specialty groups or other professional groups.

An example of an HHA's nursing standard of care is as follows:

Every HHA patient shall have a nursing assessment that is comprehensive, addresses specific patient needs, is performed by a registered nurse on admission, and is documented in the clinical record. Through complete, effective documentation, HHA nurses demonstrate that the standard of care has been met.

Emphasis on Effectiveness and Efficiency in all Health Care Settings

As HHAs and hospice organizations continue to streamline their operations, administrative tasks historically performed by nurses are being reconsidered for their effectiveness. Repetition or duplication of documentation has been an area of appropriate concern to both home care nurses and their managers. Some organizations have moved toward automation, such as laptop or notebook computers for nurses, to help prevent the duplicative nature of much clinical and administrative information needed for effective daily HHA operations. Quality, not quantity, is now emphasized with regard to documentation. Effective documentation does not need to be lengthy or wordy—it only needs to support appropriate and covered care.

All of the previously discussed factors have created an environment in which the home care nurse has increased responsibilities to be completed in a shorter time period.

THE IMPORTANCE OF THE CLINICAL RECORD IN HOME CARE

The clinical record is important because it is:

- The only written source for reference and communication among members of the home care team.
- The primary source (written or verbal) for reference and communication among the members of the home care team.
- The only text that supports insurance coverage and/or denial.
- The only evidence of the basis on which patient care decisions were made.
- The only legal record.
- The primary foundation for the evaluation of the care provided.
- The basis for staff education or other study.
- The objective source for the HHA's licensing (where applicable), accreditation, and state surveyor review.

Because home care and hospice nurses often need to meet a number of needs simultaneously, they are appropriately concerned about their ability to do so. HHA nurses in practice today can meet these needs and produce clear, effective documentation (Box 7-1).

BOX 7-1   DOCUMENTATION TIPS

Do...

Write legibly or print neatly. The record must be readable.

Use permanent ink.

For every entry, identify the time and date; sign the entry and include your title.

Describe care or interventions provided and the patient's response to care.

Write objectively when describing findings (e.g., behaviors).

Write notes in consecutive and chronological order with no skipped lines or gaps.

Write visit notes either at the patient's home (if safe and appropriate) or as soon as possible after care is provided.

Be factual and specific.

Use patient, family, or caregiver quotes.

Use the patient's name (e.g., "Mr. Smith").

Document patient complaints or needs and their resolutions. (Remember to also discuss the complaint with your manager, who may also document it in the HHA Complaint Log and note the resolution or follow-up actions taken.)

Make sure the patient's name is listed and correct on the visit record, daily note, or other HHA form.

Be accurate, complete, and thorough.

Write out what you are saying if anything is questionable. (Avoid potentially confusing abbreviations.)

Chart only the care that you provided.

Promptly document any change in the patient's condition and the actions taken based on such a change.

Write down the patient's, family's, or caregiver's response to teaching or any other care intervention.

To correct an error

1. Draw a line through the erroneous entry.
2. Briefly describe the error (e.g., wrong date, spilled coffee on visit record).
3. Add your signature, date, and time.

Don't...

Rely on memory.

White out or erase entries; such changes may appear to be an attempt to cover up incriminating entries.

Cross out words beyond recognition.

Make assumptions, drawing conclusions, or blaming.

Leave blank spaces between entries and your signature.

Wait "too long" to record entries.

Leave gaps in documentation.

Use abbreviations, except when they are clear and appear on the HHA's list of approved, acceptable abbreviations.

DOCUMENTATION
Home Care Documentation

It is important to remember that Medicare is a medical insurance program, and, as with any insurance program, there are both covered services and exclusions. For payors, documentation is the only paper trail of the care provided and the patient's response to that care.

When admitting patients to the HHA, the nurse should ensure that the patient meets the particular insurance requirements. For example, with Medicare, the patient must meet the homebound criteria, as well as other criteria. How the patient specifically meets the homebound criteria must be reflected in the clinical documentation. It is a good idea to document this on the note to visit record every visit.

The nurse should always try to read her or his documentation objectively after writing it and ask, "Does this form 485/486 or visit record reflect why the patient is homebound and how (or why) the skills of the home care nurse are needed?"

When writing clinical documentation, keep in mind that effective documentation simultaneously does the following:

1. Demonstrates the care provided and the patient's response to that care
2. Shows that the current standards of care are maintained
3. Meets documentation requirements for Medicare and other payors

Box 7-2 shows ways to ensure that quality and reimbursement requirements are being met. Remember that writing effective documentation is a learned skill and, as with any skill, improvement comes only with practice.

Remember that effective documentation does not have to be lengthy or wordy. However, it should convey to any other reader the status of your patient, the POC, and the consistent movement toward predetermined patient-centered goals.

Hospice Documentation Considerations

The HCFA, which manages the Medicare programs, also instructs the fiscal intermediaries about administering the Medicare hospice program. These instructions have implications for hospice nurses who provide care to patients covered under the Medicare hospice benefit. There are specialized fiscal intermediaries called regional home health intermediaries (RHHIs). These insurance companies have contracts with the HCFA to process and make payment determinations on all hospice (and home care) claims from across the country.

BOX 7-2   **CHECKLIST FOR EFFECTIVE
              HOME CARE DOCUMENTATION**

✔ Recognize that in home care, at the first visit, the nurse initiates the process of claims payment (or denial) with the initial forms 485/486.

✔ Try to read your documentation objectively. Ask yourself if the form 485/486 or visit record reflects why the patient is home-bound (if the patient has Medicare or another insurance that has that criteria) and how or why the skills of a nurse or therapist are needed. (Many HHAs have a peer review process that significantly helps home care nurses objectively review and create their own documentation.)

✔ Emphasize the following:

✔ 1. The reason the care was initiated

✔ 2. What the skilled nursing interventions are

✔ 3. Where the patient's plan is going (patient-centered goals)

✔ 4. What the plans are for discharge (rehabilitation potential)

✔ Try to complete your patient documentation as soon as possible. Try to document in the patients' home, when safe. Explain to your patients that the last few moments of every visit are for complet-ing the documentation required by Medicare or another payor. Patients and their families understand. In fact, it is during this quiet time that patients may think of questions and thus save un-necessary phone calls once you are gone. Careful, timely comple-tion of documentation is particularly important when working with new admissions because the patient must sign so many forms, the information on the form 485/486 must be correct, and the initial and daily visit notes must be complete. It can be difficult and of-ten unsafe to rely on memory or rough notes after seeing many patients at the end of a long day.

✔ Remember that the POC is the most important part of the home care clinical record. All other information flows from the identified skilled needs ordered on the plan. The HCFA form 485 is the home health certification and POC. The POC must be complete, and the content clear. There can be no gaps.

✔ Make sure that your patients meet the admission criteria of the organization and the insurance program requirements. This is im-portant from both a risk management and a reimbursment per-spective. Be able to clearly identify the skilled, covered service. Although the patient may not meet a particular insurer's require-ments, she or he may still have needs that another program can safely provide.

continued

BOX 7-2   **CHECKLIST FOR EFFECTIVE**
               HOME CARE DOCUMENTATION—cont'd

✔ Focus on the patient's problems in your documentation. They are why home care is being provided, and the payors must see evidence of such to justify reimbursement.

✔ Demonstrate through your documentation that the care provided is patient centered. For example, make your patient goals quantifiable and your outcomes realistic and specific to the patient's unique problems and needs.

✔ Remember that anyone who picks up your patient's clinical record does not have the depth of information and knowledge that you have from actually being there and seeing the patient in his or her own home setting. Because of this, document information that is objective and clearly paints a picture of the patient and his or her problems and needs and how the care is directed for goal achievement and discharge.

✔ Remember that effective documentation does not have to be lengthy or wordy. However, it should convey to any reader (e.g., your manager, a state surveyor nurse) the status of your patient, the adherence to the ordered POC, and consistent movement toward predetermined patient-centered goals.

✔ Check that the information on the clinical record flows well and that anyone can understand, by objective evidence, the patient's situation, including the problems and the skilled services that are needed.

✔ Remember that the record and nursing entries need to be legible, neat, and organized consistently.

✔ Try to look at the documentation objectively. Does it tell the story of the patient's progress (or lack of progress) and the interventions implemented based on the initial assessment and POC?

✔ Make sure telephone calls and other communications with physicians, community agencies, and other team members are documented. Do they explain what occurred with the patient; what actions were ordered, modified, and implemented; and what the patient's response was to these interventions?

✔ Demonstrate the nursing process in the record. Look for the nursing diagnoses, the assessment, evidence of care planning, implementation of ordered interventions and actions, movement toward patient-centered goals, assessment of the patient's response, and continued evaluation.

✔ Document goal achievement and/or progress toward goals and outcomes. Are the goals realistic, quantifiable, and patient-centered?

BOX 7-2   **CHECKLIST FOR EFFECTIVE**
                 HOME CARE DOCUMENTATION—cont'd

✔ If progress has not occurred as planned, explain the reasons in the documentation. If a patient is too ill for a rehabilitation service or refuses the service, is there evidence of communication with the doctor about this? Has an order been made to place the service on hold or to discharge the patient from that service?

✔ Documentation should include family/caregiver teaching and their responses to and demonstration of behavior and learning.

✔ Document the patient's response to care interventions and nursing actions.

✔ Modify the interventions based on the patient's response, when appropriate.

✔ Document evidence of intradisciplinary team conferences and discussions.

✔ The chart should show continuity of care planning goals and consistent movement toward goal achievement by all members of the health team.

✔ Generally the record should tell the story of the patient's care, needs, and progress while he or she was receiving home care services.

✔ The nursing entries and overall information are to reflect the level of care expected by today's health care consumers and their families.

✔ The clinical documentation should demonstrate compliance with regulatory, accreditation, licensure, and quality standards.

The RHHIs can *only* pay for hospice care under Medicare that is covered by law. They look to the clinical documentation in the medical record of the hospice to either support or not support covered care (Box 7-3).

Because of the high volume of claims, the RHHIs cannot individually look at each hospice claim. The RHHIs direct their medical review efforts toward areas and claims where there is the greatest risk of inappropriate payment. This process is called focused medical review (FMR), and hospice claims are subject to FMR based on the RHHI initiatives and findings identified in claims processing. FMR entails the screening of claims with the greatest risk of overuse of program payment. This happens through data base analysis and referrals.

BOX 7-3   **A HOSPICE DOCUMENTATION CHECKLIST**

The following documentation checklist will help ensure that clinical records are complete:

✔ Are the physician's certification, assessments, and recertification of terminal illness included in the record?

✔ Are visit notes of all disciplines/caregivers present?

✔ Has the physician provided written material or a written summary of the patient's course?

✔ Are all supporting laboratory or test results included?

✔ Is the election form signed and dated by the provider and patient/caregiver/responsible party?

✔ Overall, does the documentation support coverage of hospice services as defined in the *HCFA Medicare Hospice Manual-13*? (For more information, see Chapter 16.)

Medicare Hospice and Documentation

To qualify for the hospice benefit, a patient must have Medicare and be terminally ill, the physician must certify that the patient is terminally ill, the patient must choose to receive hospice care instead of the standard Medicare benefits for the illness, and the care must be provided by a Medicare-participating hospice program.

For documentation purposes, the patient is considered terminally ill under the Medicare guidelines if the following conditions apply:

- The medical documentation meets the criteria in the National Hospice Organization (NHO) guidelines and supports that the patient is terminally ill (i.e., there is no conflicting or inconsistent information in the record that would lead one to believe that, even though the guidelines are met, the patient is not terminally ill).
- The medical documentation in the record supports that the patient is terminally ill, even though criteria in the NHO guidelines are not met or the patient's condition is not covered by the NHO guidelines.
- The patient dies from the illness for which he or she elected the hospice benefit.
- Medical documentation is insufficient to make a decision, but the hospice medical director or attending physician provides clinical documentation to support the certification of terminal illness. (The documentation should be clear and in the records.)
- Documentation may include results of tests or narrative descriptions of the clinical indicators or progression of disease.

DOCUMENTATION: THE KEY TO HOSPICE COVERAGE AND QUALITY

Documentation is critical to the positive outcome of the focused medical review process. Paint a picture with your documentation from the onset of care through continuation of hospice services. Distinguish clearly in your documentation between the chronic and terminal phases of a disease, especially if the disease is long and chronic in nature. Specify any patient periods of exacerbation, stabilization, and further deterioration. Document how treatments and medication play a palliative role in the POC. Notes from all caregivers are usually reviewed in FMR. Documentation in all notes should complete the picture of the terminally ill patient. Box 7-3 contains a sample hospice documentation checklist. Remember that what is "normal" and "stable" to a hospice nurse or other team member may still indicate a clearly terminal patient if the details are provided in the documentation. Avoid generalizations such as "no change" or "as tolerated." The payors must pay for covered care, and the nurse's documentation plays an important role in determination to pay.

CLINICAL PATH CONSIDERATIONS

As health care generally and home care specifically seek to become more efficient, new models of care and documentation are emerging. Clinical paths or care maps are a way to ensure that all team members are literally "on the same page" as they work together to achieve patient goals. They are initiated to improve quality of care, since the main focus must be on the patient. Paths are available to all the staff involved in the POC, as well as the patient and family. Clarifying the expectations for care, integrating standards of care into the path, and identifying quantifiable patient goals at the onset create an environment for improved communications and care.

Clinical paths are one way of defining a clinical budget or the amount of resources needed to care for a particular patient or group of patients. They are tools that organize, sequence, and time the major interventions of clinicians for a particular case type, medical condition, diagnostic category, or functional diagnosis. They identify and standardize tools and information, interventions, and processes for achieving predetermined outcomes (quantifiable goals of care). The development and operationalization of clinical paths are similar to project management wherein certain key processes are mapped out schematically that can be used to monitor the effectiveness of the plan and determine progress through a process of quality improvement to positively impact and improve patient care (Marrelli and Hilliard, 1996).

Clinical paths demand the standardization of care and care processes. For example, goals are clearly defined, and all care to be provided is specifically explained, laid out in a linear design, and based on the organization's historic data. Your organization may have paths for certain groups of patients or diagnoses as a way to ensure quality care for patients with that particular problem. Not all patient problems will have a path because some medical problems do not fit a projected course for care. Common clinical paths include joint replacement surgery patients and patients status-post coronary artery bypass graft surgery (CABG) patients.

COMPUTERIZATION AND DOCUMENTATION

There is no question that nurses need to be more effective in health care and that automation or computerization is one method to achieve more efficiency while enabling team members to provide more detailed and accurate documentation. However, computers are not the answers to all care planning and scheduling issues in home care. Whether data are documented on paper or keyed into a computer, they need to be correct for the entire process to flow toward billing and discharge. It is imperative that we all hone our computer skills as patient lengths of stay in home care decrease but admissions increase as managed care penetration continues. This means operationally that there will be more work for the schedulers and clerical team members than before. The clinicians can have an important impact by entering documentation and other data correctly the first time. This must be the goal of data management as organizations move toward automated tracking systems and benchmarking with other organizations across the country. To be able to compare apples to apples, organizations all must be collecting the same information in the same format and in the same manner, using the same glossary in communications. The following section addresses the Outcome and Assessment Information Set (OASIS), a process for tracking home care patient information in the hope of comparing data across agencies in the future for benchmarking and other reasons.

OUTCOME-BASED QUALITY IMPROVEMENT

The HCFA is reviewing the reimbursement system and trying to improve the quality of care provided by organizations to Medicare beneficiaries. To this end Medicare has rewritten the Medicare Conditions of Participation (COPs) to be a more outcome-focused and quality driven process.

Currently a pilot project is ongoing with 50 participating home care organizations from across the country. In 1973 the Center for Health Services at the University of Colorado was established to analyze and review health policies, as well as provide technical assistance on such topics as quality assurance, cost containment, and regulation. HCFA funded the Research Center to administer a quality assurance demonstration program with the 50 pilot HHAs. One of the hallmarks of the research program is the use of the 90-item OASIS. The OASIS data items address sociodemographic, environmental, support system, health status, functional status, and health service utilization characteristics of home care patients. Besides being used for assessment, OASIS is used for reassessment of the patient at 60-day intervals and on discharge from home care services. The data collected under this project will create agency outcome data, as well as produce data for comparative data across agencies and geographic areas. The most important aspect of this study is that HHAs will be able to evaluate the effect of care provided in terms of patient outcomes and identify areas for improving care. Many home care organizations are integrating the elements of OASIS into their organization's assessment forms. See the Appendix for the OASIS-B in its entirety.

Only through standardized data collection tools, methods, and definitions will the home care industry be able to compare apples to apples for cost and care efficiencies. Documentation forms for the skilled or nursing notes vary across home care and hospice programs. They may be checklist formats, narratives, or a combination. Many times they are in duplicate or triplicate to facilitate communication among team members. Usually different disciplines have their own specialized note. For example, the speech-language pathologist, rehabilitation therapist, dietitian, and social worker would all have their own assessment tool and revisit forms for completion.

Examples of nursing documentation are found in Figures 7-1 and 7-2. The skilled visit note cues the home care nurse to complete information that supports coverage or meeting other requirements every visit (see Figure 7-1). It includes elements such as homebound reason, care planning revisions, home care aide supervisory visit information, and a list of interventions/instructions that are usually covered care. Although many organizations would use both the skilled nursing visit and the clinical notes, a narrative note used as the clinical note can be used to provide additional information (see Figure 7-2). Note that at the bottom of both of these forms there is an entry marked "care coordination"—this is a requirement in quality home care or hospice that connotes communicating and the working together of the entire team toward common patient goals.

Form 3570/3P
BRIGGS, Des Moines, IA 50306 (800) 247-2343
PRINTED IN U.S.A.

SKILLED NURSING VISIT NOTE

DATE OF VISIT ____/____/____
TIME IN ________ OUT ________

NURSING DIAGNOSIS/PROBLEM ______________________

TYPE OF VISIT: ☐ SN ☐ SN & Super. ☐ Super. Only ☐ Other________
HOMEBOUND REASON ________

NURSING ASSESSMENT AND OBSERVATION SIGNS/SYMPTOMS
(Mark all applicable with an "X". Circle appropriate item(s) separated by "/".)

CARDIOVASCULAR
- Fluid retention
- Chest pain
- Neck vein distension
- Edema (specify)- ☐ RUE ☐ LUE ☐ RLE ☐ LLE
- Peripheral pulses
- Other:

RESPIRATORY
- Rales/Rhonchi/Wheeze
- Cough
- Dyspnea/SOB
- Orthopnea
- Other:

DIGESTIVE
- Bowel sounds
- Nausea/Vomiting
- Anorexia
- Epigastric distress
- Difficulty swallowing
- Abdominal distension
- Colostomy
- Diarrhea
- Constipation/Impaction
- Bowel incontinence
- Other:

GENITOURINARY
- Burning
- Distension/Retention
- Frequency/Urgency
- Hesitancy
- Hematuria
- Bladder incontinence
- Catheter
- Urine- Color: ____ Consistency: ____ Odor: ____
- Pain
- Discharge
- Diabetic urine testing
- Other:

SKIN
- Color:
- Jaundiced
- Temperature
- Chills
- Decubitus/Wound
- Rash/Itching
- Turgor
- Other:

PAIN
- Origin:
- Location:
- Duration:
- Severity:
- Other:

MUSCULOSKELETAL
- Balance/Unsteady gait
- Weakness
- Other:

NEUROSENSORY
- Syncope
- Headache
- Grasp- Right: ____ Left: ____
- Movement ☐ RUE ☐ LUE ☐ RLE ☐ LLE
- Pupil reaction- Right: ____ Left: ____
- Tremors
- Vertigo
- Speech impairment
- Hearing impairment
- Visual impairment
- Decreased sensitivity
- Other:

EMOTIONAL STATUS
- Disoriented
- Lethargic
- Agitated
- Oriented
- Comatose
- Forgetful
- Depressed
- Other:

VITALS

T° ________ Wt. ________
Resp. ________ ☐ Reg. ☐ Irreg.
Pulse: A ________ R ________ ☐ Regular ☐ Irregular

B/P	LYING	SITTING	STANDING
Right			
Left			

Denote Location / Size of Wounds / Pressure Sores / Measure Ext. Edema Bil.

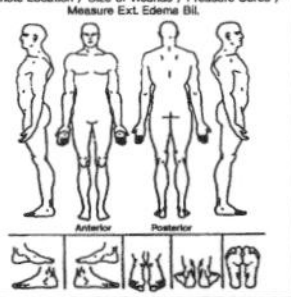

	#1	#2	#3	#4
Length				
Width				
Depth				
Drainage				
Tunneling				
Odor				
Sur. Tis.				
Edema				
Stoma				

INTERVENTIONS/INSTRUCTIONS (Mark all applicable with an "X". Circle appropriate item(s) separated by "/".)

Skilled observation & assessment (A1)	Chest physio./Postural drainage (A10)	IM injection (A13)	Evaluate diet/fluid intake
Foley care (A2)	Change NG/G tube (A17)	Psych. intervention	Diet teaching
Urine testing	Admin. of vitamin B_{12} (A11)	Observe S/S infection	Safety factors
Wound care/dressing	Prep./Admin. insulin (A12)	Diabetic observation	Prenatal assessment
Decubitus care	Teach/Admin. IVs/Clysis (A14)	Teach diabetic care (A25)	Post-partum assessment
Venipuncture (A6)	Teach ostomy/ileo. conduit care (A15)	Observe/Teach medication (N or C) effects/side effects	Teach infant/child care
Post-cataract care (A8)	Teach/Admin. tube feedings (A16)		Other:
Bowel/Bladder training (A9)	Teach/Admin. care of trach. (A20/A21)	Physiology/Disease process teaching	
Digital exam with manual removal/ Enema	Teach/Admin. inhalation Rx (A22/A23)		
	Teach care - terminally ill	Observe ADLs	

ANALYSIS OF FINDINGS/INTERVENTIONS/INSTRUCTIONS ________

EVALUATION AND PATIENT/CLIENT/CAREGIVER RESPONSE ________

APPROXIMATE NEXT VISIT DATE ____/____/____ PLAN FOR NEXT VISIT ________

CARE PLAN: ☐ Reviewed/Revised with patient/client involvement ☐ Outcome achieved ☐ PRN order obtained
MEDICATION STATUS: ☐ No change ☐ Order obtained
DISCHARGE PLANNING DISCUSSED? ☐ Yes ☐ No ☐ N/A
BILLABLE SUPPLIES RECORDED? ☐ Yes ☐ No
CARE COORDINATION: ☐ Physician ☐ PT ☐ OT ☐ ST ☐ SS ☐ SN ☐ Other (specify)________

SIGNATURE/DATE—Complete TIME OUT (above) prior to signing below.
X ________ ____/____/____
Nurse (signature/title) Date

AIDE SUPERVISORY VISIT (Complete if applicable.)
AIDE: ☐ Present ☐ Not present
SUPER. VISIT: ☐ Scheduled ☐ Unscheduled
AIDE CARE PLAN UPDATED? ☐ Yes ☐ No
OBSERVATION OF ________
TEACHING/TRAINING OF ________
NEXT SCHEDULED SUPER. VISIT ____/____/____

PART 1 — Clinical Record PART 2 — Care Manager PART 3 — Care Coordination

PATIENT/CLIENT NAME — Last, First, Middle Initial ________ ID# ________

Form 3570/3P

SKILLED NURSING VISIT NOTE

2438 p1 f1 one color hh

FIGURE 7-1 Example of a skilled nursing visit note. *(Reprinted with permission of Briggs Health Care Products, Des Moines, Iowa.)*

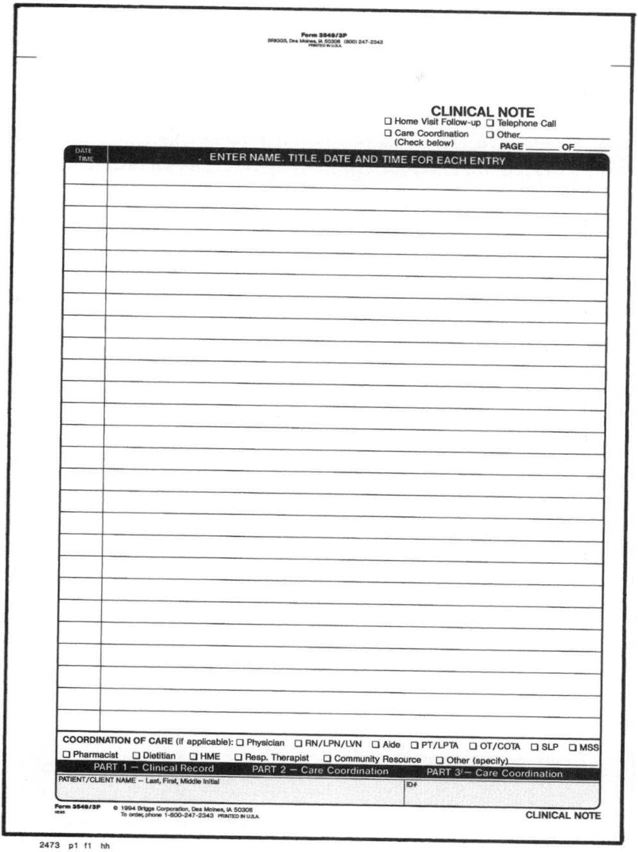

Form 3549/3P
BRIGGS, Des Moines, IA 50306 (800) 247-2343
PRINTED IN U.S.A.

CLINICAL NOTE

☐ Home Visit Follow-up ☐ Telephone Call
☐ Care Coordination ☐ Other______
(Check below)
PAGE _____ OF _____

DATE TIME	ENTER NAME. TITLE. DATE AND TIME FOR EACH ENTRY

COORDINATION OF CARE (if applicable): ☐ Physician ☐ RN/LPN/LVN ☐ Aide ☐ PT/LPTA ☐ OT/COTA ☐ SLP ☐ MSS ☐ Pharmacist ☐ Dietitian ☐ HME ☐ Resp. Therapist ☐ Community Resource ☐ Other (specify)______

PART 1 – Clinical Record PART 2 – Care Coordination PART 3 – Care Coordination

PATIENT/CLIENT NAME – Last, First, Middle Initial ID#

Form 3549/3P © 1994 Briggs Corporation, Des Moines, IA 50306
To order, phone 1-800-247-2343 PRINTED IN U.S.A.

CLINICAL NOTE

2473 p1 f1 hh

FIGURE 7-2 Example of a clinical note. *(Reprinted with permission of Briggs Health Care Products, Des Moines, Iowa.)*

SUMMARY

Home care is the fastest growing segment of health care. Nurses are acutely aware of the changes and advances in technology that have influenced the kinds of patients now seen in the home setting. The home care and hospice nurse of the present and future must be service oriented, flexible, and strong clinically. Payors and insurers must continue to address spiraling health care costs; the customary way to address rising costs has been to decrease authorized visits/services or to add additional review levels. It is the professional nurse who can validate the need for skilled home care and back it up by effective documentation. Nurses must know the coverage criteria for insurors, as well as the required documentation needed to support covered care. The importance of the documentation and the related coverage criteria go hand-in-hand and cannot be overstated, since they assist in meeting patient's needs, marketing services, safeguarding the nurse and her or his organization against alleged Medicare fraud or abuse claims, and ensuring reimbursement for services; they are the baseline for community education related to home care services and provide a benchmark for reviewing visit utilization.

Clinical documentation continues to be an important indicator of the quality of care provided in home care. In home care, where a reviewer or surveyor cannot walk down halls and see patients receiving care, the clinical record, including the format, organization and timeliness of filing, become important as the link to the care provided. From this perspective, and with the spiraling cost of home care and health care, the clinical record reflects the organization and its belief that "excellence is in the details." In home care and hospice the details of the clinical documentation are a driving force toward both payment and certification but, most important, toward reflecting that patients are receiving high quality care.

REVIEW EXERCISES

1. Outline the Medicare requirements for coverage and integrate those requirements into a coordinated plan of multidisciplinary care.
2. State three important skills needed for effective documentation.
3. Describe the documentation required to support covered care.
4. Review a peer's documentation and analyze why it does or does not support covered care.
5. List the hallmarks of effective documentation.

REFERENCES

Guide GW: *Legal issues in nursing: a source for practice,* Norwalk, Conn, 1985, Appleton & Lange.

Marrelli T: *Handbook of home health standards and documentation guidelines for reimbursement,* ed 3, St. Louis, 1998, Mosby.

Marrelli T, Hilliard L: Documentation and effective patient care planning, *Home Care Provider* 1(4):198-201, 1996.

FOR FURTHER READING

Jaffe M, Skidmore-Roth L: *Home health nursing care plans,* St. Louis, 1996, Mosby.

Sperling R: Outcomes-based quality improvement, *Home Care Nurse News* 3(4):1-5, 1996.

Sperling R: Outcomes-based quality improvement: OASIS update, *Home Care Nurse News* 3(7):1-3, 1996.

Sperling R: Outcomes-based quality improvement: OASIS update, *Home Care Nurse News* 3(11):1-3, 1996.

chapter

8

CONTINUING CARE: HIGHLIGHTS FOR PRACTICE

Tina M. Marrelli, MSN, MA, RNC

"True teamwork and collaboration occur when we know that none of us is as smart as all of us."

Tina M. Marrelli

CARE COORDINATION: IMPLEMENTING THE PLAN OF CARE

Once patients are admitted to home care or hospice, there are continuing care responsibilities. For example, Mr. Smith, our patient example in Chapter 6, is now officially admitted to home care and needs ongoing activities that support his plan of care (POC) and treatment goals related to congestive heart failure (CHF) and chronic obstructive pulmonary disease (COPD) being met by the team. These activities will be provided by the nurse and other team members as Mr. Smith is followed across his length of stay (LOS). This chapter highlights information and activities that occur during the patient's LOS in home care.

Communications: Key to Effective Care Coordination

From Medicare, accreditation, and quality perspectives the patient's clinical records must reflect effective interdisciplinary communications. All personnel furnishing services must maintain liaison to ensure that their efforts are coordinated effectively and support the objectives outlined specifically outlined in the POC. In addition, the clinical record or minutes of case conferences must demonstrate that effective interchange, reporting, and coordination occur. When surveyors visit an organization, they usually ask: "What is the organization's policy related to facilitating exchange of information among staff (both employee and contractor)?" or "How does coordination of care among staff and/or contract personnel providing services to individual patient's occur?" Accurate and timely communication is necessary to ensure continuity of care and to address patients' continuing care and care planning changes and needs. Many organizations have a special form for care coordination, but care coordination takes many different shapes and activities (Box 8-1).

The actual "how-to" of interdisciplinary communications varies across programs. The team includes the patient and/or caregiver, home health or hospice aide, nurse, agency case manager, therapists, physician, social worker, dietitian, pharmacist, the insurance case manager, and others who become involved in the patient's care. For hospice patients there will be the physician, volunteers, the volunteer coordinator, the chaplain, the hospice nurse, and others.

Litmus Test of Care Coordination

Remember that the litmus test of care coordination is in the outcome—that all team members know the patient's condition and are on the "same page" working toward common predetermined goals. An example of whether or not care coordination is occurring effectively follows: can another team member, a nurse, pick up from reading my written clinical documentation what is happening with my patient or caseload, what interventions should occur, and what the goals for care and discharge are? If you can answer yes, then you will have met care coordination standards. Most commonly home care and hospice organizations achieve this needed level of communication through team meetings and care or case conferences.

Whatever structure they take in your organization, these meetings and communications are the key to effectively caring for patients through their length of stay. Because our patients are not "down the hall" but are in a different county or many miles away, these activities take on more significance, as does the documentation related to them.

CASE MANAGEMENT AND HOME CARE

Many of the activities related to care coordination are managed by the patient's nurse. Figure 4-1 visually portrayed that nursing is the most frequent service in home care. Successful nurses in home care relinquish task orientation and focus on the coordination of patient care. In many care delivery models in home care and hospice, the clinician functions as a true case manager who manages the patient and his or her POC, as well as the details across the home care stay. Her or his role in these communications cannot be overstated. There has been much discussion about the many roles of the case manager, and it can be confusing (Box 8-2). For example, one patient could have three case managers:

BOX 8-1   **TWELVE EXAMPLES OF CARE
          COORDINATION ACTIVITIES**

These examples of communications occur in effective care coordination:
✔ Calling the therapist(s) to update them on your findings.
✔ Meeting the home health aide at the patient's home at the initial visit and completing the aide's assignment sheet so that any questions can be addressed and the role can be clarified and defined to the patient and family while the aide is also present. (This decreases miscommunication from the onset such as "the nurse said the aide would do the laundry for our family of 10").
✔ Team meetings at which the therapists, nurse, aide, and other team members are present or have called in their specific report to their manager or another team member who can update the team on the patient, or set phone conference times to discuss patients and care planning.
✔ Calling the physician with a change in the patient's condition and taking verbal orders to change the POC (such as a medication or a catheter size)
✔ Calling the home care or hospice social worker to identify changes in the patient's home environment related to finances or other impediments to effectively implementing the POC.
✔ Calling the home health aide when the patient graduates from bed bath to an assisted-shower status and simultaneously updating the "Home Health Assignment" sheet and documenting this change in the patient's clinical record.
✔ Documenting all the above communications, as well as other phone calls, meetings, and communications related to your patient's care and POC.
✔ Identifying needed changes to the POC based on the patient's condition. For example, the home health aide makes a visit to a patient and sees that the patient is sweating profusely and complains of chest pain and that the patient's color is different. Clearly the home health aide will not provide the assigned therapy activities nor personal care, but will contact the supervisor and call 911 as per agency policy. The nurse would communicate with all involved in this patient's care and document these calls.
✔ When a nurse goes to a patient's home, the patient is not home. She later finds out that the patient was readmitted to a community hospital during the night. This information would be provided to all team members involved in the patient's care for both care coordination and scheduling purposes and would be noted in the clinical record.

BOX 8-1   **TWELVE EXAMPLES OF CARE
             COORDINATION ACTIVITIES—cont'd**

✔ A scheduled meeting about patients. These may be called care
  or case conferences, team meetings, clinical meetings or updates
  or numerous other names. The meetings may be held weekly or
  bi-weekly based on the size of the agency and organized alphabetically by patient names, geographically by nurse team or patient location, based on service specialty lines such as cardiac,
  maternal-child, orthopedic, etc., or a number of other ways.
    At these meetings charts have been pulled and are updated by
  team members as they discuss the case. At this time a chart review
  occurs: medication sheets are updated, follow-up occurs on outstanding orders, referrals are initiated to therapists or other present team members, recertifications are discussed and initiated,
  POCs are updated, and plans are documented for continued care
  and agreed-on team goals directed toward patient discharge.
✔ Voice mail systems to report/update admissions, discharges, or
  changes to staff during off hours or for report that does not require feedback or discussion.
✔ Other communications, as unique as the patient and organization.

---

1. The case manager from the insurance company (managing resources, care needs across care settings)
2. The hospital case manager (providing essentially discharge planning and follow-up telephone support)
3. The home care case manager who cares for the patient while he
   or she is provided care through the home care program

A case manager then is the identified person in a system who focuses
on providing quality care and services to a given group of patients and
who works toward achieving outcomes within effective and appropriate
time frames and defined resource utilization parameters. The patient is an
equal partner in care and care planning and is motivated toward self-care
and self-management in the best of these models (see Box 8-2).

Referrals and Communication with
Other Team Members
Many times it is the nurse who identifies that the patient needs a referral to another specialist or service. Although the roles of the other team
members were described in the Medicare section related to covered ser-

BOX 8-2   **ROLE OF THE CARE OR CASE MANAGER IN HOME CARE**

The following are the roles of the case (or care manager) in home care:

1. Assumes responsibility for care from intake (sometimes will meet new patients in the hospital or other care site before discharge) through home care discharge
2. Performs initial assessment and related documentation and care coordination activities (e.g., form 485 series, physician summary, discharge)
3. Communicates effectively and on an ongoing basis with the patient and caregiver, the physician(s), the home care manager, and other team members involved in the care
4. Assumes accountability for projected outcomes for patients, including resources, time on service, and others
5. Identifies variances in standardized care and care processes to identify areas for improved performance related to patient care and the organization
6. Advocates for needed patient services or resources, based on clearly communicating quantifiable information
7. Documents communications and clinical findings in the patient record per organizational requirements and standards that support quality standards, coverage, and reimbursement
8. Acts as a positive role model or preceptor for team members new to home or hospice care
9. Coordinates care with others involved in patient care (e.g., insurance company nurse, lifeline volunteer, home medical equipment company representative)
10. Provides care, supervises, and teaches aide team member, collaborates with all team members, and otherwise provides services and activities needed to achieve patient and program goals

vices, it is very important that all nurses new to home care spend time with the rehabilitation team (occupational therapist, physical therapist, speech-language pathologist), as well as the pharmacist, dietitian, enterostomal and respiratory therapists, and others. The insight provided through these observations will prove invaluable as the nurse assesses patients and their needs. At the end of this chapter are resources related to these specialties.

Medicare is an entitlement program; thus it is only fair that the patient be referred appropriately and early for the services the debility or problem demands. This early and appropriate intervention by members of the rehabilitation team directly contributes to more positive outcomes in home care patients. Ethical and care practice issues are raised when a patient is referred and needs immediate therapy or other intervention and is expected to wait until a therapist can be located or has an opening in a case load. It is imperative from a quality and risk management perspective that patients who are admitted can realistically expect the resources, which include qualified trained team members, to be available to care for them safely and effectively and in a timely manner.

Subsequent Visits or Revisits

There usually are two types of visits in home care and hospice—initial visits and revisits. Clearly the initial visits always take more time and for good reason. The information elicited by the nurse and provided by the patient and family becomes a part of the comprehensive data base on which the care planning is based. Revisits are just as important, but there is a shorter time frame in which to accomplish usually well-defined tasks or activities. The nurse's organizational standards of care or practice prioritize and define the care to be provided during revisits, which becomes the framework for the care provided at every visit by your organization. For example, on every visit vital signs (including the fifth, pain) are obtained or assessed, a reassessment and history update occur, and plans and the date of the next visit are noted on the patient's home care calendar that remains in the home to support care coordination.

All nurses have heard the story about the nurse who did not ask and proceeded to dress the wrong wound site (the other was worse, but the patient figured the agency knew best!) Clearly, all wound sites are looked at, and complaints are followed up and addressed. The documentation is completed in the home at the end of the visit, and any physician-related communications that need to occur may be facilitated from the patient's home. This also contributes to the patient's active participation in the care.

Productivity Considerations

There has been much discussion about productivity in home care. Some organizations pay hourly, per visit, or salary their nurses. Still others "weigh" certain activities such as hospice visits, infusion visits, and admission visits to try and equal out the work load. After you have practiced in home care for some time, you will see that this all usually evens out.

Your organization may have standards for the number of initial or revisits to be done in a week. Daily productivity standards can be difficult because the work varies day to day but usually evens out over a span of a week or two. Productivity ranges from five to seven visits a day to 25 to 35 visits a week, depending on geographical locations and the acuity of patients. In areas of high managed care penetration, where the visits are longer and the nurse case manager is on the phone half the day, the number of visits may actually be fewer then the current norm. In addition, where there is more managed care, there are usually more admissions and more discharges since patient turnover increases proportionally (just like the hospitals with decreased LOSs but increased admissions and discharges). What this means to the home care organizations is that there is the same amount of work (e.g., admission paperwork, billing systems) and less time to get it accomplished. Know that the entire health care industry is "riding this wave" of change as the paradigm shift continues for inpatient to home and community-based care.

CONTINUATION OF CARE
The Dilemma of 60-Day Recertification

If your patient is a Medicare patient, there must be a recertification to continue care past the initial 60 to 62 day period. The recertification is the process of continuing to plan and project your patient's care needs for the next 60- to 62-day period. This decision to discharge or recertify a patient is usually made 2 weeks before the end of the prior certification period and is an important part of home care operations and practice. The decision is based on a reassessment, physical findings, and an overall review of the patient's trajectory to date.

Like the initial certification process, the Health Care Financing Administration (HCFA) form 485 is the form to be used. The information and the process related to the decision is made with the input of the team, following home care and clinical standards of practice. The physician and patient are also very important members of the team related to recertification. *In fact, it is a Medicare standard that the total POC must be reviewed by the physician and home care personnel as often as the severity of the patient's condition requires but at least once every 62 days.* Of course, changes in the patient's condition that require a change in the plan of care should be documented in the patient's clinical record.

The decision to recertify or move toward discharge is an important one for the organization and the patient. Thoughtful consideration and analysis of the information/data obtained creates an environment for making the best decision while supporting individualized quality patient care.

The following information is a checklist of questions that may be helpful as you recertify a home care patient.

- ✔ Does the patient continue to meet the Medicare eligibility and other required criteria (e.g., Medicare, skilled care)?
- ✔ Identify the reason for homebound status.
- ✔ Briefly identify the skilled care needed.
- ✔ Are there multiple medical problems and medications? Have there been medication or other changes to the POC during the past certification period; and do they support continued observation, management, and teaching?

  Note: For the preceding question it may be helpful to review 15 skilled nursing services in the Medicare Manual, beginning with the "Observation and Assessment of Patient's Condition When Only the Specialized Skills of a Medical Professional Can Determine a Patient's Status" and through to the last covered Medicare skilled nursing service, "Psychiatric Evaluation and Therapy."

- ✔ Is the patient frail and does he or she have a history that suggests further episodes of exacerbation or deterioration? Are you arranging, coordinating, and managing the services? Are there deficits in thought processes, nutritional/hydration problems? Is there no support system or are there deficits in it (e.g., abuse, unsafe, unkempt)? Does the patient have multiple or restrictive functional limitations? Are there safety concerns that support continued care? Consider if your patient meets the coverage criteria for management and evaluation (M&E) of a patient POC.
- ✔ What are the current medications, and what changes have been made (e.g., dosages, additional or new drugs)? What are their side effects and the implications for self-care and management? Are there implications for drug/food and drug/drug interactions? Have there been any adverse side effects noted? What were they, and what was the intervention? Can the patient articulate his or her medications and what they are for?
- ✔ Has the patient had a hospitalization or other medical health-threatening event, such as an emergency room visit or a fall during the prior certification period? If yes, to what was it attributed? Episodes of dehydration? Does the patient tell you that "his nephew comes every Tuesday with food," but, when you ask if you can prepare a snack, you note that there is no food in the refrigerator?
- ✔ Has there been a change in caregiver or caregiver status such as ability, availability, and willingness to provide care that has impacted your patient?

✔ Has the patient's status deteriorated? How and in what ways?

✔ Have other team members such as the physician, home health aide, therapists, or social worker identified changes or needs?

✔ In reviewing your documentation and the clinical record objectively, does the picture painted generally point toward discharge or recertification?

✔ Does your patient continue to be homebound and have continuing needs, based on accepted medical standards, for a Foley catheter, vitamin B_{12} injections, daily insulin injections, or other intervention(s) that originally initiated the care?

In reviewing your patient with your supervisor before recertification, identification of the above information will assist in the decision about continuing care for patients who meet the criteria from payor, quality, and organizational perspectives.

Items to Remember When Recertifying

Once the decision is made to recertify or continue care for your patient, the following three regulatory processes must occur:

1. A new, updated form 485 is generated (and there can be no gap in orders as discussed in a prior chapter). It is a Medicare standard of practice that the total POC be reviewed by the patient's physician as often as the severity of the patient's condition requires, but at least every 62 days (hence, the recertification).

2. A written summary report or care summary is sent to the physician about the patient, also every 62 days (Figure 8-1).

3. An HCFA form 486 may be generated (Figure 8-2). Your organization will have guidelines about the information and specific format that communicates to the physician the patient's status and course of care to date in home care. Sometimes the HCFA form 486 is the information also sent to the physician, and sometimes it is another form. This format of communicating to physicians varies across organizations.

The correct completion of the form 486 may be found in the *Handbook of Home Health Standards and Documentation Guidelines for Reimbursement* (Marrelli, 1998). This form simply updates what has occurred with your patient during the prior certification (62-day) period. It is also used by the regional home health intermediaries (RHHIs) to perform medical review functions and to make sure they are paying for covered care, as required by law. There are also the guidelines for complet-

Form 3583/3P
BRIGGS, Des Moines, IA 50306 (800) 247-2343
PRINTED IN U.S.A.

CARE SUMMARY

☐ Transfer/Referral
☐ Recert. Summary/Order Renewal
☐ Discharge Summary

PATIENT/CLIENT ______ ID# ______
ADDRESS ______
PHONE ______
SOC __/__/__ Most Recent Recert. __/__/__ (If applicable) Last Date of Service __/__/__

PHYSICIAN ______
☐ Notified __/__/__
☐ POT 485 Attached for Signature
☐ Copy Sent __/__/__

SUMMARY

THIS SUMMARY AREA MUST BE COMPLETED IN ALL CASES

REASON FOR ADMISSION (describe condition) ______

DISCIPLINES INVOLVED
☐ SN ☐ PT ☐ SLP
☐ HHA ☐ OT ☐ MSW
☐ Other ______
☐ Other ______

SUMMARY OF CARE (to date) ______

DISCHARGE

If Discharge Summary checked in upper right, indicate reason and date below.

☐ Patient/Client-centered goals achieved __/__/__
☐ Patient/Client expired __/__/__
☐ Geographic relocation __/__/__
☐ Transfer/Admit to other agency/organization/facility (Complete Transfer/Referral section below.) __/__/__
☐ Patient/Client refused further care __/__/__
☐ No longer home bound __/__/__
☐ Agency/Organization decision __/__/__
Explain: ______

☐ Patient/Client/Family request __/__/__
☐ Physician request __/__/__
☐ Repeatedly not home/not found __/__/__
☐ Patient/Client refused to accept care/treatments as ordered __/__/__
☐ Persistent noncompliance with POC __/__/__
☐ Failure to maintain services of an attending physician __/__/__
☐ Other (specify) ______ __/__/__

CONDITION AT DISCHARGE (describe) ______

DISCHARGE PLANNING (specify future follow-up, referrals, etc.) ______

Written instructions given to patient/client/caregiver: ☐ Yes ☐ No, explain ______
Patient/Client/Caregiver demonstrates understanding of instructions: ☐ Yes ☐ No, explain ______

TRANSFER/REFERRAL

UNIQUE NEEDS AND/OR BIO-PSYCHOSOCIAL PROBLEMS (specify) ______

Medication information attached ☐ Yes ☐ No
Advance directive exists ☐ Yes ☐ No Copy attached ☐ Yes ☐ No

Signature/Title: ______ Date: __/__/__

PART 1 — Clinical Record PART 2 — Physician or Transfer Organization PART 3 — Care Coordination

PATIENT/CLIENT NAME — Last, First, Middle Initial | ID#

Form 3583/3P © 1994 Briggs Corporation, Des Moines, IA 50306
To order, phone 1-800-247-2343 PRINTED IN U.S.A.
CARE SUMMARY

2451 p1 f1 hh

FIGURE 8-1 Written summary reports are sent to the physician about each patient. *(Reprinted with permission of Briggs Health Care Products, Des Moines, Iowa.)*

Form 3486R/3P
BRIGGS, Des Moines, IA 50306 (800) 247-2343
PRINTED IN U.S.A.

Department of Health and Human Services
Health Care Financing Administration

Form Approved
OMB No. 0938-0357

MEDICAL UPDATE AND PATIENT INFORMATION

1. Patient's HI Claim No.	2. SOC Date	3. Certification Period From: To:	4. Medical Record No.	5. Provider No.

6. Patient's Name and Address

7. Provider's Name

8. Medicare Covered: ☐ Y ☐ N

9. Date Physician Last Saw Patient:

10. Date Last Contacted Physician:

11. Is the Patient Receiving Care in an 1861 (J)(1) Skilled Nursing Facility or Equivalent? ☐ Y ☐ N ☐ Do Not Know

12. ☐ Certification ☐ Recertification ☐ Modified

13. Dates of Last Inpatient Stay: Admission Discharge

14. Type of Facility:

15. Updated information: New Orders/Treatments/Clinical Facts/Summary from Each Discipline

16. Functional Limitations (Expand From 485 and Level of ADL) Reason Homebound/Prior Functional Status

17. Supplementary Plan of Care of File from Physician Other than Referring Physician: ☐ Y ☐ N
(If Yes, Please Specify Giving Goals/Rehab. Potential/Discharge Plan)

18. Unusual Home/Social Environment

19. Indicate Any Time When the Home Health Agency Made a Visit and Patient was Not Home and Reason Why if Ascertainable

20. Specify Any Known Medical and/or Non-Medical Reasons the Patient Regularly Leaves Home and Frequency of Occurrence

21. Nurse or Therapist Completing or Reviewing Form

Date (Mo., Day, Yr.)

Form 3486R/3P BRIGGS, Des Moines, IA 50306 (800) 247-2343 PRINTED IN U.S.A.

PROVIDER

Form HCFA-486 (C3) (02-94) (Print Aligned)

FIGURE 8-2 HCFA form 486 medical update and patient information form. *(Reprinted with permission of Briggs Health Care Products, Des Moines, Iowa.)*

FIGURE 8-2, cont'd   For legend, see opposite page.

ing the HCFA form 487, which acts as an addendum to either the form 485 or the form 486. It is an overflow tool and can be either the continuation of the POC or the medical update. You can choose how to use the form by completing the appropriate box. If it is used as an overflow for physician orders, it must be signed by the physician, like any other orders or POCs.

Physician Communications

In home and hospice care, physicians are accustomed to communication via phone, fax, and mail. Because the form 485 is the POC, as well as the physician's certification, there are sometimes additional communications in efforts to retrieve this needed form. Medicare-participating agencies must have the signed certification before billing; thus not only is the document the clinical tool for care and care planning, but it is also an administrative and legal requirement for obtaining reimbursement. This is why in home care, unlike in the hospital and all other health care settings, the clinical documentation and the administrative billing requirements go hand-in-hand.

In addition, the actual care provided must follow or mirror the POC. Home care staff must promptly notify or alert the physicians to any changes that suggest a need to amend or change the patient's POC (e.g., the number of home care visits, the kinds of dressings, or new services). These changes comprise the bulk of communications with physicians in home care and hospice. Any change in the patient's condition that necessitates a change in the POC must be documented in the clinical record. The nurse must also obtain a verbal order for the change because it is also a change in the POC, which is the physician's orders in home care. Many of these changes will be related to medications and their management.

Physicians in home care are actively involved in the POC. They must be involved from both a practical and regulatory perspective. Usually when the nurse calls or meets with physicians about a patient, she or he should have clearly and objectively identified the problem and have a recommendation or suggested solution for resolution. This makes sense—it is the nurse and the home care team who see the patient and his or her environment. Physicians will usually do their best to keep the patient at the lower-cost setting for care—home. The nurse should trust her or his judgment about when physicians need to be called, but remember that nurses must notify the physician of any changes and any findings that necessitate a change in the POC. The nurse should talk to an experienced home care colleague or listen as she or he addresses a patient problem on the phone with the physician.

This will help the nurse increase assertiveness to be an advocate for the patient and family.

More physicians are making home visits to their patients. This makes sense—particularly for hospice or very ill or frail patients for whom it is very difficult to leave home without discomfort and an ambulance. Encourage physicians to make these visits when it is warranted. The nurse should speak with her or his supervisor about any problems related to obtaining physician orders or other patient needs. The supervisor may have the organization's medical director intervene in certain cases to facilitate physician communication and safe patient care.

Medication Management

A major responsibility in home care is determining your patient's medication regimen and tracking his or her course though medication management. It can feel overwhelming when a patient brings out a shoe box full of medications and is not capable of articulating his or her medications. In addition, many of the patients in home care are elderly or otherwise have compromised renal or liver functions, which contributes to drug problems such as toxicity. The nurse's role in medication management includes observation and assessment, obtaining venipunctures such as peaks and troughs, checking digoxin or theophylline levels, administering injections, infusion therapy, and administering oxygen and aerosol medication.

Some programs have interdisciplinary reviews by a pharmacist of patient medications to identify possible adverse reactions or potential problems. Whatever the system and forms at your organization, the medication sheet must be accurate and kept up to date. Remember that drugs and treatments are administered or provided by staff only as ordered by the physician and that all of these and other physician orders must be included in the documentation in the patient's clinical record. In all circumstances verbal orders must be countersigned by the physician as soon as possible.

Many home care patients are also taking over-the-counter drugs. These must also be noted in the record, and when the nurse determines that the over-the-counter drugs could be detrimentally affecting the patient, the physician should be notified. Your organization may have specific policies related to these drugs. The nurse must know what actions to take should he or she identify a patient sensitivity or other medication problems.

Patient Teaching

Home care and health care in general are being redirected, whenever possible, toward goals of self-care and self-management for our patients. What this means is that we all need to rethink how "we have always done things." Consider the patient who goes from an inpatient hospital to a skilled nursing facility to a home care program. You are the nurse coming to make the initial visit to a 86-year-old patient who has been given multiple teaching handouts related to his cardiac disease. They include:

1. How to check his pulse
2. How to sit slowly up in the mornings because he's on a medication that can cause orthostatic hypotension
3. Two different sheets on the same drug; one for digoxin and one for lanoxin; he thinks he takes both, and the print is so small that the prescription is difficult to read!

The importance of patient education is finally getting the press it needs—everyone needs to value it more across all care sites. Education really makes our patients and their families equal partners in care. In home care there are no secrets—patients are part of a mutual participant model. Family supports who work with the home care or hospice team are significant to what we can or cannot accomplish.

Experienced nurses in community health and home care have been teaching lay caregivers such as family members for years, including how to insert a Foley catheter; perform a straight catheterization; administer insulin, calcitonin (Calcimar), or B_{12}; and pack a wound. But educating the public, as well as patients and their families, is most important in home care—hopefully nurses will be discharging the patient to a home care site where the patient will be more independent in self-care and working toward health and self-maintenance.

Remember that Medicare values the nurse's higher-level skills, not just tasks performed, and that patient teaching and training are skilled covered services. Nurses need to be more astute about honing their teaching skills and documenting the specific teaching provided. Some forward-thinking organizations make standardizing patient education materials as a performance improvement activity across the entire organization. The nurses, therapists, and other team members gather "favorite" patient education tools. A work group is established, and consensus is reached on the "best" tools or handouts. "Best" can be defined as up-to-date, legible, large print, and understandable. Keep this in mind when you want to volunteer for a project and know that this is a long-term project. Forward-thinking organizations are trying to work with their referral sources, again to standardize the patient education tools so the patient has the same form and the nurse does not confuse him or her by bringing out another that sometimes contains conflicting information. Practice and use your teaching and training skills—they'll get a lot of practice in your new chosen specialty!

Bowel and Bladder Management

From a quality perspective, no patient in home or hospice care should have undetected constipation. Bowel patterns and habits are an important part of the initial assessment, as well as the continued care of patients. The nurse and the home health aide are in the key positions to follow up and identify problems. High-risk patients may be automatically placed on a bowel management regimen. Some organizations, particularly hospices, may have standing orders to decrease the possibility of avoidable impaction and discomfort for patients.

Some of the patients who are at risk for these problems and who require a plan for a continued regimen after discharge from services include:

- Patient following hospitalization or nursing home stay
- Patient who cannot remember last bowel movement
- Patient taking pain medications
- Patient has been enema or laxative dependent for years
- Patient immobile or with significantly decreased activity level
- Patient unable to eat many foods
- Patient with swallowing problems
- Patient with diarrhea of unknown etiology
- Patient with a history of impaction
- Patient who complains of pain or bleeding when having bowel movements
- Patient who has hemorrhoids
- Patient who has a history of hemorrhoids or bowel surgery
- Other reasons, based on the patient's unique history

The nurse's role in bowel management is important to the comfort and health of the patient. As the nurse's "eyes and ears," many times it will be the home health or hospice aide who identifies a bowel problem. Like pressure ulcers, prevention is the best treatment for constipation and bowel problems.

SUMMARY

Continuing care demands all the skills of the home care nurse. The ongoing assessment and planning are the case management functions of home care. The future of nursing is the nurse as case manager, whatever shape home care practice and reimbursement takes. Nurses also know that home care and all health care settings must be more productive. All clinicians in home care must be able to effectively prioritize and maximize sometimes limited interventions and authorized visits. The multifaceted roles of teacher, medication manager, coordinator, collaborator with other team members, and case manager will only increase in importance as home continues to be the preferred site for health care in the coming decades.

REVIEW EXERCISES

1. What function(s) does the HCFA form 486 serve in your organization?
2. Describe the mechanism and timelines for recertifications in your organization.
3. List some activities that are examples of care coordination.
4. Define and describe care coordination.
5. Discuss the roles of case manager in home care.
6. Define a case manager.
7. Explain the process in your organization to facilitate timely referral of patients to other disciplines.
8. Describe the rationale for and the processes involved in recertification.

RESOURCES

The Agency for Health Care Policy and Research (AHCPR) has free guidelines for patients related to urinary incontinence and other patient problems and are available in English and Spanish, (800)358-9295.

Dantone J: Bridging the gap: procedure and instructional manual for dietary and nursing interventions, Nutrition Education Resources, 1993, (601)226-3250.

REFERENCE

Marrelli T: *Handbook of home health standards and documentation guidelines for reimbursement,* ed 3, St. Louis, 1998, Mosby.

FOR FURTHER READING

Arensberg, M, Schiller R: Dietitians in home care: a survey of current practice, *J Am Diet Assn* 96(4)347-353, 1996.

Bower K: *Case management by nurses,* Washington, DC, 1992, American Nurses Association.

Broussard M, Pitre S: Medication problems in the elderly: a home healthcare nurse's perspective, *Home Healthcare Nurse* 14(6):441-443, 1996.

Harrah S: Meeting communication standards among staff, *Home Care Nurse News* 3(3):1-3, 1996.

Krulish L: Identifying physical therapy needs, *Home Care Nurse News* 1(5):6, 1994.

Marrelli T: 20 drugs generally considered inappropriate for the elderly, *Home Care Nurse News* 3(6):1-3, 1996.

Redman B: *The practice of patient education,* St. Louis, 1993, Mosby.

Stanhope M, Knollmueller R: *Handbook of community and home health nursing—tools for assessment, intervention, and education,* St. Louis, 1992, Mosby.

Tonore M: Screening patients for nutrition risk, *J Home Health Pract* 6 (3):23-36, 1994.

Zink M: Social support systems in elder homebound clients, *J Home Health Pract* 6(3):1-10, 1994.

DISCHARGE

Tina M. Marrelli, MSN, MA, RNC

"It ain't over 'til it's over."

Author unknown

Discharge from home care should always be a planned event. The only kind of patients who may be chronic and stable for home care purposes and who may not be discharged for lengthy periods are the homebound long-term Foley catheter patient who, because of bladder atony, may have the catheter for the rest of his or her life, the homebound patient who needs vitamin B_{12}, the blind diabetic patient who is unable to self-inject, homebound venipuncture patients who meet the coverage criteria, and a few others. For most patients, discharge planning truly starts on admission, when the nurse and the rest of the team determine the desired goals and outcomes and project time frames for completion. It goes without saying that discharge from home care should never be a surprise to your patient and/or his or her family.

As discussed in the previous chapter, care coordination occurs throughout the patient's length of stay in home care and occurs among all team members. A projected discharge date is usually addressed during patient case conferences. This may be changed or further defined as goals are achieved. Throughout the care, however, it is imperative that team members prepare patients for discharge at some point. *Clinicians do patients no favors by having them become dependent on their assistance for things they could do safely (if somewhat slower) themselves.* The organization will have a discharge policy that usually lists the reasons for discharge from home care. The following is an example only; refer to your organization's specific policy.

1. Patient is no longer homebound.
2. Patient moves out of the organization's geographical catchment area.

3. Patient is admitted to the hospital for more than ___ hours (e.g., 48 hours); this is up to the organization.
4. Patient has met the goals as defined on admission.
5. Patient is noncompliant.
6. Other reasons.

The physician is also kept apprised of the projected discharge, again so everyone is on the same page. Several steps occur when discharge is pending, including the following:

1. The patient has been notified in advance and has been given a specific last visit date by the nurse (assuming there are no unforeseen changes or complications).
2. The home health aide also needs to know the discharge date so this can be shared with schedulers who can assign the aide to a new patient. Usually the aide and the nurse or the therapist both visit on the last day.
3. Teaching is reviewed one last time, and the nurse ensures that the patient has the teaching materials for reference. In addition, patients are reminded of whom to call for problems (e.g., the physician).
4. Make sure that the physician is notified of the actual projected last visit date before it occurs. After the nurse has determined the last visit date, it is not unusual for patients to call the physician to ask him or her to order more care. It is important to remember that the physician does not have the relationship with Medicare and the responsibility to know the rules; these belong to the home care organization and its team members. When the physician gets this call, he or she can say that they were aware of the discharge and that follow-up care will be provided in the office since the patient is no longer homebound (or whatever the reason).
5. A specific discharge summary needs to be completed when a patient is discharged from home care (the organization has a policy defining when discharge occurs). An example of a discharge summary would be one for Mr. Smith, who was discharged as his congestive heart failure and chronic obstructive pulmonary disease stablized and returned to self-care. An example of a discharge summary is found in Figure 8-1. Some organizations also provide discharge instructions to patients and their families (Figure 9-1).

FINAL RECORD REVIEW

Documentation responsibilities include reviewing the clinical record for completeness before closure and final billing. Check that the med-

Form 3585/2P
BRIGGS, Des Moines, IA 50306 (800) 247-2343
PRINTED IN U.S.A.

DISCHARGE INSTRUCTIONS

Date of Discharge ____/____/____

We are pleased to have provided service to you. The following discharge instructions were reviewed with you and/or your caregiver(s) during the final visit(s) by organization staff. You are to:

❑ Keep your scheduled appointment with Dr. ____________________

Day ________________ Date ____/____/____ Time ________

❑ Continue to take medications as prescribed by your physician.
- ❑ Instructions attached
- ❑ Additional comments/instructions: ____________________

❑ Continue with home program as instructed by therapist.
- ❑ Instructions attached
- ❑ Additional comments/instructions: ____________________

❑ Follow the diet as prescribed by your physician and instructed by your nurse/dietitian.

❑ Continue with skin/wound care as instructed by your nurse.
- ❑ Instructions attached
- ❑ Additional comments/instructions: ____________________

❑ Follow through with community resource or other organization to which you have been referred (describe):

❑ Other instructions (describe): ____________________

If you have questions concerning these instructions, please call your care manager at (_____) ____________. We hope that if you have need for home care in the future, you will contact us.

Care Manager Signature/Title ____________________ Date ____/____/____

PART 1 — Clinical Record	PART 2 — Patient/Client
PATIENT/CLIENT NAME - Last, First, Middle Initial	ID#

Form 3585/2P © 1994 Briggs Corporation, Des Moines, IA 50306
To order, phone 1-800-247-2343 PRINTED IN U.S.A.

DISCHARGE INSTRUCTIONS

2420 p1 f1 hh

FIGURE 9-1 Sample discharge instructions form. *(Reprinted with permission of Briggs Health Care Products, Des Moines, Iowa.)*

ication sheet is updated, the care plan problem list is reviewc completed, verbal or form 485 orders that were outstanding arc turned and filed in the record, and, in general, that your clinical noι and findings tell a story about the patient's care from admission througl. discharge. Check that visits match the exact order for visit frequency. If they do not, check if there was a day that the patient was at the doctor (e.g., there should be a note stating why a patient is not home when you make a visit).

Remember that the Medicare intermediary may come back a year later to review a record; this is why discharge is the time that the nurse must review the case and complete the record. Every organization has a process related to clinical records and closure. At some organizations a sample of completed discharge records is reviewed by peers (1) to improve documentation through seeing other ways to document more effectively, and (2) to ensure that clinical records are complete so that timely and accurate billing occurs.

SATISFACTION SURVEYS

Most home care and hospice organizations elicit feedback from patients or caregivers about care that has been provided. These customer satisfaction surveys may be mailed or conducted through telephone calls. Whatever the route, what customers think is how clinicians and the organization are perceived to have performed. Customers in home care and hospice are varied but usually include the referral sources (e.g., discharge planners, case managers), the patients and/or family members, and physicians. An example of a customer satisfaction survey is shown in Figure 9-2. It may be sent out 2 weeks after discharge or immediately on discharge. All customer satisfaction tools are created, sent out, and analyzed and trended in the hopes of using this information to improve performance in the organization.

SUMMARY

Discharge in home care usually means that patients have achieved their goals and that the team assisted the patients in the goals of self-care. Discharge can be a problem area in organizations in which there is poor communication and patients and their family members are not apprised on an ongoing basis. The home care nurse and other team members play an important role in the patient's satisfaction or dissatisfaction with the care provided. This customer service area will only increase in importance as an indicator of excellence and as competition for patients increases and cost-effectiveness and positive customer relations become large parts of the definition of quality.

SATISFACTION QUESTIONNAIRE

DATE ____ / ____ / ____

Thank you for allowing us to provide care for you or your family member. We are interested in your ideas or opinions about our care/services. Please take a moment to answer the following questions. Additional comments are welcome and can be recorded on the back of this form. If you need assistance in completing this form, please feel free to contact our office.

For questions 1 - 10, please circle the appropriate number that best describes your opinion.
1-Strongly Agree   2-Agree   3-Disagree   4-Strongly Disagree   5-No Opinion or Not Applicable

1. I was satisfied with the care provided by the:					
a. Nurse(s)	1	2	3	4	5
b. Physical Therapist	1	2	3	4	5
c. Occupational Therapist	1	2	3	4	5
d. Speech/Language Pathologist	1	2	3	4	5
e. Medical Social Worker	1	2	3	4	5
f. Home Health Aide(s)	1	2	3	4	5
2. I was involved in decision-making regarding my plan of care.	1	2	3	4	5
3. My opinions were considered in the planning for discharge.	1	2	3	4	5
4. Staff treated me, my family, my home and belongings with respect.	1	2	3	4	5
5. Staff explained my conditions, rights and responsibilities, and other procedures related to the care I received.	1	2	3	4	5
6. The staff generally arrived as scheduled.	1	2	3	4	5
7. I was able to reach my nurse/therapist promptly and my phone calls were returned.	1	2	3	4	5
8. When I called the agency, office staff were courteous and available and directed my call correctly.	1	2	3	4	5
9. I would use this agency again.	1	2	3	4	5
10. I would recommend this agency to friends and relatives.	1	2	3	4	5

11. Suggestions for improvements/additional comments:

12. What most impressed me about the agency's care/service was:

Thank you for your valuable feedback. This confidential information will be used only in efforts to improve care/service.

Sincerely,

I ☐ would/☐ would not like to discuss my responses further.

Please return the completed questionnaire in the enclosed, self-addressed, stamped envelope.

____ / ____ / ____

Organization Director or Administrator Signature   _Optional Signature of Person Completing Form_   _Date_

Form 3584   © 1994 Briggs Corporation, Des Moines, IA 50306
To order, phone 1-800-247-2343   PRINTED IN U.S.A.

SATISFACTION QUESTIONNAIRE

2417   p1 f1   one color

FIGURE 9-2   Sample customer satisfaction survey. *(Reprinted with permission of Briggs Health Care Products, Des Moines, Iowa.)*

REVIEW EXERCISES

1. Describe the process for planning discharge among team memb
2. List the reasons for discharge in your organization's policies.
3. Discuss the process for clinical record review (ongoing and on discharge).
4. Review and complete your organization's discharge summary form.
5. Discuss the rationale and process for customer satisfaction questionnaires or telephone interviews for feedback.

FOR FURTHER READING

Reeder PJ, Chen SC: A client satisfaction survey in home health care, *J Nurs Qual Assur* 5(1):16-24, 1990.

part III

SPECIALTY CONSIDERATIONS IN HOME CARE

10

PSYCHIATRIC CARE IN HOME CARE

Gail Ohlund, RN

"Mental illnesses such as panic disorders, depression, and schizophrenia affect approximately 40 million Americans a year."

The American Pharmaceutical Research Companies, 1996

HISTORICAL PERSPECTIVE

Psychiatric home care nursing services have been available to clients with Medicare since the 1970s. These services were primarily delivered to medically diagnosed clients who exhibited accompanying psychiatric symptoms such as a depressed mood, anxiety, or psychotic thoughts. The psychiatric home care nurse was expected to manage the client's many medical problems and any secondary psychiatric symptoms. If the nurse was able to provide nursing services for both the medical and psychiatric problems, the home visits were usually 2 or more hours. However, most of the clients were medically very ill, and the nurse had little or no time to identify and treat the client's secondary psychiatric symptoms.

By 1989 psychiatric home care nursing became clearly defined by Medicare in the *Home Health Agency (HHA) Manual—Pub. 11,* Revision 222, Section 205.1, Paragraph 15 (HCFA) and was further identified as the "15th skilled nursing service" reimbursable by Medicare. With the regulations more clearly defined and understood, psychiatric home care nurses in HHAs began visiting clients with primary psychiatric diagnoses and concurrent secondary medical diagnoses. Psychiatric inpatient discharge planning began to include psychiatric home care services for Medicare recipients. Many of the referred clients had a secondary medical diagnosis or history of one, although some of the clients were younger with a diagnosis of schizophrenia and no medical diagnosis. Following Medicare's lead, indemnity insurance plans and health maintenance organizations (HMOs) also began authorizing and paying for psychiatric home care.

QUALIFICATIONS FOR PSYCHIATRIC REGISTERED NURSES

Medicare requires that a psychiatric registered nurse (RN) have experience and/or training beyond the standard curriculum required for an RN. Psychiatric RNs must meet one of the following qualifications:

- A registered nurse with a master's degree in psychiatric or mental health nursing who is licensed in the state where practicing and has recent nursing experience in a psychiatric or mental health unit of a hospital, a partial hospitalization program, or an outpatient psychiatric clinic.
- A registered nurse with a bachelor's degree in nursing who is licensed in the state where practicing and has 1 year of recent nursing experience in a psychiatric or mental health unit of a hospital, a partial hospitalization program, or an outpatient psychiatric clinic.
- A registered nurse with a diploma or associate's degree in nursing who is licensed in the state where practicing and has 2 years of recent nursing experience in a psychiatric or mental health unit of a hospital, a partial hospitalization program, or an outpatient psychiatric clinic.
- On an individual basis, other combinations of education and experience may be considered.
- The employing agency must send the RN's resumé to the Medicare regional home health intermediary (RHHI) for review and approval of the psychiatric RN's qualifications.

A psychiatric RN might possess additional training and experience (although not required by Medicare) that would enhance his or her career in home health (e.g., the American Nurses Association (ANA) Certification for Mental Health Nursing, mobile crisis nursing experience and experience in assessing psychiatric emergencies, expert knowledge regarding psychotropic medications and their administration, home care experience, independent and autonomous thinking and a belief in promoting client independence along the continuum of care, supervisory and program development experience, and client teaching and community educational skills).

APPROPRIATE PSYCHIATRIC DIAGNOSES

The psychiatric diagnosis must match the diagnosis that the ordering physician is treating and, when appropriate, the reason for which the client was hospitalized. Some acceptable primary psychiatric diagnoses might include, but are not limited to: depressive disorders, bipolar disorders, schizophrenic disorders, anxiety disorders, psychotic disorders, dementia of the Alzheimer type with delusions, and delirium or depressed mood. For an in-depth listing of potential psychiatric diagnoses, ICD-9 codes, and associated interventions, see the *Handbook of Home Health Standards and Documentation Guidelines for Reimbursement* (Marrelli, 1998).

Medicare has stated that diagnoses such as active substance abuse, uncomplicated dementia, Alzheimer's disease, and personality disorders may sometimes be unacceptable primary psychiatric diagnoses that may be subjected to an in-depth medical review process. It is important to note, "A finding that care is not reasonable and necessary must be based on information provided on the forms (HCFA 485) and in the medical record with respect to the unique medical condition of the individual beneficiary" (HCFA, Section 203.1).

CLIENT EXAMPLES

Most clients on psychiatric home care services are elderly Medicare beneficiaries. Their primary diagnosis is frequently major depression. However, managed care and Medicaid are referring to psychiatric home care in hopes of reducing health costs and decreasing frequent rehospitalizations. Some examples of clients who may be appropriate for psychiatric home care services follow.

Client Example 1

A 74-year-old male with a diagnosis of generalized anxiety and depressed mood and acute congestive heart failure (CHF) was referred to psychiatric home care services. The client had one psychiatric inpatient admission, but numerous medical and emergency room (ER) admissions for CHF associated with anxiety and panic attacks in the last year. The client lived alone in an apartment, which exacerbated his panic attacks, which in turn exacerbated his CHF. The client was referred by his psychiatrist to reduce the ER and hospital readmissions, allow the psychiatric home care staff to teach the client to manage his diseases and medications and learn positive coping skills, and relocate the client to a more structured, safe environment.

Client Example 2

A 30-year-old male client eligible for Medicare who has schizophrenia and delusions of paranoia was referred to psychiatric home care services following discharge from a 7-day stay in a psychiatric inpatient hospital. The client was being relocated to a new home (a licensed residential personal care facility). The client was referred by his psychiatrist with orders for psychiatric nursing to administer haloperidol decanoate (Haldol) IM every 2 weeks (there was no one available to be taught administration of the medication) and observe and assess medication dosage and effectiveness and patient's mental status for increased signs of paranoia secondary to the relocation.

Client Example 3

A 40-year-old female with private insurance and bipolar disorder was referred to psychiatric home care services. The client had over 10 admissions to a psychiatric inpatient hospital and frequent ER visits in the last year. The client was married and had a supportive family network, but the husband had been staying home from work a great deal of the time when the client was depressed and potentially suicidal and was concerned about losing his job. The client's psychiatrist ordered psychiatric nursing services to teach the client and family how to manage the cycles of bipolar disease, monitor compliance with medications, teach the client positive coping skills, and attempt to reduce the frequent hospital admissions. A social worker was ordered to assist the family in finding a homemaker to stay with the client during stressful times.

Client Example 4

A 16-year-old male with a private insurance plan and an adjustment disorder diagnosis was referred to psychiatric home care services following discharge from a 2-week stay in an inpatient adolescent unit. The client had five admissions to the unit in the last year, had been truant from high school, and was getting in trouble with the law. A treatment plan was drawn up with the client and family with agreed-on goals. The psychiatrist had started the client on a new medication while in the hospital, and the psychiatric nurse was evaluating the effectiveness of the medication. The psychiatric nurse was providing supportive therapy, disease instruction and management, and client and family counseling. The client saw the psychiatrist twice a week, and the nurse stayed in close contact with the physician regarding the treatment plan.

STANDARDS OF PRACTICE

The ANA published Standards for Home Health Nursing Practice in 1986 and a Statement on the Scope of Home Health Nursing Practice in 1991, which included the concept of nurses applying a holistic approach to the client's health and illness that emphasizes the use of a client-focused nursing care plan with goal attainment. The ANA has not published Standards for Psychiatric Nursing Home Health Practice; however, ANA's Standards for Psychiatric Nursing are used in psychiatric home care nursing.

Most of the State Nurse Practice Acts do not differentiate home care nursing from other types of nursing. All states have regulations regarding home health practice, job descriptions, and requirements for the home health nurse; however, most states do not have specific guidelines for psychiatric home care nursing.

The Joint Commission on Accreditation for Healthcare Organizations (JCAHO) has Standards for home care. For all specialty programs the JCAHO requires policies and procedures, demonstrated competence of the practicing clinicians, a standardized orientation program, and specific forms and criteria for the evaluation and assessment of specific client populations, such as the mental health client.

HHAs use their policies and procedures as their Standards of Practice or Protocols for delivering medical and psychiatric home health care. These standards are derived from state, national nursing, physician, and other therapy standards (e.g., physical therapist, occupational therapist, medical social worker, home health aide, speech-language pathologist, and dietitian), Medicaid, Medicare, and community practice.

ADMISSION CRITERIA AND DOCUMENTATION GUIDELINES

Medicare states that any beneficiary receiving home health services must meet the conditions of participation and requirements outlined in the *HHA Manual—Pub. 11* (HCFA). Requirements for home health coverage by state, managed care organizations and Medicaid are often based on Medicare guidelines with added or deleted requirements specifically identified. The guidelines for admission criteria and documentation coverage are the same (since Medicare regulations are also the laws) for medical and psychiatric clients. The differences are the specialty interventions pertinent to each nursing program (e.g., teaching and training disease process; the importance of diet, fluid restriction, and daily weights for a client with CHF; and teaching and training disease process and coping skills as symptom management for a client with depression).

The following sections outline the requirements stated in the *HHA Manual—Pub. 11* (HCFA).

Reasonable and Medically Necessary Services and Care

In determining the conditions for coverage, Medicare states that the services or care provided must be "reasonable and medically necessary." In determining reasonable and medical necessity, information from the plan of care (POC), physician orders, and medical record outlining the unique medical condition of the client is identified. Furthermore, the client's psychiatric and medical health status and history reflect a need for services that are appropriate to treat the client and diagnosis.

Example: A client was hospitalized with major depression, despondency, and suicide ideations. The client was discharged to the home with a new antidepressant medication, experiencing anxiety regarding the short hospital stay and discharge and depressive symptoms, but no active suicide thoughts.

Example: A client was started on a new antidepressant and antianxiety medication at the psychiatrist's office. The client was experiencing moderate-to-severe anxiety attacks and depression because of decreased health status (both psychiatric and medical).

In the preceding examples, the services the client requires to manage acute symptoms, new medications, and illness may be reasonable and necessary medical services to the diagnosis and treatment of the client. It is imperative that the documentation paint a picture of the patient's unique condition and problems that necessitate skilled intervention.

Homebound Status

In determining the conditions to qualify, Medicare states that the client must be "confined to the home," that the condition of the client creates a normal inability to leave the home, and that leaving the home requires a considerable and taxing effort on the client's part. The client may leave the home for medical treatment (partial hospitalization or physician visits) or infrequently for short durations for nonmedical reasons. The absences from the home must not indicate that the client has the capacity to obtain health care provided outside rather than in the home.

Medicare further states that a client with a psychiatric problem will be considered homebound if the illness is manifested in part by "a refusal to leave the home" or is of such a nature that it would be considered "unsafe to leave the home unattended."

Example: Refusing to leave or fearful of leaving the home because of extreme anxiety, with episodes of panic attacks and accompanying tachypnea and tachycardia.

Example: Refusing to leave or fearful of leaving the home because of agoraphobic and isolative symptoms associated with depression.

Example: Unsafe/unable to leave the home unattended because of paranoia and agitation that affects the client's safety, judgment, and decision making.

Example: Finds ambulation a considerable and taxing effort with shortness of breath, has extreme fatigue after 10 feet of walking, and refuses to or is fearful of leaving the home because of paranoid delusions.

Physician-Approved and Established Plan of Care

Qualifying conditions require that home care services are provided under a "POC established and approved by a physician." The POC contains all pertinent diagnoses, mental status, types of services required, frequency of visits, prognosis, rehabilitation prognosis, functional limitations, activities permitted, nutritional requirements, medications and treatments, safety measures to protect against injury, instructions for timely discharge, and additional items the physician or HHA may choose to include. This POC is called the Medicare HCFA form 485 and is established by the treating physician or psychiatrist with the assistance of the psychiatric home care RN.

Psychiatric home care nursing services are ordered by a psychiatrist or medical physician who identifies the client's psychiatric diagnosis. Psychiatric nursing services may be provided to a client with a primary medical diagnosis, as long as the visiting psychiatric nurse provides the medical interventions required by the client and identified on the POC. Medical nurses may not visit a psychiatric client who has a primary psychiatric diagnosis identified on the POC. Psychiatric nurses are required to manage the secondary medical problems that the client presents. There are a few exceptions to this condition, and the following two examples illustrate a possible scenario.

Example: If the psychiatric client has a major wound, but the primary diagnosis remains psychiatric, a nurse specialist could visit and treat the client's wound.

Example: An unstable diabetic client requires twice-a-day insulin injections, and there is no available and willing caregiver to administer the insulin. A medical nurse may visit the client to administer some of the required insulin injections. The psychiatric nurse must also administer insulin, but may accomplish this according to the psychiatric visit frequency identified on the POC.

The POC must be reviewed and signed every 62 days by the physician who established the POC, and the psychiatric client must be under the care of the referring physician or psychiatrist. The frequency of visits on the POC must be on an intermittent basis (under 35 hours of visits in a week's time), and the psychiatric POC must be psychiatric in nature with psychiatric interventions appropriate to the primary psychiatric diagnosis. If medical problems are identified as secondary problems, the POC should also identify medical interventions that are appropriate to the medical secondary diagnosis.

Required Skills

In determining home health eligibility, "the services provided to the client must require the skills of a nurse (psychiatric RN)," must be reasonable and necessary to the treatment of the client's illness or injury, and must be on an intermittent basis. The skills of the psychiatric RN are determined by/based on the "complexity of the service, the ill condition of the client, and accepted standards of medical/psychiatric and nursing practice." The following are two examples of skilled psychiatric RN services:

Example: The psychiatric RN performs a comprehensive assessment related to depression and manages a depressed client in crisis.

Example: The psychiatric RN assesses and manages the safety of a paranoid schizophrenic client who is actively hallucinating.

These services are considered skilled because they are complex, the ill condition of the client requires the psychiatric nursing interventions, and the services are accepted standards of medical and psychiatric nursing practice. The determination of whether a client needs skilled nursing care should be based solely on the client's unique condition and individual needs, without regard to whether the illness or injury is acute, chronic, terminal or expected to extend over a long period of time. The following example illustrates a possible scenario.

Example: A client who has had schizophrenia since teenage years and is experiencing an exacerbation of the illness requires skilled teaching of a new medication regime (clozapine [Clozaril]) and the potentially problematic side effects of the drug and education regarding coping techniques to manage the illness. The psychiatric RN also draws blood levels once a week to evaluate the client's white blood count.

Applications and Skilled Nursing Services
Observation and Assessment

Observation and assessment of the client's condition by a nurse (psychiatric RN) are reasonable and necessary skilled services when the likelihood of change in the client's condition requires the skilled psychiatric RN to identify and evaluate the client's need for possible modification of treatment or initiation of additional medical/psychiatric procedures until the client's treatment regime is essentially stabilized.

Example: A client was hospitalized for 5 days with depression, severe withdrawal, and suicidal gestures. At discharge, the client was sent home on a new antidepressant medication. Skilled observation is required to assess the medication's effectiveness, dosage appropriateness, and any drug interactions; to observe client's mental status for any increased signs of depression and withdrawn behavior; and to assess the client's safety status and suicidal symptoms due to a recent suicide attempt and history of suicidal gestures.

There is a likelihood of change in the client's condition and treatment because of the new medication schedule, the probability of mental status changes, and history of suicidal gestures; therefore, as clearly stated in the documentation, the observation and assessment are reasonable and necessary skilled services.

Observation and assessment by a psychiatric RN are not reasonable and necessary to the treatment of the illness or injury when there are indications that the symptoms are part of a long-standing pattern of the client's condition and there has been no attempt to change the treatment to resolve them.

Management and Evaluation

Skilled nursing visits (psychiatric RN) for management and evaluation of the client's care plan are also reasonable and necessary when underlying conditions or complications require that only a psychiatric RN can ensure that essential nonskilled care is achieving its purpose. Further, the complexity of the unskilled services that are a necessary part of the medical/psychiatric treatment must require the involvement of a psychiatric RN to promote the client's recovery and medical safety in view of the client's overall condition.

Example: A 78-year-old female with a diagnosis of major depression with psychotic features, acute CHF, and urine incontinence was referred to psychiatric home care after two recent inpatient psychiatric hospital stays. The client remained on services, and the psychiatric RN managed the client's POC with observation and assessment, teaching and training, and direct hands-on care interventions.

The client was on multiple medications; was depressed, despondent, and paranoid; and experienced impaired reality orientation at times. The client had multiple complicating psychiatric and medical problems and lived alone in a small trailer with only a neighbor as caregiver. The client was estranged from her son and wanted desperately to remain at home. The client was 30 pounds overweight, on a restricted diet and fluid intake (which the client found difficult to follow), was ambulating unsteadily with a walker, but was instructed by the physician to ambulate around the trailer each day. The client experienced frequent urinary tract infections and skin breakdowns as a result of the urinary incontinence.

At discharge the client was evaluated for management and evaluation appropriateness. The client's underlying psychiatric and medical conditions were complex and required the skills of a psychiatric RN to ensure the client's recovery and medical safety. The nonskilled services the client required were a necessary part of the medical/psychiatric treatment. The client, caregiver (neighbor), and psychiatric RN drew up a nonskilled care plan the client and caregiver had to follow while the RN evaluated their abilities to carry through with the care plan.

When visits by a psychiatric RN are not needed to manage and evaluate the effects of the nonskilled services being provided to treat the illness or injury, skilled nursing care would not be considered reasonable and necessary to treat the illness or injury.

Teaching and Training Activities

Teaching and training activities that require skilled nursing personnel (psychiatric) to teach a client/caregiver how to manage the treatment regime constitute skilled nursing services. When teaching or training is appropriate to the client's functional loss, illness, or injury, it may be considered reasonable and necessary (e.g., teaching coping skills for depression, relaxation skills for anxiety, congruent-thinking techniques for paranoia).

When it is determined after a reasonable period of time that the client/caregiver will not or is not able to learn or be trained, further teaching and training would cease to be reasonable. Reteaching or retraining may be considered reasonable and necessary when there are changes in the procedure or the client's condition or when the client/caregiver was not properly carrying out the task. Document reasons (e.g., impaired thoughts, extreme anxiety and panic attacks, post-electroconvulsive forgetfulness).

Be specific with what techniques are being taught or leave written teaching materials. Always relate the client's psychiatric/medical condition, medications, orders, and goals to support the need for teaching.

Examples:

Teach signs and symptoms of disease state, management of disease process, and when to call MD if disease process exacerbates.

Teach new or changed medication and its management: side effects, schedule, rationale, contraindications, and compliance; observe for interactions.

Teach crisis-management regarding the grieving process and its management.

Teach coping skills, stress-management techniques, relaxation measures, communication and socialization skills, desensitization skills, and phobia/anxiety and anger-management and verbalization skills.

Teach reality orientation and congruent-thinking techniques, management of hallucinations and delusions.

Teach bowel regimen, nutritional management of weight loss, orthostatic hypotension management, tachycardia and tachypnea management with anxiety, improved sleeping techniques, and medical management of other diseases.

Teach problem-solving and positive-thinking strategies, importance of journaling, daily goal setting, and assertiveness techniques.

Teach need for limit setting, how to decrease situations that create anxiety or anger, obsessive-compulsive management, and techniques to manage manic behavior.

Teach medical management with lithium and hydration status and signs of agranulocytosis/infections with clozapine (Clozaril).

Direct Care Activities

Hands-on activities or performance of services must be reasonable and necessary to the treatment of the illness, such as covered medication administration, wound care, or catheter insertion. (See the Medicare *HHA Manual—Pub. 11* [HCFA, 1996] for specific examples related to these skills.)

Examples:

- Performance/completion of suicide assessment form, mental status examination, and depression/anxiety measurement tool.
- Performance of active listening and role-playing behavior with the client.
- Observation/assessment of the medication and effectiveness/management of medication regimen.
- Venipuncture and frequent laboratory draws for lithium, carbamazepine (Tegretol), and clozapine. Venipuncture is performed when the collection of the specimen is necessary to the diagnosis and treatment of the client's illness and cannot be performed in the course of receiving medical treatment (clozapine [Clozaril] draws every week).
- The frequency of visits for venipuncture must be reasonable within accepted standards of medical practice for treatment of the illness or injury. (See the Medicare *HHA Manual—Pub. 11* [HCFA] for specific examples related to venipuncture.)

SUMMARY

Orientation to home care and especially psychiatric home care is a crucial time for transitioning clinicians. Psychiatric nurses may be unaware of the differences between hospital nursing and home care nursing. Assessments are more detailed in the home environment and include psychiatric and medical evaluations; psychosocial, economic, environmental and home safety evaluations; and assessment of the family dynamics that affect care. Differences in the role and functioning of the home care nurse include financial, frequency and duration of services, and community resource considerations. Competent home care clinicians also coordinate referral services to other resources, provide community linkage, ensure continuity of care, communicate with the physician and other team members, and perform myriad other tasks.

Co-dependent behavior in some nurses needs to be recognized. Home care may be an ideal setting for co-dependency. Psychiatric home care nurses must understand that the rigid schedule of the hospital setting does not exist and is not appropriate in home care. Nurses need to be self-disciplined with documentation and visit schedules. Psychiatric home care nursing allows the nurse to work with one client at a time and observe the immediate and positive results of the visits and understand the rewards of psychiatric home care nursing.

Psychiatric home care nurses must be multitalented. Clients can be very sick, so nurses must be highly skilled in both medical and psychiatric interventions, have expert knowledge of psychotropic medications and crisis management, perform mental status examinations, and monitor effectiveness of the POC. Psychiatric nurses must be able to effectively communicate with the physicians and other team members. Well-developed interpersonal skills also assist in maintaining the client's independence. Nurses must establish and maintain therapeutic boundaries and relationships, enhancing family dynamics by being a positive resource and educator. The multifaceted role in home care demands attention to detail, as well as well-honed clinical and interpersonal skills. Nurses wishing to provide care for clients with psychiatric conditions will find challenging opportunities in the health care setting of the future—the client's home.

REVIEW EXERCISES

1. Describe covered care as defined by Medicare for home care nursing services.
2. List three examples of clients that would be considered homebound.
3. Define the psychiatric nurse's qualifications.
4. Identify three client examples that could be covered care.
5. Summarize the rules related to Medicare documentation.
6. Provide an example of a client that would be appropriate for this intervention.

7. List the four skilled nursing services that would be provided by the psychiatric nurse.

8. Identify the reasons for more clients being cared for in home and community-based care settings.

RESOURCES

Finkelman AW: *Psychiatric Home Care,* Gaithersburg, Md, 1997, Aspen, (800)638-8437.

Home Care Nurse News, a clinically focused newsletter for home care personnel and published monthly by Marrelli and Associates, (800)993-6397(NEWS).

Home Health Care Nurse, a professional journal for the community health nurse and published monthly by Lippincott in Hagerstown, MD, (800)638-3030.

Psychiatric Home Healthcare News, an educational quarterly for psychiatric home care professionals and published by Ohlund & Associates in La Jolla, CA, (619)551-1660.

REFERENCES

Health Care Financing Administration: *Home health agency manual—Publication 11,* Washington, DC, Health and Human Services, Revision 277, 1996.

Marrelli T: *Handbook of home health standards and documentation guidelines for re-imbursement,* St. Louis, 1998, Mosby.

FOR FURTHER READING

Black L: Development of a psychiatric home care program and the role of the CNS in the delivery of care, *Clin Nurse Specialist* 7(4):164-168, 1993.

Blue Cross of California: Medicare Bulletin, Home Health Psychiatric Care Policy, Bulletin No. 398, March 1996.

Cann R: Mental health and substance use problems of the elderly, *Home Care Nurse News* 2(2):6, 1995.

Carson V: Psychiatric home care: bridge to the community and an anchor to remain there, *Home Care Nurse News* 2(7):1, 1995.

Daudell-Strejc D, Murphy C: Emerging clinical issues in home health psychiatric nursing, *Home Healthcare Nurse* 13(2):17-21, 1995.

Dellasega C, Ling L: The psychogeriatric nurse in home health care: use of research to develop the role, *Clin Nurse Spec* 10(2):64-68, 1996.

Gerace L, Tiller J, Anderson J, et al: Development of a psychiatric home visit module for student training, *Hosp Commun Psychiatry,* 1990.

Gillis LS, Koch A, Jarji M: The value and cost-effectiveness of a home-visiting program for psychiatric clients, *S Afr Med J,* 1990.

Helwig K: Psychiatric home care nursing: managing clients in the community setting, *J Psychosocial Nurs Mental Health Serv* 31(12):21-24, 1993.

Krach P: Assessment of depressed older persons living in a home setting, *Home Healthcare Nurse* 13(3):61-64, 1995.

Lear G: Managing care at home, *Nurs Times,* 1993.

McDaniel C: Reorganization of community psychiatric services by professional nurses, *Issues Mental Health Nurs,* 1990.

Miller M, Duffey J: Planning and program development for psychiatric home care, *J Nurs Admin* 23(11):35-41, 1993.

Quinlan J, Ohlund G: Psychiatric home care: an introduction, *Home Healthcare Nurse* 13(4):20-24, 1995.

Stuart GW, Sundeen JJ: *Principles and practice of psychiatric nursing,* ed 5, Baltimore, 1995, Mosby.

Task Force on DSM-IV: *Diagnostic and statistical manual of mental health disorders,* ed 4, DSM-IV, 1995.

Ward-Miller S: The psychiatric clinical specialist in the home care setting, *Nurs Clin North Am* 31(3):519-525, 1996.

Wykle M: Geriatric mental health interventions in the home, *J Nurs Mental Health Serv* 33(1):50, 1995.

chapter

11

CARDIAC HOME CARE NURSING

Dana Ellis, RN, CCRN

"Treatment costs for heart failure, including physician visits, drugs, and nursing home stays, were more than $10 billion in 1990."

The National Heart, Lung, and Blood Institute

Cardiac failure is a major public health problem and a serious condition. The National Heart, Lung, and Blood Institute has estimated that more than 2 million Americans have heart failure and that about 400,000 new cases of heart failure are diagnosed each year. Mortality is high, with 1-year mortality rates of 10% and 50% after 5 years. In addition, quality of life is reduced for many cardiac failure patients, who often experience physical symptoms and reduced functional status. Total treatment costs for heart failure, including physician visits, drugs, and nursing home stays, were more than $10 billion in 1990. The Heart Failure Guideline Panel believes that many of these hospitalizations could have been prevented by improved evaluation and care, both in the hospital and the home care setting (Box 11-1).

Skilled home care has existed for many years, but presently, with the advent of health maintenance organizations and managed care, patients are not receiving the majority of their skilled care and education while still hospitalized. Instead, the average hospital stay has been reduced, dramatically in some cases, and patients can be sent home weak, tired, and often ill prepared to successfully complete their recovery and again become independent, contributing members of family and society.

Even home care is moving toward more self care. Skilled home care nurses have a big responsibility to educate patients in all aspects of their disease processes. By doing so, nurses empower patients with the knowledge they need to take a more active, consistent role in their health maintenance.

BOX 11-1   MOST COMMON MEDICAL DIAGNOSES

As reported in a Health Care Financing Administration–sponsored study conducted by Georgetown University School of Nursing in 1991, the five most common medical diagnoses and their respective ICD-9 codes found in the Medicare home care population are as follows:

Congestive heart failure	428.0
Cerebral vascular accident	436.0
Chronic obstructive pulmonary disease	496.0
Pneumonia	486.0
Hypertension	401.9

The objective of this chapter on cardiac home care is to prepare the nurse to manage the cardiac patient in his or her home environment. At the end of this chapter the nurse should be able to:

1. List several drugs used in the treatment of heart failure.
2. List the steps in a cardiac assessment.
3. List five standards of practice for cardiac home care nursing.
4. List six risk factors for the development of heart disease.

CARDIAC DISEASE

This section reviews several cardiac disease processes that impact on cardiac output (CO). CO is the amount of blood (in liters) ejected by the heart in 1 minute. It is the product of the heart rate (HR) and stroke volume (SV) and is represented by the formula $CO = HR \times SV$. Stroke volume is the amount of blood ejected with each ventricular contraction. Factors that affect either HR or SV will alter CO. Signs and symptoms of these various disease processes are covered, as well as some of the medications the nurse can expect to see prescribed by the primary care physician or cardiologist.

Heart Failure

Symptoms suggestive of heart failure include the following:

- Paroxysmal nocturnal dyspnea
- Orthopnea
- Dyspnea on exertion
- Lower extremity edema
- Decreased exercise tolerance
- Unexplained confusion, altered mental status, or fatigue in an elderly patient

- Abdominal symptoms associated with ascites and/or hepatic engorgement (e.g., nausea or abdominal pain)

Heart failure can be left sided and/or right sided and includes the cardiomyopathies, which are abnormalities of the heart muscle itself. Patients with heart failure and signs of significant volume overload should be started immediately on a diuretic, and dosages titrated to achieve resolution or improvement of signs and symptoms of volume overload. The next level of pharmacological management is the addition of an angiotensin-converting enzyme (ACE) inhibitor such as captopril or enalapril. Clinical improvements that are related to ACE-inhibitor use are a decreased peripheral *resistance,* an increased cardiac output, and a decreased left ventricular end-diastolic pressure. Next, digoxin is used routinely in patients with severe heart failure since it can prevent clinical deterioration in patients with heart failure because of left-ventricular systolic dysfunction and improve patients' symptoms. And, in patients with contraindications or intolerance to ACE inhibitors, hydralazine/isosorbide dinitrate (Isordil) therapy may be used. Additional pharmacological management might include beta blockers such as metoprolol and nitrates other than isosorbide.

Coronary Artery Disease, Myocardial Infarctions, and/or Dysrhythmias

Symptoms of coronary artery disease, myocardial infarctions, and/or dysrhythmias may include the following:

- Angina pectoris, can be mild to severe
- Easy fatigability
- Dyspnea, with or without activity
- Syncope
- Palpitations
- Sudden death

Coronary artery disease (CAD) is caused by atherosclerosis in approximately 90% of the cases. With continued accumulation of lipids on the intima of the coronary arteries, the myocardial cells can suffer ischemia, which, if severe or prolonged, can lead to irreversible injury or infarction of cardiac tissues. Finally, following an acute myocardial infarction (MI), patients may develop a variety of conduction disturbances, or dysrhythmias. Drugs used in the treatment of CAD and post MI are directed toward reducing the myocardial demand for oxygen and improving myocardial oxygen supply. Medications that can reduce myocardial demands are beta-adrenergic blocking agents such as propranolol (Inderal) and nadolol (Corgard); calcium channel blockers such as diltiazem (Cardizem), nicardipine (Cardene), and verapamil (Calan); and nitrates such as isosorbide dinitrate (Isordil) and mononitrates (isosorbide [Ismo] and Imdur). Nitrates and calcium channel blockers can also be used to *increase* myocardial oxygen supply. Finally, CAD with or without MI may need to be treated pharmacologically with antilipemics. These include drugs that can reduce low-density-lipoprotein cholesterol levels (cholestyramines) and those that lower serum triglyceride levels and increase high-density-lipoprotein cholesterol levels, such as gemfibrozil.

Management of cardiac arrhythmias is based on correcting the deleterious effects of the arrhythmias, primary of which is the resulting inability of the heart to maintain adequate circulation of blood to the body. A cardiac rate that is extremely rapid or slow or a cardiac rhythm that is grossly abnormal results in a decrease in cardiac output. Ventricular arrhythmias are common in patients with heart failure, and death is sudden in up to half of patients. Examples of oral antiarrhythmics include the following:

- Amiodarone (Cordarone) for recurrent ventricular fibrillation and hemodynamically unstable ventricular tachycardia refractory to other antiarrhythmics
- Disopyramide phosphate (Norpace) for symptomatic premature ventricular contractions; ventricular tachycardia not severe enough to require cardioversion
- Flecainide acetate (Tambocor) for paroxysmal atrial fibrillation or flutter; life-threatening ventricular arrhythmias
- Also for life-threatening arrhythmias the following brand name drugs may be used: Mexitil, Ethmozine, Procan SR, Betapace and Tonocard

Hypertension

More than 20 million people in the United States suffer from systemic hypertension. Over one half of these cases are undiagnosed and untreated. It has a very insidious course, noticeable symptoms can take years to develop, and the patient often refuses to recognize them because he or she "feels good." Hence, the nickname, "silent killer." Hypertension is the most common complicating factor in heart failure.

The first symptoms of hypertension can include:

- Headache
- Retinal changes
- Stroke
- Symptoms associated with heart failure

The goals of treatment for hypertension include reducing the elevated blood pressure and maintaining normal blood pressure levels, as well as prevention of complications of both the treatment and the disease process. There are numerous hypertensive drugs available for prescription. Some of these are, by brand name, Tenormin, Lotensin, Capoten, Catapres, Vasotec, Monopril, Trandate, Zestril, Cozaar, Aldomet, Lopressor, Minipress, Accupril, Altace, and Hytrin.

Pulmonary Edema

The most extreme form of left-sided heart failure is pulmonary edema. The principal symptom is acute shortness of breath, and treatment must often be rapid if the patient is to survive.

Other symptoms include the following:

- Extreme anxiousness and restlessness
- Diaphoresis
- Cool and clammy skin
- Frothy sputum, cyanosis and hemoptysis

Treatment goals include increasing the cardiac output, decreasing venous return, and improving oxygenation. Cardiac glycosides are used because they have positive inotropic and negative chronotropic effects. (Some of these drugs were listed under heart failure.) Intravascular blood volume is reduced through the use of diuretics. In acute cases, intravenous diuretics are used, followed by maintenance on PO diuretics. Some commonly used brand names are Bumex, Diuril, Lasix, Zaroxolyn, and Aldactone.

ELEMENTS INVOLVED IN CARDIAC HOME CARE
Physical Assessment

At each skilled nursing visit, begin by observing your client. Never underestimate the "powers of observation." Follow then with a head-to-toe assessment of all systems, asking questions as you proceed (Table 11-1).

A physical examination of the cardiac patient is never complete unless it includes a complete examination of the precordium. It is essential to have an understanding of the gross anatomy of the normal heart, its topographic relationship to the anterior chest wall, and the cardiac cycle as it relates to valvular physiology.

For inspection and palpation, have the patient lie supine with the head of bed at 30 degrees. Inspect and palpate the precordial area for abnormal pulsation, lifts, heaves, and thrills at the five areas shown in Figure 11-1.

TABLE 11-1 **PHYSICAL ASSESSMENT**

STEPS	RATIONALE
Neurological	
Assess mental status, cognition, memory	Can be affected by HTN, decrease in cerebral blood flow caused by pump failure
Headaches? Dizziness?	
Any decreased sensation, numbness, tingling sensations?	
Pupillary checks for equal size and reactivity	You're assessing for stroke or cerebral ischemia
Evaluate extremities for strength, assess for facial symmetry	
Assess gait, coordination; any weaknesses?	Deviations from normal can have a neurological pathology
Cardiocirculatory	
Inspection for changes in skin color, pulsations, skeletal deformities and labored breathing	You're looking for signs/causes of diminished circulation
Palpation to evaluate texture, moistness, areas of tenderness, masses, and edema	
Percussion to determine density and to detect superficial lesions; to locate boundaries of various organs and tissues	Enlarged organs can be due to cardiac failure
Auscultation	Used to detect abnormalities of the cardiovascular system
Take a blood pressure and full set of vitals at each visit	Causes of increased pulse pressure are increased stroke volume, a decrease in peripheral vascular resistance and aortic distensibility, and increased intracranial pressure; decreased pulse pressure is caused by mechanical obstructions (aortic and valvular), peripheral vasoconstriction and decreased stroke volume
Assess for	
(a) an increased or decreased pulse pressure or	

TABLE 11-1 PHYSICAL ASSESSMENT—cont'd

STEPS	RATIONALE
(b) pulsus alternans, which is alternating intensity of sound produced with each beat	This phenomenon can be indicative of left-sided heart failure
Take orthostatic readings at admission and prn	To help determine the effects of drugs, as well as volume status
Inspect and palpate extremities	Can reveal important data concerning patient's status
Palpate for temperature, color, moisture and vascularity	Skin that is warm and dry is a sign of adequate cardiac output; cyanosis is evidence of poorly oxygenated blood
Inspect nails	Splinter hemorrhages and clubbing are frequent signs of cardiovascular dysfunction
Assess for edema, pitting, and nonpitting	Is considered a late sign of congestive heart failure; there are multiple noncardiac origins of edema
Assess arterial pulse for rate, rhythm and quality	Bounding pulse can be produced by complete heart block, aortic insufficiency; weak pulse is present in low-output failure such as post-MI
Examine neck, inspect jugular venous pulse and palpate carotid artery	Provides information about the hemodynamics of the right side of the heart

The only normal pulsation is at the apical area. This is referred to as the point of maximal impulse. Visible pulsations in the third, fourth, and fifth intercostal spaces along the sternal border indicate right ventricular enlargement. Abnormal prominent pulsations over the epigastric area may indicate an aneurysm.

Auscultating the precordium can provide the cardiac home care nurse with valuable information about the clinical status of a patient. During the normal cardiac cycle, two distinct sounds should be heard.

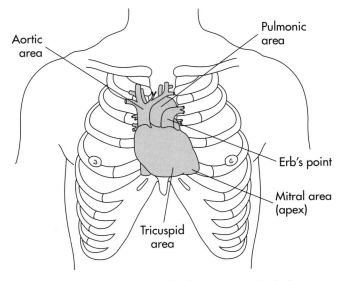

FIGURE 11-1   The five areas of cardiac inspection and palpation.

Systole begins with the closure of the mitral and tricuspid valves, known as S1, and ends with the closure of the aortic and pulmonary valves, known as S2. Diastole begins with S2 and ends with the next first sound. A third heart sound, or S3, occurs soon after S2, and, in those over 30 years of age, is considered abnormal and indicative of heart disease. An S4, which also occurs just before the first sound, is believed to be related to a decrease in left ventricular compliance or an increase in ventricular volume.

The following are the most common clinical situations in which an S4 is present:

- Hypertensive cardiovascular disease
- Myocardiopathy
- Aortic stenosis
- Myocardial infarction
- Anemia
- Elevated left end-diastolic pressure

Other sounds that might be auscultated are a murmur, which is the result of turbulent blood flow within the heart; a pericardial friction rub, which is a characteristic finding in pericarditis; and/or a click, which is probably a transplanted man-made heart valve.

Do not forget to ask the patient if he or she is having any pain, and, if so, have him or her describe it by location, type, and intensity. Ask what activities, if any, cause the pain to appear.

This is a basic review of heart tones; it is beyond the scope of this chapter to provide an all-inclusive discussion of cardiac sounds. For further information, please access the numerous books, periodicals, and audio tapes available on the subject.

Respiratory Assessment

The functions of the cardiac and respiratory systems are interdependent, and because of this, disorders of one system can precipitate disorders in the other. Perform a complete physical examination of the patient's respiratory status at each visit. Many of the same techniques used to assess the cardiac system are also used to assess the pulmonary system. Remember, the cardiac home care nurse should have a good mental image of the underlying structures, plus lung and diaphragm locations to describe any abnormalities found (Table 11-2).

Standards of Practice

Caring for the cardiac patient at home includes following certain standards of practice. These are skilled nursing actions that should occur at the initial evaluation visit and/or at each subsequent skilled nursing visit. For the cardiac patient, nurses should follow the standards of practice listed in Table 11-3.

It is very important to remember and practice the Nursing Process when caring for the cardiac patient at home. Start your skilled visits with a complete **A**ssessment, and while doing that, **P**lan on the **I**nterventions you will undertake, and, finally, **E**valuate the effectiveness of your interventions. Table 11-4 contains the Education and Instruction (E&I) for the cardiac home care client (i.e., interventions, listed according to nursing diagnosis, that help the patient recover and empower him or her with the knowledge and information to maintain more independence and/or quality of life), together with corresponding goals for these interventions. Some of this E&I is specific to the cardiac patient, and some is not.

Thorough patient education also involves discussion of risk factors for developing heart disease. Several classification systems for risk factors exist; Box 11-2 contains the three categories the American Heart Association uses.

TABLE 11-2 **RESPIRATORY ASSESSMENT**

STEPS	RATIONALE
Begin by inspecting the color of the skin, lips and nailbeds	Cyanosis of nailbeds is a late sign of hypoxemia; it is better to look at the oral and mucous membranes
Assess the breathing pattern, rate, and depth; look for evidence of respiratory distress Dyspnea? Shortness of breath?	Prolonged or shortened inspiration or expiration may be an early sign of respiratory dysfunction
Inspect for orthopnea or difficulty breathing in a recumbent position	Can be evidence of various cardiac and pulmonary disorders
Inspect the chest for symmetry and shape	The normal chest should move symmetrically with inspiration and expiration
Palpate position of the trachea	Deviation could mean pleural effusion, tumor, atelectasis
Percuss to identify lung boundaries	Dull resonance can signify fluid or solids in the normal air-filled lung; hyperresonance can be air trapping as in emphysema
Auscultate the quality and clarity of the breath sounds; develop a pattern for thoroughly auscultating over the anterior, posterior, and lateral chest walls and follow this pattern always to ensure that no area is missed.	Rales can indicate pulmonary edema, pneumonia, atelectasis; rhonchus is caused from sputum production, and wheezes are indicative of airway narrowing; familiarity with the various breath sounds and patterns usually comes with much experience in cardiopulmonary assessment; remember, audiotapes are available to assist you in familiarizing yourself with these sounds

TABLE 11-2   **RESPIRATORY ASSESSMENT—cont'd**

STEPS	RATIONALE
Gastrointestinal Assessment	
Inspect the abdominal surface Percuss all four quadrants Auscultate all four abdominal quadrants and the epigastrium Do they have any abdominal pains? Discomforts?	As heart failure worsens, edema occurs and can affect various body organs; you are assessing for hepatomegaly and splenomegaly (liver and spleen enlargement)
Genitourinary Assessment	
How much urinary output (UOP)? Any changes in UOP—color, clarity, quantity?	Decreased CO decreases flow to the kidneys, thereby decreasing UOP and causing anuria in worst cases
Musculoskeletal Assessment	
While doing a complete muscle and skeletal assessment, also observe the client's gait and assess for strength and balance Does he or she feel weak? Tired? Is there unequal strength between bilateral extremities?	If there is a decreased CO, the hypoxia in the tissues causes weakness and fatigue with little exertion

Cardiac home care nursing involves many of the same principles as in-hospital cardiac nursing, but there are also many differences between the two. In the hospital setting patient medications are administered by the nurse. The greatest problem in management of the home cardiac patient lies in compliance with the medication and treatment regime. Once patients begin to feel better and can no longer identify the effects of the disease processes, some stop taking the prescribed medications. Another example is the lack of an immediate support system in an emergency or for double-checking any questions or problems the nurse may have. There are no doctors close by, no laboratories, none of your peers. Although hospital and home care nurses share a certain autonomy in their patient care delivery, the home cardiac nurse must make treatment decisions based on a knowledge of many disciplines, none of which are

TABLE 11-3   **STANDARDS OF PRACTICE FOR CARDIAC PATIENTS**

AT INITIAL EVALUATION VISIT	AT EVERY SKILLED NURSING VISIT
Take a complete medical history	Full set of vital signs, take apical and radial pulse; compare for rate differences
Get complete set of baseline vital signs, including pain, the "fifth vital sign"	Evaluate compliance and effectiveness of medications and other therapeutic regimes
Get a weight; try to get a "dry weight" if client currently has any evidence of volume overload	
Write down all medications patient is currently taking	
Call physician to give current condition and to get orders for care that will comprise the plan of treatment (POT)	Call physician as needed concerning changes in patient's condition

standing close by for support. Also, in the home, family or caregiver support can be a deciding factor in the patient's successful recovery. And finally, financial and environmental constraints can impact on successful nursing care in the home.

Clinical Documentation

All nurses have heard the saying, "If you didn't chart it, you didn't do it." With the increasing costs of health care delivery, both in the hospital and out, charting is being scrutinized closely to justify the medical necessity of skilled interventions and to justify reimbursement. It is the home care nurse's documentation that is the basis for covered or denied care.

When charting the cardiac home care patient, develop a format that includes all of the following; then follow it closely so that nothing is forgotten. The following is a checklist for review:

- Full set of vital signs, including cardiopulmonary auscultation findings
- Education and instruction done at that visit

TABLE 11-4 EDUCATION AND INSTRUCTION

PROBLEMS/INTERVENTIONS	GOALS OF TREATMENT
Knowledge deficit regarding disease, condition, and limitations Teaching of disease process, signs/symptoms (S/S) exacerbation, reporting of significant changes to RN or physician, and activities permitted within	Increased patient/caregiver knowledge of disease process, S/S reportable to RN/physician Patient to return to predisease state/prior level of functioning Increased understanding of limitations of condition
Impaired cardiac status Assess vital signs, lung fields, edema, and peripheral circulation Teach S/S reportable to RN/physician Assess response to medications Supervise and assess (S&A) compliance Education/teaching medication administration Instruction in symptom management Teaching of prescribed diet Report significant clinical findings to physician Venipunctures as ordered	Stable cardiac status Achieve symptom management Increased patient/caregiver knowledge of diet, medications, and S/S reportable to RN/physician Increased patient/caregiver knowledge regarding limitations
Altered respiratory status Assess respiratory status Evaluate effectiveness of respiratory treatments Assess response to pulmonary medications Instruction in respiratory S/S reportable to RN/physician Instruction in use/care of respiratory equipment	Stabilize pulmonary status to maximum level Increased patient/caregiver knowledge of respiratory system Increased patient/caregiver knowledge of equipment use/care Increased patient/caregiver knowledge of changes necessary to report to RN/physician

continued

TABLE 11-4   EDUCATION AND INSTRUCTION—cont'd

PROBLEMS/INTERVENTIONS	GOALS OF TREATMENT
Unstable medical condition, frequent changes in medication regimen	
Teaching of medication administration and compliance	Increased patient/caregiver knowledge of medication administration, actions of medication, and possible side effects
Assess for effectiveness and complication effects	
Teaching of medication regimen	Increased patient/caregiver knowledge of S/S reportable to RN/physician
Teaching of S/S reportable to physician	
RN to report these S/S to physician	Patients condition to be monitored while medications are regulated; there will be no adverse reactions from the medications
Teaching of emergency procedures, home safety	
	Patient knowledgeable in emergency resources and indication for need
Alteration in comfort/pain	
Assess for pain and pain control	Pain will be controlled/minimized/eliminated
Teaching use and administration of pain medications	Increased patient/caregiver knowledge regarding alternatives for pain control
Teaching alternative methods for pain relief	
Altered bowel elimination	
Assess abdomen and elimination pattern	Normal elimination pattern restored
Teaching and management related to bowel elimination	Increased patient/caregiver knowledge/understanding of bowel function
Instruction regarding appropriate bowel regimen	Increased patient/caregiver knowledge/understanding of ostomy care
Teaching stoma care PRN	
Teaching management of diarrhea/ constipation	Patient independent in ostomy care
Teaching S/S of GI bleeding	
Guaiac stool PRN	

TABLE 11-4 EDUCATION AND INSTRUCTION—cont'd

PROBLEMS/INTERVENTIONS	GOALS OF TREATMENT
Altered urinary elimination	
Teaching and management in bladder training	Patent Foley without complications
Teaching and management of self-catheterization	Increased patient/caregiver knowledge of S/S reportable to RN/physician
Teaching and management of S/S reportable to RN/physician	Patient independent in Foley care
Assess for S/S of urinary tract infection	Management of incontinence without skin breakdown
Report significant clinical findings to physician	Stable urinary tract function
Impaired skin integrity	
Assess skin for breakdown at each skilled nursing (SN) visit	Wound/pressure ulcer will heal without complication
Teaching and management of wound/pressure ulcer care, dressing changes, and S/S of wound complications reportable to RN/physician	Patient/caregiver to be independent in wound/ pressure ulcer care
Assess/evaluate wound/decubitus at each SN visit	Increased patient/caregiver knowledge of signs/symptoms reportable to RN/physician
Perform skilled wound/pressure ulcer care at each SN visit	Skin integrity will be maintained and/or restored
Implement measures to promote healing	Patient/caregiver to be independent in skin care
Teach patient/caregiver in measures to decrease pressure over bony prominences	
Teach patient/caregiver in skin care regimen	
Knowledge deficit regarding dietary regimen and restrictions:	
Teach about prescribed diet	Increased patient/caregiver knowledge of proper dietary/fluid components and restrictions
Teach about any fluid restrictions	
Teach patient to take weight daily	

continued

TABLE 11-4 **EDUCATION AND INSTRUCTION—cont'd**

PROBLEMS/INTERVENTIONS	GOALS OF TREATMENT
Assess for weight gain/loss	Improved fluid and electrolyte balance
Teach S/S reportable to RN/physician	Increased patient/caregiver knowledge of S/S reportable to RN/physician
Evaluate for dietary compliance	
Assess nutritional status at each SN visit	Improved nutritional status
Impaired physical mobility and activity tolerance	
Teach therapeutic positioning, range of motion, transfers	Complications of immobility will be minimized/prevented
Teach progressive ambulation program	Increased patient/caregiver knowledge of home exercise program/safety
Teach home safety program to prevent falls and injuries	Patient will experience improved strength and activity tolerance
Teach graded activity regimen	
Assess activity tolerance level	
Evaluate for PT/OT referral	Patient will be functional in activities of daily living
Alteration in social/emotional/ mental status	
Assess mental and emotional status at each visit	Stabilize mental status at maximum level
Assess for signs of depression, anxiety, psychosis	Increased use of family/ community supports
Assess/teach S/S of depression, anxiety, psychosis	Increased patient/caregiver problem-solving ability and coping skills
Facilitate ability to ventilate fears, and so on	
Evaluate effectiveness of medications	Patient/caregiver will be familiar with the grieving process
Assess family dynamics	Patient behavior management at home
Evaluate for MSW referral	

BOX 11-2   HEART DISEASE RISK FACTORS

Nonmodifiable Risk Factors
Age
Sex
Race
Family history

Modifiable Risk Factors
Cigarette smoking
Hypertension
Increased cholesterol levels
Diabetes

Contributing Factors
Obesity
Physical inactivity
Personality and stress

- Nursing interventions at that visit (chart using recognized Nursing Diagnosis)
- Patient's compliance with instructions/patient education received (remember to refer to the POC)
- The reason the patient is homebound
- Show evidence of care coordination and communication
- Supplies used
- Safety concerns, safety education
- Plan for and date of next SN visit
- Any laboratory draws or test results
- Case conferences with other team members
- Any communication with MD, new orders received
- End with goals or outcomes for this cardiac patient

Some home care organizations are developing and using clinical paths as tools to standardize care and care processes for cardiac patients. For an in-depth discussion of clinical paths, refer to *Home Care and Clinical Paths: Effective Care Planning Across the Continuum* (Marrelli and Hilliard, 1996).

Cardiac Home Health Care Team Members

The patient's physician has the primary responsibility of referring his or her client for skilled home health services. The physician orders the interventions and sets the medical parameters for treatment. The SN must follow these orders, communicate any changes in patient condition to the physician, and receive and follow new orders. Other members of the home health team are:

- Therapists; physical, occupational and speech-language pathologists
- Home health aides
- Medical social workers
- Dietitians
- Family members, caregivers
- Pharmacists
- Others, based on the patient's unique needs

These other team members services are often ordered by the physician based on the skilled assessment of the patient by the RN. Remember, the RN guides the care given by the home health organization and provides supervisory visits regularly.

Cardiac Rehabilitation

Cardiovascular disease is the leading cause of morbidity and mortality in the United States, accounting for almost 50% of all deaths. The almost 1 million survivors of MI each year and the more than 7 million patients with stable angina pectoris are candidates for cardiac rehabilitation, as are patients following coronary artery bypass graft, percutaneous transluminal coronary angioplasty, and several other millions of people with coronary heart disease. *Heart failure is the most common discharge diagnosis for hospitalized Medicare patients and the fourth most common discharge diagnosis for all hospitalized patients in the United States.* Cardiac rehabilitation services for patients with heart failure and after cardiac transplantation has gained increasing recognition and acceptance as its benefits and safety are documented. Educational materials regarding rehabilitation are sometimes given to patients while still hospitalized, but it is often the home health nurse who is instrumental in beginning the rehabilitation process by the education and instruction she provides to recovering patients. As stated, she or he is evaluating the client at each visit, assessing the effectiveness of exercises and other therapeutic regimes, discussing cardiac risk factor modification, and assisting with behavioral modifications. These are all characteristics of cardiac rehabilitation, according to the Agency for Health Care Policy and Research (AHCPR). Patients just discharged from the hospital are often homebound for long periods before they are able to go to hospital-based cardiac rehabilitation programs; therefore the home care nurse has an important responsibility in "strengthening the heart that is still at home."

Cardiac Care: A Case Study

A 45-year-old man was diagnosed as having significant CAD. He underwent coronary artery bypass graft × 4 and had a stable course in the hospital; after 5 days he was discharged to cardiac home health by his physician. Your initial assessment at admission indicates that your client has a knowledge deficit because this is his first hospitalization for coronary disease. Risk factors include smoking (two packs per day), sedentary life-style, type A personality, very stressful occupation, and a father who died at age 43 of an MI:

1. What medical POC can you expect the doctor to order?
2. What other multidisciplinary team members might be involved in his care?
3. What enhances compliance with a treatment plan that requires life-style modifications for a patient such as this?

You can expect the medical POC to include progressive ambulation according to cardiac rehabilitation protocol; low-sodium, low–saturated fat diet; monitoring full set of vitals at each SN visit and routine monitoring of weight. Other team members might include a registered dietitian to assist in meal planning and a social worker or counselor to help assist this patient with behavior modification and psychological support. Compliance is enhanced by giving the patient the education he needs to understand his disease process and the various therapeutic regimes he must follow. Always include the spouse/significant other in as many aspects of rehabilitation as possible.

FUTURE TRENDS IN CARDIAC HOME CARE NURSING

If there were any doubt that home care nursing is becoming increasingly more acute and high tech, read on! The new buzzword in home health is *telemedicine,* also called *televisits.* Telemedicine, one of the newest technologies in health care, is based on a simple premise: move the information rather than the people. It involves transmitting digitized bits of information such as video and audio, thus eliminating in many instances the need for physical proximity. Telemedicine has strong implications for caring for ill cardiac patients in the home, particularly in rural areas.

SUMMARY

The area of cardiac nursing is a fast-growing specialty and an area in which all home care nurses should have competency related to assessment and care planning. This chapter addressed some of the information needed to effectively care for cardiac patients at home. The review exercises, resources, and bibliography contain information that assists in acquiring more knowledge about this large component of clinical practice in home care.

REVIEW EXERCISES

1. How is the cardiac output measured?
2. What are five symptoms suggestive of heart failure?
3. What clinical improvements are related to ACE inhibitors?
4. List five drugs used to treat cardiac arrhythmias.
5. What are three causes of an increased pulse pressure?
6. What are five standards of practice for a cardiac home care assessment?
7. What are the four steps in the nursing process?
8. What are five risk factors for the development of heart disease?
9. List six areas of cardiac home care that should be written on each visit chart.
10. What is the basic premise for telemedicine?

RESOURCES

Agency for Health Care Policy and Research (AHCPR) (1996). Free resource: Cardiac Rehabilitation Guidelines. Call (800)358-9295. The patient guide is available in English and Spanish.

American Heart Association (800)AHA-USA-1

Mended Hearts (214)706-1442

REFERENCE

Marrelli T, Hilliard L: *Home care and clinical paths: effective care planning across the continuum,* St. Louis, 1996, Mosby.

FOR FURTHER READING

Brent N: Cardiac rehabilitation in the home: legal implications for the home health-care nurse, *Home Healthcare Nurse* 13(2):8-9, 1995.

Carroll T: Home care of severe heart failure with intravenous diuretics and inotropes, *Infusion* May:13-26, 1996.

Franz A: The cardiac care step-down unit at home, *Caring Magazine* October: 42-48, 1994.

Green K, Lydon S: Home health cardiac rehabilitation, *Home Healthcare Nurse* 13(2):29-39, 1995.

Groer M, Shekleton M: *Basic pathophysiology,* St. Louis, 1979, Mosby.

Konstam M, Dracup K, Baker D, et al: Heart failure: evaluation and care of patients with left-ventricular systolic dysfunction, Clinical Practice Guideline No. 11, AHCPR Publication No. 94- 0612, Rockville, Md, June 1994, Agency for Health Care Policy and Research, Public Health Service, U.S. Department of Health and Human Services.

Marrelli T: *Handbook of home health standards and documentation: guidelines for reimbursement,* ed 3, St. Louis, 1998, Mosby.

Marrelli T: AHCPR releases cardiac guidelines, *Home Care Nurse News* 3(2):6, 1996.

Murray T: Switching from hospital-based practice to home care, *Home Care Provider* 1(2):79-82, 1996.

Parmely W: Cost-effective management of heart failure, *Clinical Cardiology* 19(3):240-242, 1996.

Saba V, Coopey M: Develop and demonstrate a method for classifying home health patients to predict resource requirements and measure outcomes, Health Care Finance Administration Cooperative Agreement No. 17-C-98983-3-01, Washington, DC, February 1991, Georgetown University School of Nursing.

Villaire M: Telemedicine: tuning in critical care's future? *Crit Care Nurse,* vol 16, no 3, June 1996.

Wenger NK, Froelicher ES, Smith LK, et al: Cardiac rehabilitation as secondary prevention, Clinical Practice Guideline, Quick Reference Guide for Clinicians, No. 17, AHCPR Pub. No. 96-0673, Rockville, Md, October 1995, Agency for Health Care Policy and Research and National Heart, Lung, and Blood Institute, Public Health Service, U.S. Department of Health and Human Services.

Yee B, Zorb L: *Cardiac critical care nursing,* Boston, 1986, Little, Brown.

WOUND CARE IN HOME CARE

Bonnie Bolinger, RN, CETN and Janice Cuzzell, RN

> *"By the year 2000 the volume of chronic and acute wounds is expected to reach 39,000,000 in the United States. Of this number, 7 million will be chronic, nonhealing wounds requiring long-term care."*
>
> *Medical Data International (MDI), 1996*

Although the actual percentage of wounds and skin care problems managed in the home is not well documented in the literature, trends reflect that both the acuity and severity of these problems have increased considerably in the home care setting. Subsequently, the demand for knowledgeable home health providers who are also skilled in wound management can be expected to rise proportionally. A study of home care consumers further supports the need for increased wound care knowledge and skills. In 1993 Georgetown University College of Nursing surveyed 9000 home health care enrollees to categorize the types of nursing intervention needed. Pressure ulcer management and incisional care were requested by over 30% of those surveyed. *The cost of treating complex wounds has traditionally been high, with the average cost to treat one pressure ulcer estimated between $14,000 and $40,000.* Continued escalation of wound care costs is expected, with costs as high as 6.9 billion dollars by the year 2000.

These numbers and the associated care have important implications for clinicians in home care practice today. With continuing initiatives for more productivity, more cost-effectiveness, and improved performance, it is the clinician providing the wound, skin, or ostomy care who may be in the pivotal role to assist in these efforts. This chapter seeks to provide information about common wound and skin care problems seen in home care, as well as provide helpful tips related to regulatory compliance, infection control, and outcome-driven patient care.

WOUND CARE IN THE HOME SETTING: THE REASON IT IS DIFFERENT

As discussed in previous chapters, the home setting is different from other health care settings, creating unique challenges for the clinician. Management in the home of such issues as infection control, wound irrigation, and débridement; the logistics of transporting dressing supplies or wound cultures; and many other patient care activities must be implemented without the benefit of the many resources and support systems that are readily available in the acute care setting. Taking health care into the home not only requires a different approach to providing comprehensive patient care, but demands careful planning and a working knowledge of regulatory issues.

The "best" home care organizations are those that others want to emulate and benchmark themselves against. In all settings, continued improvement in the quality of wound care requires a consistent approach to patient assessment and intervention. Some of the "best practices" related to wound care in the home include the following:

1. *Measure and document vital signs every visit.* Routinely, vital signs include temperature, pulse, respirations, and blood pressure. Some home care programs have added pain as a fifth vital sign, valuable information when assessing a patient with a wound. Slight elevations in body temperature accompanied by increased pain in and around the wound site may be the first sign of an impending wound infection.

2. *Perform a thorough wound assessment at the start of care and reassess the wound every visit.* Specifics of what should be included in a wound assessment, such as how often to measure wound size, are usually defined by organizational policy. However, an in-depth reassessment of both the patient and wound should be repeated, at least every 10 to 14 days. If clinical outcomes aren't being met or the wound appears to be deteriorating, notify the physician and have the plan of care reevaluated.

3. *Check to make certain there are written and signed orders from the physician for all wound care services and products provided.* Orders should include the frequency of dressing changes, type of dressing to be used, special dietary considerations to promote healing, and any other parameters needed to ensure a positive clinical outcome.

4. *Provide and document "critical wound-care services" at every skilled nursing visit.* The three critical skilled services related to wound care and covered by Medicare are: (1) hands-on care (dressing removal, wound cleansing/débridement, dressing application), (2) observation and assessment of wound progress, and (3) patient/family teaching and skills training to promote self-care behaviors. Remember that from a payor perspective, anyone can be taught to pack a wound. It is the professional nurse's use of critical thinking and other analytical skills that enables her or him to evaluate progress toward healing, recognize signs and symptoms of impending complications (such as infection or dehiscence), and provide individualized patient education. Documentation of each skilled visit must clearly reflect assessment of the patient's progress toward predetermined outcomes, as well as the patient's response to treatment and changes in the plan of care.

5. *Document clinical observations at the bedside, while at the patient's home.* While this "best practice" may not always be possible, it ensures that important observations and data are captured immediately. This is particularly important when caring for complex chronic wounds. Quantitative data such as wound measurements, as well as subtle changes in wound appearance or the condition of the surrounding skin, may herald impending complications. Such observations should be thoroughly documented and never trusted to memory.

6. *When performing a patient assessment, consider any co-morbidities or underlying pathology that could delay healing.* Effective wound management depends not only on treatment of the underlying cause of the wound, but attention to factors such as poor nutrition and inadequate circulation. Remember, the visit is more than a dressing change. Effective wound management requires a comprehensive approach to patient assessment and intervention.

7. *Describe wound location in specific anatomical terms.* Avoid using general terms such as hip, buttocks, or thigh. For example, a pressure ulcer should be described as being located over the left trochanter or right ischial tuberosity. Use of "left hip" or "right buttock" as descriptors may be both imprecise and misleading.

8. *After each visit, critically evaluate the patient's medical record to determine if your documentation ensures continuity of care.* Remember that the "litmus test" for well-coordinated care is

documentation that allows for a smooth transition to a new care-giver when you are ill or unable to make a visit. Look at your records from the perspective of a nurse unfamiliar with the patient and wound status. Are the expected clinical outcomes well-defined and measurable? Does the documentation reflect whether or not the expected outcomes are being met? Are changes in wound appearance and patient response to treatment clear to the reader? Are wound care orders and medications up-to-date? Can you tell which wound care supplies or products are being used? Would you be able to continue patient education and follow through with the plan of care based on the information in the record?

9. *Use photographs of the wound to supplement written observations.* Although wound photographs should never replace written documentation, they provide a visual reference of wound progress that can be kept in the clinical record and shared with both the patient and physician as needed to communicate progress. Instant print cameras are available that are specially designed for wound documentation purposes. Before taking a photograph, a consent form must be signed and kept as part of the permanent record. Legal experts advise taking a full-body photo with the wound in the picture and a second close-up photo of the wound. The patient's medical record number and the date the photo is taken should be visible within the close-up photo. This can be accomplished by recording this information on a small piece of white paper and lightly taping it to the skin near the wound.

10. *Use wound care experts as resources to assist you with establishing realistic outcomes, assessing wound progress, and planning care.* Many programs have an enterostomal therapist or clinical nurse specialist available to the team for consultation. The information and expertise they share will not only enhance patient care and contribute to improved outcomes, but will also help you increase your knowledge and skill level.

11. *Incorporate professional guidelines of care into wound care policies and procedures.* The Agency for Health Care Policy and Research (AHCPR) has published national guidelines for the care of patients with pressure ulcers. These guidelines help ensure consistency in care and care processes. (This information is listed in the Resource section at the end of the chapter.)

12. *Store wound care supplies safely in the home.* Wound care supplies left in the home should be always stored in a clean, dry

area. Refrigeration may be required for some biological dressings and compounded pharmaceutical solutions.

13. *Before ordering a specialty bed, check to make certain the home can accommodate the equipment.* Many specialty beds have load-bearing limits or electrical requirements that can't be accommodated in some homes. Likewise, the dimensions of some beds are too large to move through standard size doorways. Call a manufacturer's representative or the home medical equipment company to verify equipment specifications and determine the safest and most compatible product for your patient.

14. *Before beginning a dressing change, always clarify whether the physician has ordered clean or sterile technique.* Unless otherwise ordered, clean or "no touch" technique using good hand-washing technique and nonsterile supplies may be acceptable for some chronic wounds. All chronic wounds are considered contaminated and colonized. As a result, unless the patient is immunocompromised or at risk for infection, the use of sterile supplies may be both unnecessary and costly.

15. *Screen **all** patients for pressure ulcer risk at the start of care, on recertification, and when there is any significant change in condition.* Most elderly, debilitated patients are at risk for pressure-related skin breakdown, particularly those that are homebound. Therefore early identification of risk factors and prevention of skin breakdown should be the goal of every home care clinician. Valid and reliable risk assessment tools are available that are easy to use in the home setting. Once high-risk patients are identified, measures should be taken to reduce or relieve pressure. These measures include use of pressure-relieving devices, frequent repositioning, and patient/family education.

16. *When performing wound care in the home, use Universal Precautions to prevent the spread of potentially infectious organisms.* For example, remember to use goggles during wound irrigation when there is risk of splash-back. In some instances you may need to take additional measures to contain excessive and potentially infectious wound drainage, by either increasing the frequency of dressing changes or asking the physician to order a more absorbent dressing material.

17. *Identify measures to reduce excess skin moisture and the corrosive action of perspiration, stool or urine.* Excessive perspiration and incontinence can interfere with dressing adherence and, more important, lead to additional skin problems. The home health aide, or whoever is providing personal hygiene for the

patient, should be taught measures to minimize complications. For example, instruct caregivers to keep the skin clean and dry at all times. Having the patient wear loose cotton clothing helps promote air circulation to the skin and discourages the growth of yeast in skin fold areas. Regular use of skin barrier ointments and creams helps protect the skin from contact with the corrosive chemicals in urine and stool. Every effort should be made to use skin barriers as a preventive measure, *before* the skin becomes macerated and irritated.

18. *Obtain dietary consultations or evaluations as needed to maintain adequate nutrition and hydration.* Adequate protein, calorie, and fluid intake is essential for normal healing and needs to be closely monitored. Vitamin and mineral supplements may also be indicated, especially in the elderly population.

19. *Do not forget to address psychosocial issues that may impact clinical outcomes.* Wounds are often associated with concerns about body image, offensive odor, and activity limitations. Home care nurses may identify difficulties with coping mechanisms and interpersonal relationships or alterations in mental-emotional-spiritual well-being that need to be addressed as part of the plan of care. If living conditions are poor or place the patient at risk for wound infection, a social services consultation may be indicated.

20. *Work with the patient's physician to design a wound care regimen that promotes an optimal environment for healing.* Currently accepted standards of wound care include timely débridement of necrotic tissue, avoidance of harsh wound cleansers and disinfectants, and use of moisture-retentive dressings to promote healing. Many physicians are unfamiliar with recent advances in wound care and continue to use products that are proven detrimental to healing. Take some time to educate yourself in the principles of moist wound healing by reading professional journals and attending in-services. Many wound dressing manufacturers provide educational sessions and published articles free of charge. Share scientifically based articles and photographs of successfully treated wounds with physicians to help inform them of new and better approaches to wound management.

INFECTION CONTROL IN THE HOME SETTING

Infection control is always a concern when the patient has a wound or any alteration in skin integrity. In the home, infection control measures

---

BOX 12-1   **SUPPLIES NEEDED**

The following checklist of supplies can be used when planning a
visit to a patient with a virulent wound infection:
- Disposable "splash" gown
- Disposable mask
- Splash shield or goggles (for wound irrigation)
- Clean examination gloves
- Plastic bags for trash disposal
- Germicidal spray (for cleaning contaminated surfaces)
- Disposable wound cleansing and dressing supplies
- Blood pressure cuff and stethoscope (to be left at bedside)
- Intravenous (IV) supplies (if IV antibiotics ordered)
- Others, based on the patient's unique needs and physician
  orders

---

are based on the same principles as in the hospital setting (Box 12-1).
However, in attempting to follow these principles, the home care nurse
often faces challenges of inadequate handwashing facilities, limited
space, and frequent schedule changes.

The cardinal rule of infection control, thorough handwashing before
and after patient contact, is equally important in home care and of even
greater importance in wound care (Box 12-2). If you're entering the patient's home for the first time, ask where you can wash and dry your
hands. Some homes may have dirty or inadequate handwashing facilities. Others may not even have the luxury of running water. It is good
practice to carry some form of skin disinfectant in your bag to be used
in place of soap and water should the need arise. Do not use the patient's bar soap and towels. Use liquid soap and paper towels.

Patients with open wounds are sometimes colonized with virulent
organisms that can be spread to other patients and even family members if proper precautions aren't taken. A virulent organism such as
methicillin-resistant *Staphylococcus aureus* (MRSA) is best managed
in the home by first establishing a clean "prep" area. This area allows
the nurse to gown, glove, and mask before coming in direct contact with
the patient.

To minimize cross-contamination, use disposable items whenever
possible. Leave your bag in the clean area, and only take items to the bedside that are needed for patient care. Contain soiled dressings and used
protective gear in a plastic bag for disposal according to local regulations
and organizational policy. Whenever possible, leave a blood pressure cuff,

---

BOX 12-2 **INFECTION CONTROL TIPS**

Remember that cross-contamination can be prevented by effective handwashing technique. In addition to washing your hands before and after contact with the patient:

- Always use Universal Precautions when caring for a patient with a wound or weeping skin condition.
- Use clean or sterile gloves per physician orders.
- If there are multiple wounds, proceed from the cleanest wound to the dirtiest wound; change gloves between wounds.
- Dispose of soiled supplies and dressings according to local regulations and organizational policies.
- Follow organization policies and accepted standards of practice.

---

stethoscope, intravenous therapy equipment and other nondisposable items at the bedside until the patient is discharged. On discharge, double bag nondisposable items for disinfection at a later time.

Because the potential for cross-contamination is higher with virulent organisms, it is always best to schedule infected patients as the last visit of the day. If twice-a-day dressing changes are ordered, schedule immunocompromised patients and patients with clean wounds before the first "infected" dressing change. In some cases, having patients who are unusually susceptible to infection reassigned to another nurse may be the only alternative to ensure safe patient care.

The extra precautions required for patients with virulent infections can be frightening to both the patient and family members. Before implementing these measures, educate both the patient and family on the reasons for the special precautions and how to limit exposure to other "susceptible" family members such as newborns or the very elderly. In most cases family members need only be taught to follow Universal Precautions to prevent spread of virulent organisms. However, depending on the infectious agent and susceptibility of those in close contact, additional precautions (such as masking) may be warranted. If unsure, check with an infection control nurse at a local hospital for patient-specific recommendations.

PATIENT ASSESSMENT

Wound healing involves a complex series of physiological events that results in predictable changes in wound appearance (Cuzzell, 1995). Assessment of a patient with a wound requires an understanding of these events, as well as the many factors that can delay the healing process (Cuzzell, 1995).

Although wound healing is often described as occurring in three separate "phases," it is important to note that many of the cellular and biochemical events in these phases overlap or occur simultaneously. Likewise, when discussing the healing response, it is important to differentiate between superficial wounds with minimal tissue destruction and deep wounds with extensive tissue destruction. Superficial wounds generally heal within 10 to 14 days, primarily by re-epithelialization from intact epidermal cells at the wound margins and skin appendages. Deep wounds take much longer to heal, requiring granulation and wound contraction to promote closure. The following table outlines the natural physiological response that occurs whenever there is an alteration in skin integrity and indicates the expected time frames for each phase when healing progresses normally (Table 12-1).

There are many health-related factors that can delay natural healing and extend the time to complete wound closure. This is particularly true in the case of chronic wounds, such as pressure ulcers and leg ulcers. Chronic wounds become "stuck" in one of the phases described in Table 12-1, and, even with appropriate local care, healing may be delayed indefinitely. *In fact, a healed wound may not even be a realistic outcome for some patients with multiple medical problems.* The medical history and initial physical examination can provide valuable clues about a patient's general health status and help guide the nurse in identifying potential obstacles to healing (Box 12-3).

WOUND ASSESSMENT

Effective wound assessment requires a systematic collection of information that is measurable and clearly reflects progress toward or away from the expected outcome. It is extremely important to quantify your observations of the wound so that you have reliable information with which to compare subsequent assessments. For example, the subjective documentation "healing well" has different meanings to different people and begs the question, "Compared to what?" On the other hand, documentation of wound dimensions, amount and type of necrotic tissue, and amount of wound drainage gives objective information that facilitates accurate evaluation of changes in wound status from visit to visit. Box 12-4 summarizes key information that needs to be gathered when performing a wound assessment.

The baseline observations and subsequent changes in wound status that are reflected in quantitative wound documentation should reflect

TABLE 12-1   **PHASES OF WOUND HEALING**

PHASE OF HEALING	PHYSIOLOGICAL EVENTS	CLINICAL MANIFESTATIONS	EXPECTED TIME FRAME
	Hemostasis Vasodilation Increased capillary permeability and leakage of serum	Blood clot/scab/eschar forms Blanchable erythema Warmth on palpation Localized edema Pain Copious serosanguineous exudate leaks from the wound	Injury to approximately 3 days
INFLAMMATION	Blockage of lymph channels with fibrin Leukocyte (neutrophil and macrophage) migration into the wound to destroy bacteria and serve as a first defense against infection		
PROLIFERATION	Capillaries bud and grow into the wound space to revascularize the tissue Fibroblast proliferation is initiated by natural growth factors released by the macrophage	Granulation tissue begins to form (deep wound only)	Superficial wounds—injury to 10 to 14 days Deep wounds—injury to 21 days+

continued

TABLE 12-1   **PHASES OF WOUND HEALING—cont'd**

PHASE OF HEALING	PHYSIOLOGICAL EVENTS	CLINICAL MANIFESTATIONS	EXPECTED TIME FRAME
	Fibroblasts secrete collagen to replace damaged tissue	Granulation tissue thickens	Three weeks to several years
	Bacteria proliferate in dead tissue, and macrophage activity increases proportionally	Eschar begins to slough, and exudate becomes purulent	
	Epithelial cells replicate and migrate once the necrotic tissue is removed and the granulating base is clean	New skin growth is seen at the margins (superficial wounds have minimal tissue damage and heal primarily by reepithelialization from the margins and skin appendages)	
MATURATION	Certain fibroblasts change into myofibroblasts and migrate into wound	The wound contracts or shrinks (deep wound only)	
	Fibroblast and macrophage activity decrease	Granulation tissue formation ceases	
	Collagen is broken down and redeposited in a more organized fashion to increase wound strength	The wound closes	
		Scar tissue flattens and softens	
	Blood vessels and fibroblasts recede	Scar color gradually changes from pink to white	

BOX 12-3   **PATIENT ASSESSMENT CRITERIA: SYSTEMIC AND PSYCHOSOCIAL FACTORS THAT CAN ALTER THE HEALING RESPONSE**

Nutritional Status
General appearance
Recent weight loss/obesity
Skin turgor
Total protein/calorie intake
Intake and output

Chronic Illness/Conditions
Chronic obstructive pulmonary
  disease
Arteriosclerotic heart disease
Venous hypertension
Diabetes
Renal failure
Collagen disorders
Sensory deficit

Oxygenation/Circulation to the Tissue
Respiratory impairment
Circulatory impairment
Peripheral vascular disease
Smoking

Corticosteriods
Chemotherapy

Immune Status
Cancer
Human immunodeficiency virus
Septicemia

Continent Status
Urine
Feces

Psychosocial Factors
Coping mechanisms
Interpersonal relationships
Mental/emotional/spiritual status
Compliance with the treatment
  plan
Living conditions

Other
Age
Activity/mobility limitations

---

forward progress along a predictable path toward wound closure. Lack of forward progress alerts the nurse of the need for reevaluation of both the patient and the plan of care. Table 12-2 outlines predictable changes in wound status and the implications of those changes.

WOUND CARE DOCUMENTATION

In most settings, including home care, wound documentation is facilitated by the use of documentation forms or flow sheets. These forms may either be designed to document healing progress of a specific wound type such as pressure ulcers, or they may have generic application to all wound types (Figure 12-1).

BOX 12-4 **WOUND ASSESSMENT CRITERIA**

Type of Wound
Acute
Surgical incision
Burn
Skin tear/abrasion
Chronic
Pressure ulcer
Leg ulcer
Diabetic ulcer
Other

Anatomical Location

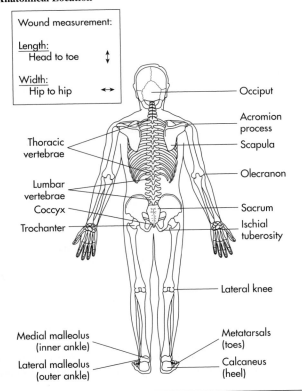

Wound measurement:

Length:
Head to toe ↕

Width:
Hip to hip ↔

Occiput
Acromion process
Scapula
Thoracic vertebrae
Olecranon
Lumbar vertebrae
Coccyx
Sacrum
Trochanter
Ischial tuberosity
Lateral knee
Medial malleolus (inner ankle)
Metatarsals (toes)
Lateral malleolus (outer ankle)
Calcaneus (heel)

Figure from Johnson & Johnson Medical, Arlington, Texas.

BOX 12-4   WOUND ASSESSMENT CRITERIA–

Depth of Tissue Damage
Stage (pressure ulcers only)
Partial thickness
Full thickness

Size of Wound
Greatest length measured head to toe
Greatest width measured hip to hip
Greatest depth

Exudate
Amount
Color
Consistency
Odor

Amount and Type of Tissue
Percent red (healthy granulation and/or epithelial tissue)
Percent yellow (soft, stringy necrotic tissue)
Percent black (thick, adherent eschar)

Condition of Wound and Surrounding Skin
Presence/absence of sinus tracts
Presence/absence of undermining
Condition of surrounding skin
  Signs and symptoms of infection (local versus systemic)
  Presence/absence of maceration, irritation, rash, etc.
  Presence/absence of pain

Home care nurses are encouraged to refer to the AHCPR guidelines for a more in-depth discussion on accepted wound care interventions, including:

- Categories of débridement
- Wound cleansing principles
- Moisture-retentive dressings
- Bacterial colonization and infection
- Operative repair of chronic wounds
- Adjunctive therapies (e.g. electrical stimulation, hyperbaric oxygen)

Text continued on p. 240.

TABLE 12-2 WOUND ASSESSMENT/DOCUMENTATION GUIDELINES

EXPECTED OUTCOMES	ASSESSMENT GUIDELINES	WHAT TO DOCUMENT	DOCUMENTATION TOOLS
Wound location will remain unchanged	✔ The location of the wound provides information about the possible cause of skin/tissue breakdown	**On admission:** ✔ Anatomical location of the wound(s) ✔ Distribution or percent body surface area involved if large wound (burn), rash, or multiple sites ✔ Proximity of the wound to a bony prominence	✔ Body line drawing ✔ Photograph
Wound size will decrease with healing at a rate dependent on the amount of necrotic tissue present and the patient's overall condition.	✔ Wound size increases as necrotic tissue is debrided ✔ Wound size decreases as infection is controlled and healing occurs by reepithelialization and contraction ✔ The wound changes in shape as healing occurs ✔ Large superficial wounds may become multiple smaller wounds as new skin growth occurs	**EVERY WEEK and PRN changes in wound status:** ✔ Length in cm (largest dimension from head to toe) ✔ Width in cm (largest dimension from hip to hip) ✔ Extent of undermining at wound margins in cm (circumferentially) **Daily:** ✔ Changes in plan of care	✔ Disposable measuring device ✔ Plastic "baggie" and marker (for tracing irregularly shaped wounds) ✔ Polaroid grid camera ✔ Cotton-tipped applicator stick (to measure undermining)

Wound depth will
decrease with
healing at a rate
dependent on the
amount of necrotic
tissue present and
the patient's
overall condition

✔ Wound depth increases as necrotic tissue is removed
✔ Wound depth decreases as
granulation tissue forms
✔ The amount of packing material
needed to fill deep wounds
decreases as healing progresses

On admission:
✔ Stage of pressure ulcer (if
wound base visible)
✔ Partial- or full-thickness
designation (if unable to
stage due to presence of
necrotic tissue)

**EVERY WEEK and PRN
changes in wound status:**
✔ Depth in cm at deepest
portion of wound
✔ Depth and direction of
soft tissue tunneling
✔ Amount of packing ma-
terial needed to loosely
pack deep wound cavaties
Daily:
✔ Changes in plan of care

✔ Cotton-tipped appli-
cator stick
✔ Gloved finger to
gently probe wound if
deep tunneling is
present
✔ Wound drawing using
a clock face to
describe the direction
of soft tissue tunneling

continued

TABLE 12-2 WOUND ASSESSMENT/DOCUMENTATION GUIDELINES—cont'd

EXPECTED OUTCOMES	ASSESSMENT GUIDELINES	WHAT TO DOCUMENT	DOCUMENTATION TOOLS
Tissue type (will change from a high percent of necrotic tissue to absence of necrotic tissue as healing progresses)	✔ Tissue color changes from black to yellow to red as healing progresses ✔ The percent of black necrotic tissue, yellow slough, and incidence of infection decreases with appropriate treatment ✔ The percent of granulation and new epithelial tissue increases with appropriate treatment	**EVERY WEEK and PRN changes in wound status:** ✔ Percent of black tissue ✔ Percent of yellow slough ✔ Percent of granulation tissue **Daily:** ✔ Changes in plan of care	✔ Good light source ✔ Photograph q 2 weeks
Wound exudate will decrease in amount once necrotic tissue is removed and infection is controlled	✔ Amount of serosanguineous exudate increases suddenly before surgical wound dehiscence ✔ Exudate increases in amount and viscosity with autolytic débridement of necrotic tissue using occlusive dressings ✔ Exudate decreases in amount once necrotic tissue is removed and the wound is granulating ✔ Exudate increases in amount and viscosity if wound becomes infected	**EVERY WEEK and PRN changes in wound status:** ✔ Amount of drainage as quantified by: ✔ Small, moderate, and large ✔ Frequency of dressing changes to control drainage ✔ Number of gauze pads saturated with drainage at each dressing change	✔ Patient reports of drainage on linens, etc.

Surrounding skin will remain intact and free of signs and symptoms of infection

✔ Exudate increases in amount with venous leg ulcers if compression isn't adequate or patient is non-compliant with bedrest and elevation

✔ Skin around the wound becomes macerated and colonized with yeast if drainage is excessive and not controlled by use of an absorptive dressing

✔ A pruritic "burnlike" skin reaction that has well-defined borders usually indicates an allergic reaction to the dressing material

✔ Cellulitis and tenderness extending more than 2 cm beyond the wound margins indicates possible infection

Daily:
Changes in plan of care

EVERY WEEK and PRN changes in wound status:
✔ Condition of surrounding skin (intact or not intact)
✔ Description of skin changes if present (including associated symptoms)

Daily (if infected)
✔ Extent of cellulitis (measurement in cm)
✔ Amount and type of wound drainage

✔ Good light source
✔ Palpation
✔ Patient reports of discomfort (e.g., increased tenderness, pruritus)
✔ Photograph

PRESSURE ULCER MONITORING CHART

Patient _____

Caregiver _____

Date _____

Patient _____

Caregiver _____

Date _____

1. Location of ulcer: _____

2. Present stage: □ I □ II □ III □ IV

3. Size:
   Length: _____
   Width: _____
   Depth: _____
   Description (in words): _____

4. Color (%): _____

5. Exudate (color and type):
   □ None □ Slight □ Moderate □ Large

6. Uncharacteristic odor:
   □ None □ Slight □ Marked □ Severe

1. Location of ulcer: _____

2. Present stage: □ I □ II □ III □ IV

3. Size:
   Length: _____
   Width: _____
   Depth: _____
   Description (in words): _____

4. Color (%): _____

5. Exudate (color and type):
   □ None □ Slight □ Moderate □ Large

6. Uncharacteristic odor:
   □ None □ Slight □ Marked □ Severe

7. Pain: In wound site?   ☐ Yes ☐ No
        In surrounding tissue?   ☐ Yes ☐ No
8. Is wound healing?   ☐ Yes ☐ No
   Granulation tissue visible?   ☐ Yes ☐ No
   Epithelialization in progress?   ☐ Yes ☐ No
   Necrotic tissue present?   ☐ Yes ☐ No
9. Describe surrounding tissue:

10. Symptoms of infection:
        Local?   ☐ Yes ☐ No
        Systemic?   ☐ Yes ☐ No
11. Pressure relief obtained?   ☐ Yes ☐ No
12. Braden risk score
13. Nutritional assessment   ☐ Yes ☐ No

FIGURE 12-1   Example of a wound documentation form.

7. Pain: In wound site?   ☐ Yes ☐ No
        In surrounding tissue?   ☐ Yes ☐ No
8. Is wound healing?   ☐ Yes ☐ No
   Granulation tissue visible?   ☐ Yes ☐ No
   Epithelialization in progress?   ☐ Yes ☐ No
   Necrotic tissue present?   ☐ Yes ☐ No
9. Describe surrounding tissue:

10. Symptoms of infection:
        Local?   ☐ Yes ☐ No
        Systemic?   ☐ Yes ☐ No
11. Pressure relief obtained?   ☐ Yes ☐ No
12. Braden risk score
13. Nutritional assessment   ☐ Yes ☐ No

Although these guidelines specifically address the management of pressure ulcers, the standards of care outlined in this valuable reference readily apply to other types of chronic wounds.

The following is documentation of a case study that applies both the principles of quantitative wound assessment and the intervention based on color classification.

A CASE STUDY
Assessment
Patient bedbound with multiple sclerosis. Unable to chew/swallow without assistance. Emaciated, diaphoretic, incontinent of urine and stool. Foley catheter to straight drainage. Pressure relief with closed-cell foam mattress. Diaphoresis decreased after mattress placement.

Pt. afebrile; chronic, Stage III ulcer located on (R) trochanter: (L) 3 cm × (W) 2.5 cm × (D) 1.5 cm; draining large amounts serosanguineous exudate with slight pungent odor; 75% of wound bed = thick tenacious yellow slough; 25% = pale pink granulation tissue; peri-wound skin with blanchable erythema extending 2 cm in all directions. Wound responding well to collagenase (see Figure 12-1). Consent obtained and photographs taken.

Intervention
Using clean technique and Universal Precautions, wound is irrigated thoroughly with normal saline. Apply antimicrobial powder and collagenase to wound and cover with one sterile 4 × 4 gauze. Peri-wound is protected with skin sealant before dressing application, and dressing borders are taped to prevent dislodging. Soiled gloves, dressings, and supplies are discarded in red bag and placed in biohazardous container.

Patient/Family Teaching
Daughter observes wound care procedure for first time and is instructed to call nurse if redness around wound increases or patient becomes febrile. She is instructed how to turn and reposition with return demonstration. She agrees to have family members assist with turn schedule q2h. 24-hour diet recall is done, and daughter is instructed in need for increased protein intake, vitamin C, and iron. Daughter states that she tries to supplement mechanical soft diet with 2 to 3 cans of Ensure per day. She is instructed in handwashing after care of mother. Daughter has antimicrobial soap and uses Lysol disinfectant. She states that "all this is getting too expensive." Reasons for precautions are reinforced.

On the basis of this documentation, covered services for skilled nursing include:

Observation and assessment
Resolution of diaphoresis with pressure relief
Quantification of size, necrotic tissue, drainage, odor, condition of
   peri-wound skin
Stage of ulcer
Wound photograph
Response to treatment
Diet recall
Hands-on care
Wound irrigation
Dressing change
Treatment as ordered
Teaching and training
Wound care procedure
Signs and symptoms of infection
Dietary needs to promote healing
Turning/postioning
Infection control

WOUND HEALING CONSIDERATIONS

As mentioned earlier in this chapter, many factors can interfere with the normal healing and therefore the patient's response to treatment. Most chronic wounds are "stuck" in one or more phases of the wound healing process because of inability or failure to treat the underlying cause of the ulcer, co-morbid illnesses, inadequate tissue perfusion, nutritional deficiencies, bacterial burden, or continued tissue trauma. Table 12-3 outlines some important wound healing considerations that will ultimately impact clinical outcomes.

SPECIAL CHALLENGES IN HOME CARE WOUND CARE PRACTICE
Lower-Extremity Ulcers

As a single category, arterial, venous, and diabetic ulcers of the lower extremity exceed the number of pressure ulcers treated in the home setting. Unlike pressure ulcers, lower extremity ulcers are often recalcitrant to treatment or require interventions from multiple specialists to accurately assess the underlying vascular problem and achieve acceptable outcomes. In addition, noncompliance with the treatment regimen is common in this patient population, requiring an increased emphasis

TABLE 12-3   WOUND HEALING CONSIDERATIONS

KEY CONSIDERATIONS	MECHANISM OF ACTION
Malnutrition Protein depletion with serum albumin <3 g/dl	Prolonged inflammatory phase; impaired revascularization of wound and collagen synthesis; impaired maturation phase; decreased resistance to infection
Vitamin deficiency	Vitamin C: altered fibroblast function Vitamin C and A: poor quality of healing Vitamin D: impaired healing of bone
Trace element deficiency (zinc, copper, ferrous iron, manganese)	Altered enzymatic reactions
Tissue hypoxia (from arteriosclerosis, diabetes, cardiopulmonary disease, hypovolemia, advanced age, etc.)	Impaired capillary budding; impaired fibroblast function, decreased epithelial cell regeneration; impaired white blood cell function; increased wound infection
Increased bacterial burden >10^5 organisms per gram of tissue, or less burden if organism is virulent or patient is immunocompromised	Prolonged or recurrent inflammatory phase of healing; continued tissue damage from bacterial toxins
Advanced age	Decreased epidermal cell regeneration; increased skin fragility; prolonged healing response (all phases); increased incidence of malnutrition; impaired cardiopulmonary status and immune system; decreased tissue perfusion
Steroid therapy	Prolonged inflammatory and proliferative phases (frequent cause of surgical incision dehiscence)
Diabetes	Impaired arterial perfusion (large and small vessels); impaired WBC function; increased incidence of wound infection

TABLE 12-3 WOUND HEALING CONSIDERATIONS—cont'd

KEY CONSIDERATIONS	MECHANISM OF ACTION
Necrotic tissue	Physical obstacle to epidermal cell migration and wound contraction; pablum for bacterial growth
Continued tissue trauma (from un-relieved pressure, too-aggressive cleansing; or inappropriate use of wound care products)	Cellular injury and reinitiation of the inflammatory phase of healing
Topical antiseptics and skin cleansers	Potentially cytotoxic to cells when used inappropriately
Tissue desiccation	Increased inflammation and pain response; impaired epithelial migration and fibroblast proliferation
Dead space (wound space in a deep wound that is left unfilled by dressing material)	Pooling of wound exudate and increased bacterial proliferation; formation of soft tissue abcesses

on patient education to promote healing and prevent ulcer recurrence (Table 12-4).

Clinical fact sheets developed by the Wound, Ostomy, and Continence Society outline the types of lower-extremity ulcers, assessment criteria, and usual methods of treatment. These fact sheets also contain guidelines for patient education that can be copied and distributed as needed.

Bedbound or Immobilized Patients

As one might expect, bedbound and chairbound patients are at particular risk for pressure-related skin breakdown. Risk assessment scales such as the Braden or Norton scale establish a baseline for maintaining skin integrity for these and all homebound patients. Once a patient is determined to be "at risk," timely implementation of interventions to minimize pressure and prevent skin breakdown becomes critical (Boxes

TABLE 12-4 **LOWER-EXTREMITY ULCERS**

ULCER TYPE	CAUSE	LOCATION	SIGNS/SYMPTOMS	INTERVENTIONS
Diabetic foot ulcers	Occlusion of small and large arteries leading to tissue ischemia and skin breakdown following minor trauma	✔ Weight-bearing surfaces of foot (under calluses) ✔ Areas of friction (poor-fitting shoes) ✔ Tips of toes and interdigital spaces ✔ Bony prominence of foot	✔ Poor or absent pedal pulses ✔ Diminished or absent sensation ✔ Cellulitis ✔ Dry, gangrenous "black" wounds ✔ Dry, "punched out" appearing ulcers with pale granulation tissue Signs and symptoms (S/S) of infection (local S/S may be masked in advanced disease)	✔ Control of diabetes ✔ Pressure/friction relief ✔ Avoid occlusive dressings (increased risk of infection) ✔ Topical antimicrobials as indicated ✔ Teach foot care ✔ Surgical débridement and amputation to control infection

Arterial leg ulcers	Blockage of one or more major arteries in the lower limb leading to tissue ischemia, cell death, and ulcer formation	Areas prone to trauma	Poor or absent pedal pulses	Avoid leg elevation
		✔ Lateral surface of lower leg	✔ Rubor (pale skin color with elevation of leg; red skin color when dependent)	✔ Analgesics for pain
		✔ Toes and heels		✔ Keep legs/feet warm
		✔ Bony prominences		✔ Avoid compression
			✔ Cool, shiny skin with absence of hair	✔ Prevent friction and pressure
			✔ Severe resting pain at night or when legs are elevated	✔ Prevent skin maceration or excessive dryness
			✔ Dry, pale ulcer base with well-defined margins and poor granulation	✔ Avoid occlusive dressings (increased risk of infection)
				✔ Topical antimicrobials PRN
				✔ Surgery: arterial bypass

continued

TABLE 12-4 **LOWER-EXTREMITY ULCERS** —cont'd

ULCER TYPE	CAUSE	LOCATION	SIGNS/SYMPTOMS	INTERVENTIONS
Venous leg ulcers	Damage or incompetence of the valves in the large veins leads to increased venous hypertension, dilated veins (varicose veins), leakage of serum into the tissue, and fibrin deposits around the vessels; the fibrin deposits harden, preventing the diffusion of oxygen and nutrients to the skin; anoia and malnutrition of skin cells lead to cell death and ulcer formation	✔ Medial surface of lower leg in gaitor or "sock" area ✔ Less common occurrence on lateral surface of lower leg ✔ Often located superior to the malleolus	✔ Thickening and reddish brown staining of the skin, often associated with scaling and inflammation ✔ Pitting edema ✔ Varicose veins ✔ Palpable pedal pulses ✔ Shallow ulcers with irregular flat margins ✔ Large amount of serosanguineous drainage ✔ Dark, ruby red granulation tissue ✔ Pain rare (only if very edematous or infected)	✔ Compression with elastic wraps or surgical support hose to reverse venous hypertension ✔ Elevation of legs above heart level ✔ Avoid prolonged standing ✔ Prevent pressure to heels and ankles ✔ Dressing that absorbs excessive exudate; change PRN leakage ✔ Surgery: vein stripping; valve repair; skin grafts

12-5 to 12-7). Because pressure-relieving devices are costly, home care nurses must remain knowledgeable about Medicare reimbursement for these products. A patient's access to pressure-relief devices is governed by preset Medicare criteria and requires a physician order. Within recent years Medicare rules regarding coverage have changed frequently and may continue to do so in the future.

Follow these two basic rules when investigating pressure-relief surfaces for high-risk patients:

1. *Know the current Medicare regulations for pressure-relief devices.* Reimbursement guidelines can be obtained from many home medical equipment companies or directly from the regional HCFA office.
2. *Investigate the reliability of various support surfaces.* As with wound dressings, the number of pressure reduction or relief products on the market can be confusing. If unsure of the best product for your patient, seek input from an enterostomal nurse or clinical nurse specialist.

The AHCPR Guidelines, Pressure Ulcers in Adults: Prediction and Prevention, recommends following the criteria presented in Boxes 12-5 to 12-7 for "high risk" bedridden or immobilized patients.

For bedbound individuals, the AHCPR Guidelines suggest additional pressure-relief interventions:

- Reposition the patient at least every 2 hours.
- Use pillows or foam wedges to keep bony prominences from direct contact.
- Use devices that totally relieve pressure on the heels.
- Avoid positioning directly on the trochanter.
- Elevate the head of the bed for as short a time as possible.
- Use lifting devices to move rather than drag patients across the bed linens during transfers and position changes.
- Place at-risk individuals on a pressure-reducing mattress. *Do not* use donut-type devices.
- Avoid vigorous massage over reddened bony prominence or stage 1 areas.

For chairbound individuals:

- Reposition at least every hour.
- Have patient shift weight every 15 minutes if able.

BOX 12-5   **GROUP I: PRESSURE-REDUCING
                 SUPPORT SURFACES**

A patient must fall within one of the following scenarios to qualify
for a group I pressure-reducing device.

Scenario 1: Patient Meets Criterion No.1
1. Patient is completely immobile

Scenario 2: Patient Meets the Following Criteria
2. Patient has limited mobility, or
3. Patient has any stage pressure ulcer

And Meets At Least One of the Following:
4. Impaired nutritional status
5. Fecal or urinary incontinence
6. Altered sensory perception
7. Compromised circulatory status

Primary Categories of Group I Support Surfaces
Foam, gel, water, or air mattresses (no pump)
Alternating-pressure or low-air-loss overlays (with pump)
Foam, gel, water, or air overlays

Data from AHCPR Guidelines.

- Use pressure-reducing devices for seating surfaces. Do *not* use
  donut-type devices.
- Consider postural alignment, distribution of weight, balance and
  stability and pressure relief when positioning individuals in chairs
  or wheelchairs.
- Have a written plan of care.

SPECIFIC DOCUMENTATION CONSIDERATIONS

Documentation is an area in home health and hospice that can be problematic. The clinical documentation in the patient's record is the legal
record and story of the care provided by team members and the patient
and caregiver's response to interventions. Nowhere is the topic of documentation more fraught with problems than in the area of wound care.
There are many reasons for this, including the variation in the types of
wounds, kinds of interventions and products, and different staging tools
and other factors contributing to the variations. As home care and hos-

---

BOX 12-6   GROUP II: PRESSURE-RELIEVING SUPPORT SURFACES

A patient must fall within one of the following scenarios to qualify for reimbursement of a Group II device:

Scenario 1: Patient Must Meet Criteria 1 to 3
1. Multiple stage II pressure ulcers are located on the trunk or pelvis.
2. Patient has been on a comprehensive ulcer treatment program for at least 1 month, which has included the appropriate use of a group I product.
3. The ulcers have worsened or remained the same over the last month.

Scenario 2: Patient Meets Criterion 4
4. Patient has a large or multiple stage III or IV pressure ulcer(s) located on the trunk or pelvis.

Scenario 3: Patient Meets Criteria 5 and 6
5. Patient has had a myocutaneous flap or skin graft on the trunk or pelvis within the preceding 60 days.
6. Patient has been on a group II or III product before discharge from a hospital or skilled nursing facility.

Primary Categories of Group II Support Surfaces
Low-air-loss mattress replacement units
Alternating-pressure mattress replacement units

Data from AHCPR Guidelines.

---

pice move toward more outcome-focused care, the standardization of care and care processes should contribute to less variation, which should facilitate improved data collection and evaluation of goal achievement. Five documentation problems related to wound care include:

1. Initial assessment form and information elicited during the initial visit
2. Context and descriptions of homebound status
3. ICD-9 codes, especially locator 11,12, and 13 on the HCFA form 485, Home Health Certification and Plan of Care
4. Goals, outcomes, discharge plans
5. Daily visit note or another clinical documentation form

BOX 12-7   **GROUP III: PRESSURE-RELIEVING SUPPORT SURFACES**

An air-fluidized bed is covered only if all of the following criteria are met:

1. The patient has a stage III or IV pressure sore.
2. The patient is bedridden or chair bound as a result of severely limited mobility.
3. In the absence of an air-fluidized bed, the patient would require institutionalization.
4. The air-fluidized bed is ordered in writing by the patient's attending physician, based on a comprehensive assessment and evaluation of the patient after conservative treatment has been tried without success. **Attempts at conservative treatment must be documented and should generally include:**
   a. Education of the patient and caregiver on the prevention and/or management of pressure ulcers
   b. Assessment by a physician, nurse, or other licensed health care practitioner at least weekly
   c. Appropriate turning and positioning
   d. Use of a group II product, if appropriate
   e. Appropriate wound care
   f. Appropriate management of moisture/incontinence
   g. Nutritional assessment and intervention consistent with the overall care plan
   The patient must have been on the conservative treatment program for at least 1 month before use of the air-fluidized bed with worsening or no improvement of the ulcer. The evaluation generally must be performed within a week before initiation of therapy with the air-fluidized bed.
5. A trained adult caregiver is available to assist the patient with the activities of daily living, fluid balance, dry-skin care, repositioning, recognition and management of altered mental status, dietary needs, prescribed treatments, and support of the air-fluidized bed system and its problems such as leakage.
6. A physician directs the home treatment regimen and evaluates and recertifies the need for the bed on a monthly basis.
7. All other alternative equipment has been considered and ruled out.

Data from AHCPR Guidelines.

Initial Assessment Form and Information Gathered During the Initial Visit

The initial assessment visit sets the groundwork for all care and care planning that occurs throughout the patient's length of service. Therefore the importance of the initial assessment and information obtained and recorded during this visit cannot be underestimated. The information on the assessment must be complete and accurate. The data on this form and information become the basis for the HCFA form 485 and care plan for the patient. Many comprehensive assessment tools have a picture of a patient with space for marking the wound or wounds on the appropriate part of the body. The assessment form should also include areas for an in-depth history related to vascular problems, chronic conditions such as diabetes or peripheral vascular disease, or integumentary indicators that are noted during the interview and physical examination. These assessment details assist in creating a unique, individualized picture of patients and their problems that have contributed to the wound and substantiate the need for skilled care.

Documentation Tips

Standardize the process and the order in which the information is collected from the patient. This helps to ensure that all team members gather data and create the plan in the same method. The documentation should also be standardized, including a process that requires all data elements to be completed or marked N/A, as appropriate. Once completed, review the initial assessment form and ask yourself whether this document describes the information needed to effectively create a plan for this patient and safely and adequately care for the wound in the home environment.

Homebound Status

Homebound is one of the eligibility criteria for admission to the Medicare home care program. For a Medicare beneficiary to be eligible to receive covered home health services, the law requires that the beneficiary be confined to his or her home. In practical language this means that "an individual does not have to be bedridden to be considered as confined to home. However, the condition of these patients should be such that there exists a normal inability to leave home and, consequently, leaving their homes requires a considerable and taxing effort" (*HHA Manual—Pub. 11*, 204.1 [HCFA]. Confined to the home).

Patients with wounds have many reasons for being homebound, based either on the uniqueness of the wound or other medical problems and/or findings. For example, the elderly patient with weeping cellulitis on the lower leg may be homebound because of the considerable, taxing effort it takes to walk, the pain movement and walking produces, or because the patient has been ordered by the physician to keep the leg elevated. On a recent record review, a patient with a toe ulcer and diabetes was noted to be homebound because of "unstable blood sugars." Usually, unstable blood sugars do not make a patient homebound. On further review, the documentation noted that the patient could only stand up and walk with assistance because of pain and unsteadiness on his feet because he could not bear weight on his great toe. These two reasons clearly document homebound status, thereby meeting Medicare homebound criteria.

Documentation Tips

After the initial assessment and throughout the plan of care, patients should be assessed and viewed as either homebound or not homebound. *Patients who are not homebound are not eligible for covered care under the Medicare home care program.* Always document clearly the reasons that support the homebound status. Patients with wounds may be homebound for the following reasons:

1. No, or very limited, weight bearing
2. Only up with assistance of person or assistive devices
3. Requires assistance to ambulate
4. Surgically restricted activities after débridement or flap/other surgery
5. Open, infected wound with generalized weakness
6. Bedridden or up in chair only
7. Assistance needed for all activities

Clearly, there are other reasons that are unrelated to the actual wound that may make the patient homebound, such as the stroke patient who has a pressure ulcer because of immobility and is essentially bedbound or chairbound and/or other medical problems that meet the homebound criteria.

ICD-9 Coding of Diagnoses

ICD-9 coding of diagnoses can also be problematic in patients with wounds. Many times patients with wounds have other medical conditions that may have contributed to the etiology of the wound. The ICD-code that is listed on the HCFA form 485 as the principal diagnosis needs to be the focus of the plan of care. It must relate to the services and supplies the home care organization is providing. When more than one diagnosis is being treated, a common occurrence in home care, always use the diagnosis that represents the most acute condition and requires the most intensive services. As an example, a patient with a Foley catheter who is receiving daily visits for wound care must have a realistic, projected end point to the daily wound care visits. The principal diagnosis should be the wound-related diagnosis, since that is the most acute condition requiring the most intensive (daily) services.

Documentation Tips

When choosing ICD-9 codes, consider that the communication about an individual patient's problems to the intermediary, the payor of the Medicare home care services, must be appropriate. *The choice of appropriate ICD-9 codes is a major part of effective documentation in wound care.* Use additional diagnoses that also support covered care. For example, a Foley catheter ICD-9 code supports homebound, even if it is not the principal diagnosis. Similarly, the listing of diabetes, peripheral vascular disease, or other chronic conditions as secondary or additional diagnoses that could potentially impede progress toward healing and resolution contributes to painting an overall clinical picture supporting Medicare coverage of services. Surgical treatment or V-codes also communicate patient problems. Examples may include débridement, amputation, arterial graft, and/or attention to catheter. Remember, review patient diagnoses/surgical codes during the reassessment or recertification process. Reviewers and/or payors will be able to visualize the changing status of your patient and the progress of the wound based on your documentation.

Goals, Outcomes, and Discharge Plans

Goals, outcomes, and discharge plans become more important as the home care industry moves toward outcome-based care. With this in mind, think of outcomes as quantifiable goals of care. For example, a patient with diabetes who has also had a toe amputation may have this outcome: evidence of infection-free wound healing (and the way infection-free would be defined). Next, identify measurement criteria supporting the outcome statement. For a patient with this kind of surgical wound the outcome(s) statement could include: patient verbalization of signs and symptoms of infection, oral temperature maintained at or below ___, and/or other defined parameters.

Discharge plans should always include a statement of where and/or how the patient will be cared for once home health services are discontinued. These plans need to be realistic and individualized for each patient. Once the discharge plans/goals are met, the patient should be discharged; thus the stated goals should be reviewed regularly to note if they are no longer reasonable or there has been a change in the patient's status.

Documentation Tips

Make discharge goals, outcomes, and discharge plans realistic and individualized for your patients. This kind of information may be integrated into a clinical path, using these parameters as standards for measurement, with variances being any deviations from these standards. Discharge statements become the point at which the patient outcome is measured and evaluated. As an example, a patient may be appropriate for discharge if the goal of being able to safely and effectively apply dressings has been accomplished.

Skilled Care

The daily visit note or other clinical documentation form must show that the patient is homebound and needs skilled care. Skilled care for Medicare services is defined in the Coverage of Services section of the *HHA Manual—Pub. 11* (HCFA). Remember, for wound care there are actually three separate nursing skills:

1. Observation and assessment of the wound and patient
2. Teaching and training related to the wound
3. The actual hands-on site care of the wound

Documentation Tips

For each visit, document the skilled care provided, the patient response to the intervention/care, patient homebound status, and the plans for continued care. Observation and assessment include vital signs; teaching and training include what was taught specifically that visit and the patient's response to the information/teaching. Documentation of the actual hands-on wound care should include the kind of dressing and other physician orders as specified in the plan of care.

Many forms for daily visit notes provide an area for writing why the patient is homebound. This information is very important to reviewers as they look to the provider to provide covered care and because homebound is an eligibility criteria for Medicare home care. Knowing and communicating the specific reason why the patient is homebound assists in painting a picture for any reviewer or payor and can also support medical necessity. In effective documentation forms, these kinds of activities are listed in a checklist format for the clinician. This checklist format also assists providers as home care moves toward collecting data for patient groups, as well as comparing such information. The visit note is the source in which a reviewer, including the nurses at the intermediary, should find the specificity in the information needed to support covered Medicare services.

Remember, by law Medicare can only pay for covered home care services. It is up to the clinician to make the difference between covered and reimbursed care and care that is denied. Effective documentation, particularly in wound care, can make that important difference (Box 12-8).

EVALUATION AND PATIENT FEEDBACK

Timeliness, critical pathways, outcomes, variances, and practice guidelines or standards—these are the rules nurses will live by and practice in

---

BOX 12-8   WOUND CARE DOCUMENTATION TIPS

1. Identify the location of the wound site(s) clearly in the clinical record. Many organizations use forms that have a drawing of a body for ease in identification and care coordination/communication among care providers.
2. Consider the patient's nutritional status and other factors that support wound healing and/or deterioration and refer to the dietitian or wound care specialist for follow-up and collaboration.
3. Be aware that many wound care records, especially daily wound care records, may be requested by the Medicare regional home health intermediary (RHHI). Therefore, make it a standard practice to review clinical entries for clarity and overall adherence to the ordered plan of care.
4. When your patient qualifies for daily wound care (5, 6, or 7 days of care) have the projected end point clearly stated on the HCFA form 485. The end point should be realistic to the patient's problem and supported in the clinical documentation by the other services.
5. Review the Wound Care section of the Coverage of Services section of the *HHA Manual—Pub. 11* (HCFA). For skilled nursing care to be reasonable and necessary to treat a wound, the size, depth, nature of drainage (color, odor, consistency, and quantity) and condition of the wound, as well as the appearance of the surrounding skin must be documented in the clinical findings so that an assessment of the need for skilled nursing care can be made.
6. Be sure the plan of care contains all the specific instructions for the treatment of the wound, including interventions and products or supplies ordered and used during patient care.

the 21st century. How can nurses enlist the patient and family in a partnership of care to provide the highest quality outcomes at the lowest cost? The task or challenge becomes how to predict realistic outcomes with greater accuracy using a treatment algorithm or critical pathway and convert both the patient and family to self-care behaviors.

- Can the patient verbalize the plan of care?
- Are the timeliness and expected outcomes reasonable when considering outliers or the patient's current medical status?
- Does the patient understand and accept the expected outcomes?
- Can the patient/family demonstrate safe and appropriate wound care and verbalize the expected changes in wound appearance that should occur with healing?
- Does the patient know signs and symptoms that signal wound deterioration or require immediate medical intervention?
- Does the patient/family know what is required to prevent wound recurrence?
- Can the patient's caregiver correctly provide the wound care as observed in the return demonstration?

In most cases documentation should reflect progress toward achievement of the following clinical outcomes. The time required to achieve these outcomes will be patient-specific, depending on his or her overall medical condition and ability to reverse factors that delay healing.

1. Wound is healed or shows evidence of progress toward healing.
2. Wound is clean and free of infection.
3. Patient/significant other knows protocol for and verbalizes understanding of wound care and takes preventive measures to avoid reoccurrence.
4. Patient/caregiver demonstrates behaviors related to health maintenance.

In certain instances a healed wound is not a realistic outcome. Patients who are terminal, mentally unstable, or noncompliant with treatment may never experience a healed wound.

OSTOMY MANAGEMENT

The United Ostomy Association (UOA) and International Ostomy Association (IOA) give the following estimates of the ostomy population: worldwide 1.9 million, with 887,000 residing in North America. The breakdown in types of surgery for 1991 was 56,000 colostomies, 7,000 ileostomies and 7,000 urostomies. Since that time further refinement in medical technology (i.e., creating internal reservoirs, performing low-level anastomoses, and earlier detection of cancer) has reduced these figures significantly.

Like wound care, ostomy management requires a comprehensive approach to patient education, with emphasis on self-care and prevention of complications.

TRACHEOSTOMY CARE

In most instances, a tracheostomy site has the treatment goal of protecting the site from further trauma. Nursing interventions should include the following:

- Secure the tracheostomy tube in such a way as to prevent friction or pressure on surrounding, intact skin. This may require "padding" the tracheostomy tie or strap with pieces of foam or a similar material.
- Use an absorptive dressing around the stoma site to absorb excess secretions and prevent maceration of the peristomal area. Some wound care materials have been adapted as tracheostomy site dressings (e.g., the foam products). Gauze pads may prove more cost-effective, but should be soft and nonabrasive and changed as soon as they become saturated. If secretions from around the tracheostomy site are copious or unusually viscous, the use of skin sealants or zinc oxide containing moisture barrier creams may provide added skin protection.
- Monitor fresh tracheostomy sites for signs and symptoms of infection. Like any acute wound, a fresh tracheostomy site can become infected. This is particularly true if the patient has a fulminant pneumonia. Treatment of the pneumonia (including vigorous pulmonary toilet) will usually lead to resolution of the wound infection, negating the need for local treatment.

SUMMARY

Wound care is an important part of clinical practice in home care. An essential consideration in the provision of quality care in the home is infection control. For specific wound care questions, clinicians should refer to their clinical specialists or enterostomal therapy nurses for standards within their organizations to provide the best care possible.

REVIEW EXERCISES

1. Describe the predictable changes in wound appearance that correspond with each of the three phases of wound healing.
2. Name the three skilled components of covered services under current Medicare requirements.
3. List five quantitative wound observations that reflect progress toward wound closure.
4. What governmental organization published prevention and treatment guidelines for pressure ulcers?
5. The Braden Risk Assessment Tool calculates the risk for _____.
6. When caring for a patient with a pressure ulcer, what observations signal a need for reevaluation of the treatment plan ?
7. Discuss the impact of the patient's nutritional status on wound care and wound care healing.
8. List the Universal Precautions that are specific to wound care.
9. What laboratory tests are helpful in determining wound healing potential?
10. The specialized health professional who serves as a resource for wound and ostomy care is the _____.

RESOURCES

Association for Advancement of Wound Care (AAWC)
320 E. Towsontown Blvd, Suite 207
Baltimore, MD 21286
(410)321-5557

Agency for Health Care Policy and Research (AHCPR)
Executive Office Center, Suite 501
2101 E. Jefferson Street
Rockville, MD 20852
(800)358-9295

American Urological Association Allied
11512 Allecingie Parkway
Richmond, VA 23235
(804)379-1306

Help for Incontinent People
P.O. Box 544
Union, SC 29379
(803)579-7900

Guidelines for the Prevention and Prediction of Pressure Ulcers
Agency for Health Care Policy and Research
2101 E. Jefferson St., Suite 501
Rockville, MD 20852
(800)358-9295

Guidelines for Treatment of Pressure Ulcers
Agency for Health care Policy and Research
2101 E. Jefferson St., #501
Rockville, MD 20852
(800)358-9295
National Digestive Diseases Education and Information Clearinghouse
1555 Wilson Blvd., Suite 600
Rosslyn, VA 22209
(301)496-9707
National Foundation for Ileitis and Colitis
444 Park Ave. S.
New York, NY 10016
(212)685-3440
United Ostomy Association
36 Executive Park, Suite 120
Irvine, CA 92714-6744
(800)826-0826
Urinary Incontinence Patient Guide
Agency for Health Care Policy and Research
2101 E. Jefferson St., Suite 501
Rockville, MD 20852
(800)358-9295
WOCN Clinical Fact Sheets
WOCN
2755 Bristol St.
Costa Mesa, CA 92626
(714)476-0268
Wound, Ostomy, and Continence Nurses Society (WOCN)
2755 Bristol St.
Costa Mesa, CA 92626
(714)476-0268

REFERENCES
Cuzzell JZ: Wound healing: translating theory into clinical practice, *Dermatol Nurs* 1(2):127-131, 1995.
Medical Data International, Wound Care Market Forecast, Irvine, Calif, 1996.

FOR FURTHER READING
Bryant R: *Acute and chronic wounds,* St. Louis, 1992, Mosby.
Barr JE, Cuzzell J: Wound care clinical pathway: a conceptual model, *Ostomy/Wound Management* 7(42):18-26, 1996.
Cuzzell JZ: Choosing a wound dressing: a systematic approach. In Stotts N, editor: *Clinical issues in critical care,* Philadelphia, 1990, JB Lippincott.
Cuzzell JZ: The right way to culture a wound, *Am J Nurs* 93(5):48-50, 1993.
Cuzzell JZ: Back to basics: test your wound assessment skills, *Am J Nurs* 94(6):34-35, 1994.

Cuzzell J, Krasner D: Wound dressings. In Gogia P, editor: *Clinical wound management,* Thorofare, NJ, 1995, SLACK.

Cuzzell JZ, Stotts N: Trial and error yields to knowledge, *Am J Nurs* 90(10):53-63, 1990.

Hampton B, Bryant R: *Ostomies and continent diversions,* St. Louis, 1992, Mosby.

Krasner D, Cuzzell J: Pressure ulcers. In Gogia P, editor: *Clinical wound management,* Thorofare, NJ, 1995, SLACK.

Krasner D, Cuzzell J: Treatment of pressure ulcers: A new clinical practice guideline from the AHCPR, *DME Review,* 1995, Norwell, Mass, 1995, Benkei Publishing.

Levin M: *The diabetic foot,* ed 5, St. Louis, 1996, Mosby.

Marrelli T: *Handbook of home health standards and documentation guidelines for reimbursement,* St. Louis, 1998, Mosby.

Meyers D: *Client teaching guides for home health care,* Gaithersburg, Md, 1989, Aspen.

Standards of Care: Urinary Incontinence, 1988, International Association for Enterostomal Therapy.

Standards of clinical nursing: 1991, Washington, DC, American Nurses Publishing.

Standards of urologic nursing practice: 1991, Washington DC, American Nurses Publishing.

Stanhope M, Knollmueller R: *Handbook of community and home health nursing: tools for assessment, intervention, and education,* St. Louis, 1992, Mosby.

ONCOLOGY NURSING IN HOME CARE

Marilynn Berendt, RN, BSN, EdM, CD

> *"Cancer is the number two cause of death in the United States, preceded by cardiovascular disease, but estimates indicate that by the year 2000 cancer will become the number one cause of death."*
>
> *American Cancer Society Facts and Figures, 1996*

As of 1996, death from lung cancer is the leading cause of death from cancer in both men and women. Just as trends in the disease are changing, so are the acuity levels of patients, the care settings, and delivery of care models. This chapter reviews some of the changes seen in cancer care in the home setting and offers suggestions on providing quality care for cancer patients at home.

ONCOLOGY CARE: A GROWING PART OF HOME CARE

According to Haylock, nearly 90% of all cancer care is delivered in outpatient settings, which includes home care (Haylock, 1993). In the 1995 Medical Data International Marketing Report forecasters project that revenues for chemotherapy administered at home will see a growth of 13.2% between 1997 to 1998 compared to a growth in hospitals and physician offices.

Nonhospital cancer services or outpatient care include same-day diagnostic services, minor surgery, outpatient chemotherapy and radiation therapy, day hospital, home care, and hospice. According to Yost (1995), one barrier to the receipt of needed care after hospital discharge is a patient's lack of knowledge regarding home health services. Others include a refusal by patients and families for home care service, patient's or family's inability to pay for home care services, and a lack of availability of much-needed home care services in certain areas (i.e., rural areas). Short hospital stays in which rapid discharges give health care professionals little time to assess a patient's ability to care for himself or herself, as well as the strengths of the patient's support system or the home environment to which a patient is returning, are additional reasons for lack of referrals to home care. Yost suggests that the primary barriers to patient use of home care services seem to be related to the capabilities of the health care professionals responsible for discharge planning. The top five complex problems identified among patients who did not receive home care nursing services were as follows:

- Difficulty eating (60%)
- Walking/immobility (33%)
- Breathing (27%)
- Complicated oral medicine regimens (27%)
- Pain control (27%)

Also of note in her report is that 6 of the 15 patients actually refused home care, which illustrates the importance of the discharge planning role in overcoming some of the barriers to home care. The feasibility of home care management must be individually determined by assessing the needs of the patient and the abilities of the patient and family to meet these needs (Yost, 1995).

HISTORY OF ONCOLOGY NURSING

Nurses have historically cared for patients with oncological diseases in varied health care sites, including home care. The Oncology Nursing Certification Corporation (ONCC) was founded in 1984 with the purpose of developing, administering, and evaluating a program for both the generalist and the advanced certification of oncology nurses. The society continues to provide a network of peer support and exchange for registered nurses dedicated to excellence in patient care, teaching, research, administration, and education in the field of oncology (Oncology Nursing Society, 1996a).

The evolution of oncology nursing practice in home care shares major objectives with other care issues for noncancer diagnoses. They include a comprehensive home health care program that involves health promotion and disease prevention, restoration of health, and health maintenance. Home health care also incorporates rehabilitation, long-term care, and care of the dying.

Services for the client with cancer at home may include skilled nursing services, palliative care, home health aides, dietary services, psychosocial care, services of an oncology clinical nurse specialist, speech/physical/occupational therapy, pastoral care, pharmacy, respiratory, home volunteer services, and other services.

DEFINING ONCOLOGY NURSING

Oncology nursing in the home is different from that in other care settings for a variety of reasons. The population, settings, and technical complexities found in the home are especially different.

The Population

Important patient population information for oncology home care includes the following:

- Most people with cancer (57%) are older than 65 years of age; the average age of the caregivers in the home is older than 66 years of age.
- The priority needs and expectations as identified by the nurse may differ from those identified by patients and families.
- For many caregivers the caregiving experience marks the beginning of a serious decline in their own health.
- Caregiver needs may vary according to the geographical location (e.g., urban vs. rural); in some situations the family/caregivers may have more needs than the patients. These difficulties in providing care to a family member generally fall into the following four dimensions: physical care, psychosocial concerns, role alterations, and financial alterations (Haylock, 1993).

The Setting

Those involved in home care can recite various stories and situations with which they have been faced regarding the condition of many home environments, from unsafe neighborhoods to unstable living conditions. Each situation needs to be reviewed independently, with attention to safety concerns for the patient and the nurse. For this reason, most organizations set minimal acceptance criteria that must be in place for care to be given in the home setting. Additional criteria for some specialty services or products exist. Home infusion and, more specifically, home blood transfusions have specific criteria over and above the usual home care admission criteria. Generic safety concerns and areas for assessment should be reviewed with the family before home care, and recommendations should be made on ways to clear the safety hazards, restrictions, and barriers to safe and effective care. Some of these areas include the overall environment of care; fire and safety prevention; electrical safety; the bathroom, stairs, steps, ramps, kitchen; general safety regarding storage of supplies, sharps, pump care/maintenance, pets/

plants; and emergency phone numbers. Another area of safety is related to medications, their storage, and their effects.

During the initial, comprehensive visit, the home care nurse reviews information, including the Patient Bill of Rights and advanced directives; procures appropriate consents; and completes a wide variety of forms. This may be met with some resistance by the patient and family. It may come at a time when they are unusually tired from their hospital stay and at a time when they want to regain control of their lives. Sometimes patients cannot understand the reason they must answer all the same questions again. They think that, since the hospital has a complete set of their records, the home health care team should have access to it. At a time when the nurse is attempting to establish a trusting relationship, these attitudes can make it more difficult to facilitate this goal.

Technical Complexity

Cancer patients often require infusion services, in addition to chemotherapy and pain management. Eleven of these therapies in decreasing quantitative order of revenues are colony-stimulating factors, antiemetics, home total parenteral nutrition, pain management, erythropoietin, intravenous antibiotics, home enteral nutrition, interleukin-2, alpha interferon, hydration and anti-hypercalcemic therapy (Medical Data International, 1995). The complexity of these therapies requires that nurses working for home care organizations that provide home infusion be highly skilled and have the ability to communicate the essential care issues to patients and caregivers. In addition, patients may require a variety of high-tech procedures in the home, including peripherally inserted central catheter line placement, epidural pain administration, continuous infusion chemotherapy, intraperitoneal chemotherapy, aerosol inhalation treatments, and blood drawing. These procedures require a high level of proficiency, clinical expertise, and demonstrated competence. For these reasons, the organization has added responsibility for proper training and certification of these advanced skills.

NECESSARY SKILLS FOR SUCCESS AS A HOME ONCOLOGY NURSE

Cancer is thought to be at least 100 different diseases, each with unique cellular characteristics. The progression of the disease and subsequent clinical manifestations of advanced disease make the field of oncology nursing one of the most all-encompassing. Technology has contributed in a positive way. Patients are being diagnosed earlier and treated more aggressively, and more cures are being seen than in the past. Although cancer is still thought to be a chronic disease, we are seeing acute care of clients with cancer being treated in the home care setting. To be successful in home care, the nurse must possess a variety of skills to meet the following four goals of caring for the patient with cancer at home, as suggested by Stair and McNally (1990):

1. To assist the patient and family in developing strategies to achieve optimal independence and attain client-identified goals
2. To assist patients in attaining optimal physical and psychosocial status in collaboration with other members of the home care team
3. To assist the patient and family in developing support systems to facilitate a therapeutic environment
4. To assist the individual and family in planning for the future by providing adequate information and support.

Ideally there are several qualities that professional nurses should possess. Some of these qualities include the following:

1. Ability to practice independently with confidence in one's own clinical knowledge and assessment skills
2. Ability to manage all aspects of patient's care throughout the continuum of the health care episode
3. Ability to delegate and supervise others on the home care team (e.g., home health aides) to ensure quality care that is focused to the individual and family and that is within the scope of practice for the caregiver
4. Possess an excellent clinical knowledge base that is specific to needs of the patient population served
5. Proficiency in clinical skills to provide excellent, personalized patient care
6. Ability to teach patients at their level of understanding, using the teaching tools that are appropriate
7. Excellent communication skills to collaborate with patients, families, and other members of the health care team
8. Attention to thoroughness in planning, coordination, implementing, maintaining, and evaluating all aspects of the health status and clinical outcomes of both the patient and the caretaker
9. Ability to provide the caretaker with reassurance, practical support, and emotional support
10. Thorough knowledge of community and national resources for referral to outside services
11. Recognition of the fact that the patient's and caregiver's needs change over time as their condition changes, either improving or worsening, and as they adjust to the home care routine

STANDARDS OF PRACTICE

A variety of organizations have set standards related to care of patients in the home care setting, each unique to their own domain. For example, if a home health agency (HHA) is a Medicare-certified HHA, knowledge of the following is required: Medicare Conditions of Participation, *HHA Manual—Pub. 11* (HCFA) provisions about home care coverage, and the manual section that addresses the correct completion of the Health Care Financing Administration (HCFA) 485 series form (Marrelli, 1998). The HCFA, under the Department of Health and Human Services, publishes revisions to the *HHA Manual—Pub. 11* (HCFA) that must be reviewed regularly to stay current with home care practice coverage.

In 1988 the Joint Commission on Accreditation of Healthcare Organizations (JCAHO) initiated its home care program that was developed to set standards in home care. JCAHO was established in response both to this rapidly growing segment of the health care delivery system and to public policy concerns regarding the potential for poor quality in delivery of home care services. Eligibility for accreditation for home care requires that one of the following be provided either directly or as a contracted agreement:

- Home health services provided by health professionals (i.e., nursing, physical therapy, speech-language pathology, social work, dental, medical, and nutrition counseling)
- Personal care
- Support services
- Pharmaceutical services
- Equipment management
- Clinical respiratory services
- Hospice services

In addition, services must be provided in an individual's place of residence and must be provided on an intermittent or hourly basis. To qualify, the organization applying for accreditation must be formally organized and have been servicing patients for at least 4 months. At least one patient must be active at the time of the survey (Popovich, 1995).

The ONS has published four publications that address Standards of Practice. A list and description of standards is found in Box 13-1.

Each organization sets its own policies and procedures as they relate to the nature of the organization's scope of care. Each must define the role of the registered nurse (RN) in home care. These roles include generalists and specialists such as masters-prepared clinical nurse specialists. No mat-

| BOX 13-1 | **STANDARDS OF ONCOLOGY NURSING PRACTICE** |

Standards of Oncology Nursing Practice includes professional practice standards in the area of oncology nursing and delineates professional performance standards.

Professional Practice Standards
Standard I (Theory)
The oncology nurse applies theoretical concepts as a basis for decisions in practice.
Standard II (Data Collection)
The oncology nurse systematically and continually collects data regarding the health status of the client. The data are recorded, accessible, and communicated to appropriate members of the multidisciplinary team. Data are collected on high-incidence problem areas that include but are not limited to

- Prevention and early detection
- Information
- Coping
- Comfort
- Nutrition
- Protective mechanisms
- Mobility
- Elimination
- Sexuality
- Ventilation
- Circulation

Standard III (Nursing Diagnosis)
The oncology nurse analyzes assessment data to formulate the nursing diagnosis.
Standard IV (Planning)
The oncology nurse develops an outcome-oriented care plan that is individualized and holistic. This plan is based on nursing diagnosis and incorporates preventive, therapeutic rehabilitative, palliative, and comforting nursing actions.
Standard V (Intervention)
The oncology nurse implements the nursing care plan to achieve the identified outcomes for the client.
Standard VI (Evaluation)
The oncology nurse regularly and systematically evaluates the client's responses to interventions to determine progress toward achievement of outcomes and to revise the data base, nursing diagnoses, and plan of care.

Professional Performance Standards
Standard VII (Professional Development)
The oncology nurse assumes responsibility for the professional development and continuing education and contributes to the professional growth of others.

continued

BOX 13-1　**STANDARDS OF ONCOLOGY NURSING**
　　　　　　PRACTICE—cont'd

Standard VIII (Multidisciplinary Collaboration)
The oncology nurse collaborates with the multidisciplinary team in assessing, planning, implementing, and evaluating care.

Standard IX (Ethics)
The oncology nurse uses the code for nurses and the Patient Bill of Rights as guides for ethical decision making in practice.

Standard X (Research)
The oncology nurse contributes to the scientific base of nursing practice and the field of oncology through the review and application of research.

From American Nurses Association, Oncology Nursing Society, 1987.

ter what the role within the organization, the nurse has the responsibility to consider the legal implications and areas of risk management (i.e., identification, reporting, prevention, and control of safety/security hazards in both patients and staff members). The health care provider also has a role in the area of infection control that includes surveillance, reporting, prevention, and control of infection in both patients and staff members in accordance with the Centers for Disease Control and Prevention (CDC) and the Occupational Safety and Health Administration (OSHA) guidelines, which include aseptic procedures, transmitted diseases, isolation precautions, Universal Precautions, personal hygiene, staff health, equipment cleansing/storage and supply handling, transport, and storage.

INFECTION CONTROL AND ONCOLOGY NURSING: MORE IMPORTANT THAN EVER

Infection is the major cause of morbidity and mortality among persons with cancer. Resistance to infection in people with cancer is affected by many interrelated factors, including the cancer itself. The approach of using high-dose chemotherapy, also referred to as dose intensification, can greatly affect the neutrophils and thus make the patient at high risk for overwhelming infection. Neutropenia definitions may vary across settings, but generally may be defined as an absolute neutrophil count (ANC) of less than $1500/mm^3$. The neutrophils are the body's first line of defense against bacterial infections, and the lower the ANC falls, the greater the risk from infection. For example:

ANC $>1000/mm^3$: minimal risk of infection
ANC 500 to $1000/mm^3$: moderate risk of infection

ANC <500/mm^3: severe risk of infection

Infection can be prevented or minimized if the oncology nurse implements various protective interventions. Interventions should be modified as the level of neutropenia changes. Patients with neutropenia need to be protected from actual or potential sources of infection. People who have, or may possibly have, a communicable infection should be screened from any contact with the patient. The patient with neutropenia should avoid crowds and should wear an isolation mask when out of their "protective" hospital or home environment. Depending on the level of neutropenia, the patient may be placed on a low-bacteria diet (antimicrobial) and antibacterial prophylaxis and require the addition of colony-stimulating factors to their treatment regimen (Rostad, 1991).

Mortality rates related to sepsis and septic shock range from 40% to 90%. Estimates indicate that more than 80% of infections in persons with cancer arise from endogenous microbial flora. The most common bacterial pathogens in neutropenic patients are the gram-negative bacilli *(Pseudomonas, Escherichia coli,* and *Klebsiella pneumoniae)* (Haylock, 1992).

Progression from infection to sepsis can take place in a matter of hours. The timeliness of recognition and appropriate intervention may determine the patient's outcome. Neutropenia is the *single-most important factor* in determining the risk for infection and sepsis. This is complicated by the fact that clinical signs and symptoms of infection (i.e., redness, swelling, inflammation, temperature and pus) are absent in the patient with neutropenia because there are no circulating neutrophils that normally produce these symptoms. Self-care instructions should be targeted toward prevention of infection. Handwashing remains the number one defense against the spread of microorganisms. Use of gloves as a part of Universal Precautions does not take the place of thorough handwashing with a dispenser-type antimicrobial soap and drying with disposable paper towels. The nurse should prepare the patient and family for their responsibilities in the home that impact the early recognition and care for the "at risk" cancer patient.

The trend for care of the patient with cancer-related neutropenia is changing. Neutropenia in the person with cancer is no longer an indication for hospitalization; thus many neutropenic patients are in the home setting. Although this environment can be much safer for the patient in terms of absence of hospital-associated pathogens, the patient is at high risk of not detecting and acting on subtle changes in his or her condition, which can place him or her at high risk of morbidity and mortality. For example, development of a fever requires immediate medical assessment and may or may not mean an admission to the hospital, depending on a variety of factors, one of which is the home care organization's neutropenia protocol and its ability to get to the patient's home in less than 2 hours from the time of the first spike in temperature to both assess and culture the patient. Most organizations, unless they have experience in caring for these specialty patients and administering intravenous antibiotics, do not care for neutropenic patients at home. Some specialized organizations care for neutropenic patients at home who have had bone marrow transplants. The continuing care after bone marrow or stem cell transplant includes rapid assessment, blood culturing, and immediate dosing of antimicrobial intravenous therapy. Care of this patient population at home is not a universal practice. However, this "cutting-edge" practice is changing rapidly as home care organizations change their practice focus to care for more acutely ill populations. One can see that care in this patient population demands a highly skilled and knowledgeable group of nurses and pharmacists to effectively meet the needs of this complex, fragile patient population.

THE NURSING PROCESS

Care given to patients should not differ across the different practice settings, whether the care is delivered in the hospital, in the ambulatory setting, or at home. Application of the nursing process (i.e., assessment, planning, implementation and evaluation) in home care should include the following:

Assessment
Patient History

It is necessary to include the following in each patient's history (Stair and McNally, 1990):

1. Primary site of the tumor, including stage/grade, type, and site
2. Site(s) of metastasis
3. Past and present treatment(s), dates, and response
4. Risk factors: age, gender, environmental exposure, and life-style that contribute to further risk
5. Other medical conditions
6. Chief complaint, including severity (location, pattern, quality, quantity), temporality (onset, duration, frequency, precipitators), and alleviating factors
7. Medication history and current profile

Physical Assessment

Initial physical assessment should include the following (Belcher, 1992):

1. Vital signs: To establish a baseline, vital signs should include temperature, pulse, respiratory rate and blood pressure in both arms, and height and weight whenever possible. Pain is considered part of vital signs and should be assessed in detail during every home visit.

2. Neurological status: Assess for level of consciousness, orientation (person, place and time $\times 3$); pupils equally round, reactive to light (PERRL); neuromuscular function (assess gait for steadiness and extremities for tremors); ask the patient or family if personality changes, seizures, headache, intermittent vertigo, syncope, ataxia, altered reflexes, sudden sensory/motor losses or episodes of unconsciousness, or paralysis has occurred.

3. Respiratory status: Observe rate, rhythm, movement of chest, symmetry, use of accessory muscles; auscultate breath sounds both anteriorly and posteriorly, listening for rales (crackling sounds heard on inspiration generally indicative of fluid) and rhonchi (wheezing sounds heard on expiration generally indicative of obstruction); assess skin and mucous membranes for color; observe respirations while patient is moving about to assess for dyspnea on exertion and elicit whether patient complains of cough; presence of sputum (amount, color); and if the patient has chest pain or tightness (including number of pillows used at night). Monitor use of oxygen therapy, including how many liters per minute and delivery system and supplies.

4. Cardiovascular status: Inspect anterior chest for thrills/heaves; auscultate apical rate and rhythm, abnormal sounds or murmurs and arterial palpation (i.e., rate, rhythm, intensity-carotid, brachial, femoral, and dorsal pedis).

5. Musculoskeletal status: Assess for edema/swelling, masses, lower-extremity edema and range-of-motion loss and ask patient if he or she has pain/tenderness in joints/bones, including what makes it worse and better.

6. Head/neck status: Assess for asymmetry of face (at rest and with movement); abnormal protrusion of eyes, drainage from eyes, ears, nose or mouth; presence of dentition and lesions; tracheal deviation; and presence of masses/nodules. Ask if patient has noticed any deficit in hearing vision, taste, smell, swallowing, and presence of pain.

7. Gastrointestinal status: Auscultate bowel sounds in all four quadrants, observe for evidence of ascites/masses, elicit when last bowel movement was, establish normal elimination pattern and if the patient has nausea, vomiting, anorexia, bleeding, recent weight loss/gain and amount, pain, and special diet (if any).

8. Genitourinary status: Elicit whether the patient has urgency, burning/pain on urination, flank pain, hesitation, or incontinence; if a catheter is in place, the color and clarity of urine should be observed.

9. Skin: Assess for color, warmth, moisture, integrity, turgor, lesions (including moles), rashes, scaly patches/plaques, discolorations, ulcerations, and abrasions/cuts; elicit whether the patient has itching or easy bruising/petechiae/bleeding.

10. Hematological: Inspect for pallor, petechiae, purpura, cranial nerve dysfunction, gingival enlargement, hepatomegaly, splenomegaly, and lymphadenopathy; palpate for areas of tenderness, masses, enlargement of sternum, lymph nodes, liver and spleen.

11. Pain: Evaluate pain every visit using a standardized assessment tool. Monitor pain management, medications, and successful relief measures. Pain is the fifth vital sign.

Ongoing Clinical Assessments

A physical assessment, including all vital signs, should be conducted and recorded every visit by the RN, especially with acutely ill patients. If the patient is receiving home infusion therapy, key areas per type of therapy that should be assessed include the following:

1. Total parenteral nutrition (TPN)
   - Complete vital signs, including weight and temperature
   - Lung sounds to assess for signs of fluid overload
   - Heart sounds and pulses to assess for signs of fluid overload
   - Skin, hair, and nails to assess for signs of mineral deficiency
   - Vascular access device for signs of infection
2. Hydration
   - Vital signs, including orthostatic blood pressure and pulse, weight, and temperature
   - Heart and lung sounds to assess for signs of fluid overload
   - Skin turgor and mucous membrane assessment
3. Antibiotics
   - Vital signs, including temperature
   - Infectious site assessment for response to therapy
   - Gastrointestinal assessment to assess for signs of toxicity such

as diarrhea or anorexia
- Skin assessment to assess for rash or itching indicative of allergic reaction

4. Chemotherapy
   - Complete vital signs, including temperature and weight
   - Assess for gastrointestinal side effects
   - Assess skin for bleeding, bruising, and fatigue indicative of myelosuppression

5. Pain management
   - Assessed every visit and managed through patient's course of care
   - Neurological assessment
   - Evidence of weight loss related to anorexia
   - Evidence of constipation related to narcotic use
   - Evidence of pain control or lack of with the use of a pain scale

Functional Status

A functional assessment should define the type and amount of assistance required to meet the goal of the home care interventions. For example, if the goal of home care is to promote or maintain the patient's optimal functional ability, a baseline of the current activity status should be ascertained for a basis of comparison. A variety of performance scales are used in oncology that measure function as it relates to mobility. The performance status of the patient is an important measure to assess at each encounter with the patient, whether it is in person or over the telephone. The scale provides a baseline measure to which the nurse can compare what he or she is hearing or seeing in the patient and serves as a clinical indicator of improvement or decline in function. The oldest measurement scale, named after Dr. Karnofsky, dates back to 1948 and is widely used today in combination with the Zubrod rating scale (Table 13-1) (Oncology Nursing Society, 1996c). Each organization should develop or use tools according to its preference, although there are commonly used scales that are excellent and widely used. The HCFA OASIS tool is a data set to measure patient progress toward outcomes (see Appendix).

Physical Care Tasks

To determine the needs of the patient, one must be sure to include an assessment of what specific care tasks are to be performed; who will perform the tasks and how; and what equipment, assist devices, and supplies will be needed. Stair and McNally (1990) suggest that one useful way to prioritize these tasks in the oncology patient at home is to correlate the physical care tasks using the ONS standards framework,

TABLE 13-1 PERFORMANCE STATUS SCALE

ZUBROD RATING	GENERAL CATEGORY	KARNOFSKY PERCENT	SPECIFIC PERFORMANCE
0	Able to carry on normal activity; no special care needed	100	Normal; no complaints; no evidence of disease
		90	Able to carry on normal activity; minor signs or symptoms of disease
		80	Normal activity with effort; some signs or symptoms of disease
1	Unable to work; able to live at home and to care for most personal needs; a varying amount of assistance needed	70	Care for self; unable to carry on normal activity or do active work
		60	Occasional assistance; able to care for most of needs
		50	Considerable assistance and frequent medical care
3	Unable to care for self; equivalent of institutional or hospital care; disease may be progressing rapidly	40	Disabled; special care and assistance
		30	Severely disabled; hospitalization; death not imminent
		20	Very sick; hospitalization necessary
4	Completely disabled	10	Moribund; fatal processes progressing rapidly
5		0	Dead

From Karnofsky DA et al; The use of nitrogen mustards in the palliative treatment of carcinoma with particular reference to bronchogenic carcinoma, *Cancer* 1:634, 1948. In Otto S: *Oncology nursing,* St. Louis, 1991, Mosby. Adapted with permission.

which includes care issues related to comfort, nutrition, protective mechanisms, mobility, elimination, sexuality, and ventilation (American Nurses Association, Oncology Nursing Society, 1987).

Caregiver/Family Assessment

Emphasis needs to be placed on the characteristics of the caregiver in the home as they relate to the ability, availability, and willingness to care for the patient. The nurse must recognize that many factors such as gender, marital status, education, work status outside the home and the caregiver's own health status all may impact the way he or she delivers care. Because of shorter hospital stays, nurses must begin the educational process early and continue to assess the caregiver's needs, both psychological and informational, after discharge. Linking families to volunteer and professional community service agencies is key. The nurse should also consider exactly how much the caregiver knows about the patient's condition and the expected outcomes, the responsibilities he or she is assuming, and their knowledge/understanding of when to report various symptoms to the health care team (Hileman, Lackey, and Hassanein, 1992). A detailed assessment of the family and the roles and relationships of family members is essential whenever the nurse is attempting to maximize the available resources in the home.

Psychosocial Assessment

Many factors enter into the psychosocial makeup of an individual, which makes this assessment at times more complex than the physical assessment. People all relate differently and have individual reactions to the diagnosis of cancer; therefore the nurse should attempt to find out what the diagnosis means to her or his patient and how the patient views the outcome. Frequently the manner in which people have handled other stresses in their life can provide a clue to how they handle this situation. It seems that most persons faced with a new diagnosis seem to experience the greatest stress during the work-up phase when they experience a tremendous fear of the "unknown." Individuals move at their own speed toward acceptance of what the reality of the situation is, and some never accept it. Overwhelmingly, patients express the loss of control as being the one thing that causes the helpless feeling many have. Allowing the patients to be a part of the plan of care can help to restore a small part of the helplessness they feel. The nurse should assess the patient's mood/affect, which may change from visit to visit and the causative factors, which very well may have a psychiatric or organic cause, and determine how the mood/affect will impact the person's functioning (i.e., role performance, sexual functioning, functional performance status, and activities of daily living).

The caregiver may also have health problems and/or dysfunctional relationships before the illness that may have been strained to the extent that he or she cannot or will not assume caregiving tasks. In this instance the nurse needs to explore outside support systems and community resources for help.

Environmental Assessment

Environmental assessment is an important area and one that can have great impact on the determination of whether the patient can be safely cared for at home. In general, safety areas to assess in the home should include general safety, bathroom safety, patient care safety, telephone safety, fire safety, medical equipment, supplies/drugs/gases, and waste disposal. Issues related to mobility inside the home, mobility outside the home (safety of the neighborhood), usual living arrangements, and the physical layout of the residence are additional areas to consider. The Omaha Classification System (OCS) developed by the Visiting Nurse Association of Omaha is an attempt to list client problems that nurses may encounter in various community health settings. This system covers four areas/domains: environmental, psychosocial, physiological, and health behaviors. For example, Domain 1, environmental, covers material resources and physical surroundings both internal and external to the client, home, neighborhood, and broader community. Within this classification system are subgroups for each of the following five areas: income, sanitation, residence, neighborhood, and workplace safety and an "other" category. The following is an example of elements found under the residence category (Humphrey, 1994):

- Health promotions
- Potential deficit
- Deficit
    Structurally unsound
    Inadequate heating/cooling
    Steep stairs
    Inadequate/obstructed exits/entries
    Cluttered living space
    Unsafe storage of dangerous objects/substances
    Unsafe throw rugs
    Inadequate safety devices
    Presence of lead-based paint
    Unsafe gas/electrical appliances

Inadequate/crowded living space
Homeless
Other

Financial Assessment

Because of the chronicity and longevity of life for many people with cancer, in addition to the rising health care costs, it is little wonder that more than 50% of families expressed the need for financial assistance or counseling. Stair and McNally report that an early study of the impact of home care indicated that 15% of families experienced great financial disruption, which included accepting welfare benefits, selling personal property, or accruing numerous unpaid bills and great debt (Stair and McNally, 1990). Many of the costs covered by third-party payors while the patient is hospitalized are not covered at home. The reimbursement issues and limits should be explored before the client is placed on home health service, and options should be discussed with the patient, family, physician, and social service.

Nursing Diagnosis

Using and analyzing the assessment data gained, the nurse then formulates nursing diagnoses that serve as a framework for planning, intervening, and evaluating the health concerns of clients. NANDA nursing diagnoses are often based in home care to identify patient/family problems. Readers are referred to the *Handbook of Home Health Standards and Documentation Guidelines for Reimbursement* (Marrelli, 1998), which integrates ICD-9 codes and nursing diagnoses by patient problem.

Care Planning

On receiving the referral for home care services, a plan of care is determined based on the physician's orders, keeping in mind the goals of the intervention. The initial visit includes aspects of care and teaching that need to be completed before any subsequent home care visit. This initial visit is important because it is the one that patients and families will base their initial impressions on and influences the ongoing experience. Appropriate supportive referrals to other home care providers/disciplines need to be initiated in a timely basis. Other activities include all areas of assessments, determination of the frequency of visits, planning for emergencies, and developing realistic patient and family outcomes.

Implementation (Intervention)

Determination of the division of labor such as care to be provided by the nurse and other health care professionals versus care to be provided by the family/caregiver needs to be defined. Patients and families need to know the role of the nurse (and other members of the health care team) so they know exactly what to expect from whom. A part of this process should include ways to minimize costs by working around what resources the family may have in place in the home already. Methods for minimizing costs such as teaching patients/caregivers and how to use supplies in a cost-effective manner should be introduced.

Evaluation

Evaluation is the last important component of the nursing process used in home care. The ONS *Standards of Oncology Nursing Practice* and the ANA *Standards of Home Health Nursing Practice* serve as useful models. Communication with all members of the health care team, including the patient/family, allows the nurse to evaluate the results of nursing care/interventions and helps her or him recognize the need to develop alternate plans when appropriate. Involving the patient in the evaluation of goal attainment and revision of the care plan is as essential as it was at the first home visit.

Documentation Considerations

Documentation is key in that it is a legal record that demonstrates the care provided and the patient's response to the care, provides an objective source for the organization's licensing/accreditation, shows that the current standards of care are maintained, meets the documentation requirements for Medicare and other payors, and is the primary foundation for the evaluation of care on which decisions can be made in a timely manner (Marrelli, 1998a). It is the role of the professional nurse to validate the need for skilled care and back it up with effective documentation. This is especially important so that care can be evaluated on an ongoing basis and interventions can be modified on a timely basis if needed. Patients that nurses see in home care today are more complex than ever, and quality (not quantity) documentation is the pivotal record that reflects patients' progress (or lack of), their response to care given, and their understanding of patient education issues.

PAIN MANAGEMENT IN THE HOME
Assessment

A detailed assessment, including physical examination, functional assessment, psychosocial assessment, and diagnostic evaluation should be carried out. Assessment should include a qualitative and a quantitative component of the patient in pain (U.S. Department of Health and Human Services, 1994). The Agency for Health Care Policy and Research (AHCPR) has developed guidelines for clinical practice and a variety of assessment tools that have become universally used. The assessment should include questioning the patient to determine a qualitative assessment of associated symptoms that are self-reported by the patient such as mood, fatigue, and relations with other people (Figure 13-1) (U.S. Department of Health and Human Services, 1994). The qualitative assessment component includes determining intensity of pain, which is helpful in that each person involved in managing the pain is using the same method for measuring the extent and outcome of the intervention for pain (U.S. Department of Health and Human Services, 1994). Assessment should be at regular intervals after initiation of medication, at each new report of pain, and at a suitable interval after the intervention (e.g., 15 to 30 minutes after intravenous medication and 1 hour after oral administration). The goal for pain control (i.e., where he or she wants to be on the pain scale) should be identified by the patient. If the patient identifies the goal of maintaining the level of pain under a "5" on the scale, that gives all the providers a set goal. It also gives them a qualitative measurement for reaching the desired outcome. Families/caregivers and patients should be taught in the use of pain management principles and the use of the monitoring tool and pain scale.

Nursing Diagnosis

When caring for the patient with cancer-related pain, the following nursing diagnoses may apply:

Alteration in:
    Comfort
    Mobility
    Coping
    Elimination
    Protective mechanisms
    Home management
    Anxiety
    Fear
    Fatigue
    Social isolation
    Hopelessness
    Others, based on the patient's unique condition

Brief Pain Inventory (Short Form)

Date: _____ / _____ / _____

Time: _____

Name: _____ _____ _____
             Last   First   Middle Initial

1. Throughout our lives, most of us have had pain from time to time (such as minor headaches, sprains, and toothaches). Have you had pain other than these everyday kinds of pain today? 1. Yes 2. No

2. On the diagram, shade in the areas where you feel pain. Put an X on the area that hurts the most.

Right   Left   Left   Right

3. Please rate your pain by circling the one number that best describes your pain at its **worst** in the past 24 hours.

0	1	2	3	4	5	6	7	8	9	10
No pain								Pain as bad as you can imagine		

4. Please rate your pain by circling the one number that best describes your pain at its **least** in the past 24 hours.

0	1	2	3	4	5	6	7	8	9	10
No pain								Pain as bad as you can imagine		

5. Please rate your pain by circling the one number that best describes your pain on the **average.**

0	1	2	3	4	5	6	7	8	9	10
No pain								Pain as bad as you can imagine		

FIGURE 13-1 A pain inventory form helps health care providers document the qualitative assessment of associated symptoms reported by the patient.

6. Please rate your pain by circling the one number that tells how much pain you have **right now.**

0	1	2	3	4	5	6	7	8	9	10
No pain									Pain as bad as you can imagine	

7. What treatments or medications are you receiving for your pain?

_____

8. In the past 24 hours, how much **relief** have pain treatments or medications provided? Please circle the one percentage that most shows how much relief you have received.

0%	10%	20%	30%	40%	50%	60%	70%	80%	90%	100%
No relief									Complete relief	

9. Circle the one number that describes how, during the past 24 hours, **pain has interfered** with your:

A. General activity

0	1	2	3	4	5	6	7	8	9	10
Does not interfere									Completely interferes	

B. Mood

0	1	2	3	4	5	6	7	8	9	10
Does not interfere									Completely interferes	

C. Walking ability

0	1	2	3	4	5	6	7	8	9	10
Does not interfere									Completely interferes	

D. Normal work (includes both work outside the home and housework)

0	1	2	3	4	5	6	7	8	9	10
Does not interfere									Completely interferes	

E. Relations with other people

0	1	2	3	4	5	6	7	8	9	10
Does not interfere									Completely interferes	

F. Sleep

0	1	2	3	4	5	6	7	8	9	10
Does not interfere									Completely interferes	

G. Enjoyment of life

0	1	2	3	4	5	6	7	8	9	10
Does not interfere									Completely interferes	

FIGURE 13-1, cont'd For legend see opposite page. *(From Charles S. Cleeland, Pain Research Group, Department of Neuro-Oncology, University of Texas, MD Anderson Cancer Center, Houston.)*

Care Planning

Planning follows assessment and identification of nursing diagnosis. In the home the patient/caregiver must understand the goal of the intervention (i.e., pain scale under 5) and agree to the plan. They should be a part of the plan for managing side effects such as constipation, nausea/vomiting, sedation, urinary retention, dizziness, and respiratory depression.

Intervention

Choose an appropriate analgesic for the type and level of pain. Schedule an around-the-clock routine to achieve a steady state of analgesia instead of PRN. The home care nurse should also obtain an order for any "break-through" pain before it is needed so that it is available for patient use at his or her discretion. The World Health Organization has illustrated a three-step analgesic ladder for choosing the appropriate medication type to match the type of pain, with the top of the ladder being the goal of freedom from pain (Marrelli, 1998a). For example:

- If pain exists, administer a nonopioid medication with or without an adjuvant drug.
- If pain persists or increases, administer a weak opioid with or without a nonopioid medication and with or without an adjuvant drug.
- If pain persists, use a strong opioid with or without a nonopioid drug and with or without an adjuvant drug.

Use of nonpharmacological (e.g., massage, heat, cold, distraction) interventions should be included in the plan. Last, patient and family education is an integral component of the interventions for home pain management. The patient and the providers both have responsibility for the pain control plan. Areas to be covered include causes of pain; anticipated outcomes; what to expect and what to report to the physician or nurse; and information about refills, drug interactions and dosing, and side effects and how to prevent them both verbally and in writing.

Evaluation

Caregivers need to establish the effectiveness of the present plan, need for revision, patient's level of satisfaction with the pain control, presence of side effects, and tolerance to the medications. Reassessment at regular intervals and use of patient diaries or flow charts can be useful in documenting pain relief (Figure 13-2) (U.S. Department of Health and Human Services, 1994). It is the professional nurse's moral, ethical, and legal responsibility to include patient and family education about pain and its management in the treatment plan.

Pain Management Log

Pain management log for

_____

Please use this pain assessment scale to fill out your pain control log:

0	1	2	3	4	5	6	7	8	9	10

No pain   Worst pain

Date	Time	How severe is the pain?	Medicine or non-drug pain control method	How severe is the pain after 1 hour?	Activity at time of pain

FIGURE 13-2 The pain management log is yet another tool that health care providers can use to effectively document a patient's pain relief. *(From Charles S. Cleeland, Pain Research Group, Department of Neuro-Oncology, University of Texas, MD Anderson Cancer Center, Houston.)*

SUMMARY

Oncology care accounts for a large part of home care practice today. Hospice and home care organizations and nurses care for these complex oncology patients with multifaceted needs. The well-prepared, experienced, and competent oncology nurse can contribute positively to the patient's comfort level and to more positive and pain-free patient outcomes. Throughout the years, patients have taught their nurses very valuable lessons and will continue to do so as health care providers listen. Home health providers will continue to learn more about oncology care and pain management as they listen to the experiences of other providers and to the care needs of their patients.

REVIEW EXERCISES

1. The qualities of the nurse caring for the client with cancer in the home are the same as those required for all home care patients. (True or False)
2. Neutropenia is defined as an absolute neutrophil count of less than 15,000/mm³. (True or False)
3. *Staphylococcus aureus* is the most common bacterial pathogen seen in the neutropenic patient. (True or False)
4. Fever in the neutropenic patient is an ominous sign and needs *immediate* intervention. (True or False)
5. Performance status refers to the ability of the patient to perform work-related tasks at the same level as before the cancer diagnosis. (True or False)
6. A grade 4 toxicity of the gastrointestinal system indicates that the diarrhea is minimal and needs to be monitored. (True or False)
7. Nurses caring for patients with cancer pain are legally obligated to include patient and family education about pain control measures. (True or False)
8. The AHCPR was established and primarily developed to set standards for practice such as those for pain management, incontinence care, and cardiac rehabilitation. (True or False)
9. Pain management is a key component of every visit/intervention with home care patients. (True or False)

RESOURCES

Agency for Health Care Policy and Research (AHCPR). (800)358-9295.
American Cancer Society. (800)227-2345.
Fact Sheets on Anticancer Drugs. Fact sheets are available for approximately 55 drugs
   used to treat cancer. These fact sheets are two-sided: one side is in English, the
   other is in Spanish. The sheets list information about each drug related to possible

HALLMARKS OF EFFECTIVE CARE FOR EARLY MATERNITY NURSING PRACTICE

The hallmarks of effective care for early maternity nursing practice include the following:

1. Nurses practicing in this specialty area need education and experience in addition to the standard Medicare-focused home care orientation. There are varying models for obtaining this expertise. Hospital-based home care programs may cross-train their inpatient postpartum and newborn nursery nurses to home care operations and documentation. Other organizations send interested home care nurses into the inpatient postpartum and newborn nursery areas to gain the needed experience. Home health aides also need additional education and supervision related to these specialized services. Home health aides may spend a defined amount of shifts in the inpatient area learning, observing, and caring for postpartal new mothers and infants.

2. There must be clear role differentiation concerning the care to be provided. Because there are various models of postpartum home care, there are varying roles. If you are unsure about the scope of your responsibilities or the care interventions that should be provided, ask your supervisor.

3. There must be a well-defined, research-based standardized care plan of activities, assessment areas, and teaching to be provided to each patient. Examples include whether you support and teach breast feeding or if the organization has a nurse lactation specialist who visits every new mother and the primary nurse reinforces that plan. Some programs have standardized educational tools for new mothers and infants that are initiated in the hospital and continue to be used at home.

4. Supplies are different in this specialty. The contents of the nursing bag will have additional and different supplies. These may include pediatric (and adult) stethoscopes, bulb syringe, laboratory supplies and slips for newborn metabolic screening tests, disposable measuring tape, and others such as A&D ointment. It is also important to know whether your program has well-calibrated (accurate) infant scales that can be transported safely. Phenylketonuria (PKU) sticks look easy until the nurse encounters the new mother who is upset at hearing her new infant cry. It is important to have supervised education about these specialized skills and activities.

5. A background and/or interest in pediatrics and/or perinatal nursing is very helpful. Extensive history-taking, two physical examinations, strong detail-oriented assessment skills, multifaceted documentation data elements, and communicating with pediatricians and obstetricians are components of care that are very different from adult home care practice. Certification, continuing education, and additional training are all needed in this growing specialty.

6. Nurses need an outcome-oriented focus toward assisting patients in achieving predetermined, measurable goals of care. Common outcomes for this special patient population include the collection of adequate blood sample for infant screening, observation and assessment of the mother and newborn, identification of problems and possible complications necessitating further intervention, and mother being able to provide care to infant safely and adequately and knowing where to call for assistance.

CARE PLANNING IN POSTPARTAL CARE

Care planning is initiated on referral, and data are collected during the extensive initial assessment visit. For the mother this includes her history and a physical assessment particularly related to cardiac, respiratory, and genitourinary systems. Other important areas include baseline physiological data, assessment of breast-feeding skills, and comfort level. The infant assessment may include weight, neurological assessment, and feeding activity.

Common nursing diagnoses that may be appropriate and identified when creating the plan of care include activity intolerance, anxiety, body image disturbance, breast-feeding–related nursing diagnoses, caregiver role strain, constipation, coping, fatigue, fear, family processes altered, fluid volume deficit, infection, injury, knowledge deficit, mobility, nutrition, pain, parenting, role performance changes, sexuality patterns, skin integrity, sleep, and urinary elimination.

Because the initial assessment creates the basis for the care and care planning, it is important that the interventions be standardized across all patients with a given diagnoses, yet individualized based on the composite of problems and actions needed as identified on admission and as care continues and outcomes are achieved.

Whatever the interventions, all activities are ultimately directed toward self-care health maintenance and patient education, with teaching activities related to care of self and the newborn. The nurse's role in these activities is key to meeting patient and organizational goals.

DOCUMENTATION IN EARLY MATERNITY PROGRAMS

For nurses new to home care, documentation can be a problematic area. As in other home care specialties, the documentation is the basis for coverage, quality, or denial of payment. At some level our clinical documentation (i.e., what it "looks like") represents our care and our program to any state survey, managed care nurse reviewer, or other interested party.

Education related to documentation and the importance and format may consist of a didactic component and hands-on practice in completing the required documentation. Many forms that have been developed for these early discharge programs are designed in checklist formats. Not only does this design streamline time spent on clinical documentation, it allows clear, well-defined parameters to be able to quantify and review data. Hence, when there is consensus on terms and accurate completion, checklist forms allow information to be collated. Deming, the father of quality improvement initiatives is quoted as saying: "in God we trust, all others must have data." With this in mind, clear forms and data create the environment for comparing "apples to apples." For this reason, home care is moving away from lengthy narrative notes; nurses must be able to quantify data and attribute their interventions to positive patient outcomes. Whatever the format of the forms at the organization, they must be completed accurately at the time of the assessment or when other care is provided.

SUMMARY

Although the actual models and services vary, home care has been demonstrated to be a safe and cost-effective alternative to hospitalization for new mothers and infants. This specialized care must be skillfully provided by clinicians with this background and interest to safely provide the best care. In addition, we must quantify our activities and interventions to be able to demonstrate to payors and consumers, our customer of care, that we can provide the best care at the best price and with improved outcomes.

REVIEW EXERCISES

1. List three of the skills needed to be a successful perinatal nurse in home care.
2. Identify one association that has standards related to this specialty.
3. Describe the relationship between effective documentation and data collection.

4. What areas need assessment on these special patients?
5. Describe three models of organizations that provided early maternity care.
6. List two reasons why there has been growth in this home care specialty.
7. Describe some of the areas of knowledge that a nurse desiring to transfer to this specialty should have/develop.
8. Explain the statement, "We may have come full circle."
9. List three types of specialized home care maternity or infant programs.
10. Describe the importance of clinical documentation in home care generally and in this specialty area specifically.

REFERENCES

Evans C: Postpartum home care in the United States, *J Obstetric Gynecol Neonatal Nurs* 24(2):180-186, 1995.

Jones D, Collins B: The nursing management of women experiencing preterm labor: clinical guidelines and why they are needed, *J Obstet Gynecol Neonatal Nurs* 25(7):569-591, 1996.

FOR FURTHER READING

Brooten D. (1995). Perinatal Care Across the Continuum: Early discharge and nursing home follow-up, *J Perinatal Neonatal Nurs* 9(1):38-44, 1995.

Brooten D, et al: Early discharge and home care after unplanned cesarean birth: nursing care time, *J Obstet Gynecol Neonatal Nurs* 25:(7)595-600, 1996.

Christian A: Clinical nurse specialists: creating new programs for Neonatal Home Care, *J Perinatal Neonatal Nurs* 10(1):54-63, 1996.

Evans C: Postpartum care in the United Sates, *J Obstet Gynecol Neonatal Nurs* 24(2):180-186, 1995.

Goodwin L: Essential program components for perinatal home care, *J Perinatal Neonatal Nurs* 23(8):667-673, 1994.

Mendler V, et al: The conception, birth, and infancy of an early discharge program, *MCN* 21(5):241-246, 1996.

Shapiro C: Shortened hospital stay for low-birth-weight infants: nuts and bolts of a nursing intervention project, *J Obstet Gynecol Neonatal Nurs* 24(1):56-62, 1995.

Williams L, Cooper M: Nurse-managed home care, *J Obstet Gynecol Neonatal Nurs* 22(1):25-31, 1992.

Williams L, Koechley Cooper M: Nurse-managed postpartum home care, *J Obstet Gynecol Neonatal Nurs* 22(1):25-31, 1992.

Whaley L, Wong D: *Nursing care of infants and children,* St. Louis, 1996, Mosby.

PEDIATRIC CARE IN HOME CARE

Carolyn Viall, MSN, RN and Mary Jo Savage, MSN, RN, CNS

> *"A hundred years from now it will not matter what my bank account was, the sort of house I lived in, or the kind of car I drove. . .but the world may be different because I was important in the life of a child."*
>
> *Anonymous*

Many nurses in home care provide services to both adult and pediatric patients in the course of their day. Pediatric nurses are essential to the successful implementation of a home care plan. This chapter provides guidelines to the nurse caring for pediatric patients in the home care setting. It provides the pediatric nurse, new to home care, a basis for developing, implementing, and evaluating the care of a pediatric patient in the home setting. For the nurse who has had limited experience with home care, this chapter provides information to assist in a family-centered approach to the care of children and the concepts related to pediatric care.

Pediatric home care has been an aspect of health care for children since the 1700s. There has been a dramatic increase in the use of pediatric home care in the past two decades. Much of home care includes the use of complex medical technology, most of which has increased the survival rate of infants and children who previously would not have been candidates for discharge and home care. The home would not have been considered an intensive care nursery in the 1980s, yet the availability of technology and the need for efficacious delivery of health care has fostered the discharge of patients to the home setting. Infants with birth weights of 500 g are now actively treated, and the increased survival has brought the needs of a (this) new population to the forefront (Hack et al, 1994).

PEDIATRIC HOME CARE: A SPECIAL POPULATION

Approximately 10 million children with chronic diseases live in the United States. Many require some type of episodic or chronic monitoring of their health on an outpatient basis. The improved survival of these children has not only brought a complex patient population into home care but has raised issues related to the family's abilities to provide care to children with diverse and demanding medical and psychological needs. Not so many years ago, it was unusual to transfer a patient from an intensive care unit with a central venous catheter to a general nursing unit in a hospital. The home care nurse now sees pediatric patients in the community with even more challenging technologies and therapies.

Emerging Populations

The pediatric population in the home care setting is varied. Patients may require short-term monitoring and care for acute episodes or may need long-term intervention and evaluation for multiple, complex health care problems. A growing number of neonates who once remained in the hospital for an extended period of time are now being cared for at home. Home care visits for pediatric patients may involve various skills, including teaching or reinforcement of teaching; hands-on intervention (e.g., injections, wound care); monitoring of the child's response to therapy; evaluation of compliance with the treatment plan; or other skilled nursing services.

Diagnoses for Pediatric Home Care Patients

The diagnoses for pediatric home care patients are varied. Many patients with chronic diseases need home care follow-up as their survival is improved and as their care becomes more complex. Premature or low-birth-weight infants are surviving respiratory problems as a result of the development of drug therapy to treat immature lungs; however, their long-term treatment may require monitoring or intervention for tracheal stenosis, apnea, or bronchial pulmonary dysplasia. Congenital cardiac diseases have resulted in a number of children who need home care services for an extended period of time based on the severity of their disease. Spina bifida patients have multiple needs, and their improved survival also requires the health care team to facilitate improving their function and quality of life. Other chronic diseases that frequently are referred to home care are cancer, asthma, human immunodeficiency virus/acquired immune deficiency syndrome (HIV/AIDS), chronic renal failure, diabetes, cerebral palsy, cystic fibrosis, and muscular dystrophy.

Infusion therapies are now common for a host of disease states in pediatric patients, including parenteral nutrition, enteral feedings, antibiotics, colony-stimulating factors, transfusion therapy, chemotherapy, and pain control (see Chapter 17). The equipment used in home care includes infusion pumps, monitors (e.g., electrocardiogram, apnea), suction machines, phototherapy lights, ventilators, and nebulizers. This high-technology equipment may be in addition to any number of home medical equipment (HME) needs usually associated with home care patients such as wheelchairs and hospital beds. The availability of high-technology equipment in the home has been a contributing factor to the growth of pediatric home care.

BENEFITS OF PEDIATRIC HOME CARE

The benefits of home care for the pediatric population are experienced by the patient, family, health care team, and payors. The cost-effectiveness of providing most treatments and therapies is generally less than in the acute setting. Initial costs of arranging home health care services may be high as resources and equipment are put in place to safely care for the child. This is particularly true for the complex patient. These costs usually decrease over time as the family becomes more familiar and comfortable with the technology and responsibility for caring for their child at home (Cabin, 1985). Reducing hospital readmissions is a primary goal of third party payors, and the outcomes of home care intervention should also be focused on reducing recidivism (Hill, Thompson, 1994).

The child's development can be promoted in the home care environment. The goal is to provide a setting that will most likely facilitate as normal a life-style as possible. Coordinating a plan to promote normal family relationships is central to promoting growth and development in children. The difficulties of establishing this environment in conjunction with the complexities of care can sometimes seem overwhelming for the home care nurse and family. Effective communication, care coordination, and teamwork are essential components to meet this goal.

FAMILY-CENTERED CARE

The knowledge and expertise of the family are the most important considerations in the planning of pediatric home care. Health care professionals may have episodic or long-term encounters with a child; however, everything that is central to a child is based within the context of the family. The definition of the family unit includes multigenerational, single or two-parent, extended, or significant individuals in the child's life. The primary factor is that "family-centered" care is considered the best approach to the child's health care (Ahmann, 1996).

Recognizing family-centered care also requires that one acknowledge the diversity of families and their members. Home care nurses need to incorporate strongly held cultural beliefs and values of families into the plan of care. Failure to do so inhibits communication between the nurse and the family and prevents their working toward a common goal.

A trusting relationship with the family is imperative. It is common for a conflict in authority between the nurse and the family to arise because of the differences in the sources from which their authority is derived. The nurse delivers patient care in the home setting under orders of the physician, whereas the family has their own beliefs in how to care for their child based on their perception of their child's needs. The nurse may know and understand the physician's orders, but the family knows the child. Communication between the nurse and the family is essential to continue to pursue common goals and to clarify and reevaluate the plan of care as conflicts arise. The nurse and the family need to keep the physician informed as to the child's response to care. The child is best served when interventions to accomplish care are mutually agreed upon.

Families may experience anxiety about their own abilities to care for their child. Occasionally this may manifest itself in differences in opinions with the health caregivers caring for their child. It may also affect the parents' ability to perform the necessary tasks to care for their child. Recognition of this anxiety will help the nurse to identify the issues that most concern the family. The nurse can then intervene with appropriate resources and education to address their concerns.

Working effectively with all family members is key to caring for the child. Demonstrating respect for families' time is an important first step in developing trusting relationships with them. Home health professionals can also role model to families by keeping appointments on time. It is important to teach families to be organized by being an example.

The ability to function as a team member and coordinator of care will facilitate communication with the family. Difficulty discerning the boundaries between personal vs. professional relationships may compromise the nurse's successful involvement with the pediatric patient and the family. The nurse can support family relationships by establishing boundaries and continuing to show respect for the values of the family and the role of family members in the care of their child.

The input of parents is paramount to fostering a positive relationship with the family and child. The ability to listen to a parent's concerns about or comments on the child's usual responses can assist in identifying a problem area. Collaboration with the family develops a partnership in which everyone can contribute to the plan of care to achieve the best outcomes.

HOME CARE PLANNING

Initial planning for a patient's discharge should address three questions as to the appropriateness of home care for an individual:

1. Why would the home be the best setting for this patient with his or her particular health care needs?
2. When would discharge take place and what parameters need to be met before discharge to home?
3. Who should be involved in the child's care in the home setting?

Not all pediatric patients necessarily benefit from receiving home care services. Although most patients, particularly children, recover better in the home setting, each patient needs to be assessed for the capabilities of the family and support systems to manage the patient's care. Sometimes this may require delaying a discharge for a period of time until the patient's acuity level decreases in terms of the types or number of services and care needed. The decision to discharge the patient to home should be supported by both the health care team and the family. There should be mutual agreement on the ability to provide care to meet expected outcomes.

In planning a patient's discharge, consideration should be given to the resources available to the patient to provide for continuity of care. The home care plan may need to be modified, depending on the availability of direct caregivers, emergency services, and ancillary services and equipment for the patient. The team of home care personnel involved in the patient's care should be fully informed as to their roles and responsibilities. The family should know the roles of the home care team members and whom to call for particular issues. Clarity for the family and caregivers is essential to reduce confusion and avoid misunderstandings.

A discharge assessment to determine home care needs should be done soon after admission to the hospital. The attitudes of the family toward home care and attendant caregiving responsibilities is necessary to ensure compliance and a partnership with the health care team. A determination of the family's abilities, capabilities, and knowledge of the disease process and plan of care will be instrumental in coordinating the care plan and discharge. The discharge assessment should also include the need for any specialized equipment, teaching of procedures, environmental needs in the home specific to the planned treatment, and availability of caregiving and ancillary services. For some therapies, such as parenteral nutrition or home dialysis, a home visit may be beneficial for the discharge team, home care nurse, and family to anticipate discharge needs. Frequently it

is challenging to adapt a complex medical procedure for the home setting. Successful adaptation to the home environment requires flexibility
and creativity on the part of the health care team. The home care nurse is
instrumental in facilitating this process.

PAYMENT CONSIDERATIONS FOR PEDIATRIC SERVICES

Reimbursement or payment for home care services varies by payor. For
many pediatric patients with chronic diseases, state Medicaid programs
may be the primary insurer. Each state administers the Medicaid program
individually, and coverage criteria will vary according to the specific state
requirements. Many Medicaid programs have initiated managed care programs that have enrolled the individuals in health maintenance organizations (HMO). It is important for home health nurses to understand that
the limits of covered care (e.g., number of visits) are defined by third party
payors or state-funded programs. Nurses need to know the parameters in
which they must function to provide care for their patients and families
(i.e., the amount and type of covered care).

Children's home care services may also be reimbursed under a third-
party payor of a commercial insurance company. Benefits vary according
to individual payors, and home care services are diverse. Deductibles and
co-payments for home care services need to be determined so that the family is aware of any financial impact of the services to be provided.

Many commercial insurance plans offer several insurance products
to their members. Most managed care plans, for example, HMOs and
preferred provider organizations (PPOs), have preferred providers for
services, including home care agencies, HME, diagnostic laboratories,
hospice organizations, and ancillary services. Being aware of the preferred providers for an individual payor will facilitate the discharge
planning process for the health care team and the family. Discussion of
the discharge plan for home care with the case manager representing
the insurance company will assist in expediting discharge planning. Including this case manager as an integral part of the health care team is
an important component of successful discharge planning.

There are special programs in regions of the country that will also
provide coverage of some specific services, particularly on an outpatient basis. Some states have Crippled Children's Services programs,
although it may be identified by another name, that may provide some
reimbursement for home care. Depending on the patient's primary disease state, there are also disease-specific organizations (e.g., American
Cancer Society or Cystic Fibrosis Foundation) that also may provide
services, supplies, or reimbursement for specific items. Some organiza-

tions also offer newsletters and support groups locally that provide additional information on available resources, in addition to opportunities for linkage and support among patients and families. Other funding programs include Supplemental Security Income and Women's, Infant, and Children programs. At the end of this chapter is a partial listing of some of these resource organizations.

PEDIATRIC PLAN OF CARE

The home care plan should encompass all aspects of care that are necessary to meet the expected outcomes. Goals should be established for the home care plan that are realistic and attainable and that provide a time frame for completion. The services necessary to meet the patient care goals should be outlined by the team and the family. The team includes not only the inpatient staff (case manager, staff nurses, discharge planner, clinical nurse specialist, ancillary health care professionals), but also the physician, home care nurse, and other ancillary outpatient providers. Specific criteria should be established for providers to meet in order to provide care to the patient.

The home care plan should address specific care to be provided, patient/family teaching or reinforcement of teaching needed, roles of caregivers, responsibilities of providers and family, and monitoring parameters. Provision for ongoing monitoring and follow-up is also a necessary component to the plan. As with any intervention, there should be some method to evaluate its effectiveness. If the patient is not attaining expected outcomes, the plan should be evaluated and modified as necessary, according to the patient's progress.

PEDIATRIC HOME CARE NURSE SKILLS

The pediatric home care nurse has a number of skills that she or he brings to the child needing home care. Since the needs of children who are ill may be complex, pediatric home care nurses must be able to completely assess pediatric growth and development. Well-developed physical assessment skills are needed by the home care nurse to differentiate nuances of abnormal findings or changes from the patient's baseline. Since the physical findings may vary from one age group to another, the home care nurse must know physical assessment norms and skills across the life span. Newborn assessment requires very different skills and techniques from those needed for the adolescent. The pediatric nurse often needs to comprehend subtle changes or differences in pediatric patients to determine and identify problem areas.

The growth and development of children follows certain predictable milestones. The ability to anticipate these milestones assists the health care team in determining the patient's progress. There are standards established for growth that the nurse can use to assess the patient's response to therapy and to ongoing needs (Lierman, 1996).

All home care organizations providing services or products to pediatric patients should have home care nurses competent in the care of children. This includes staff nurses and advanced practice nurses (e.g., pediatric clinical nurse specialist to plan and provide care to pediatric patients). There should be written policies and procedures that address specific care given to pediatric patients, equipment needs, intake and assessment procedure tools, and resources available for ongoing needs. The documentation of care provided to pediatric patients should include growth and development; a review of systems; family/social support; and response to therapy.

HOME CARE: A TEAM EFFORT

Coordinating patient care may be challenging to the home health organization because of the multidisciplinary nature of pediatric home care. The home health organization has a responsibility to provide effective case or care coordination across the entire health care team. Continuity of care is facilitated by consistent communication of the patient's progress to all providers. The patient receiving chronic or long-term services benefits from effective case coordination because of the need for consistent communication among multiple care providers.

ASSESSMENT: IMPORTANT BASIS FOR CARE AND PLANNING

Home care organizations administering care to pediatric patients should develop documentation forms specific to the assessment and care of infants and children. The initial intake or admission of a pediatric patient to home care should include a prenatal and health history. A review of body systems on admission provides baseline data for any subsequent assessments. Visits to a pediatric patient should always include a review of body systems and a review of the following:

- Nutrition
- Safety
- Growth and development
- Social information
- Response to therapy
- Compliance with prescribed treatment regimen
- Need for new teaching or reinforcement of teaching
- Other information based on the child's unique needs and condition

The evaluation of each visit's assessment should be compared to the data from previous visits and the baseline assessment. Particular attention should be paid to deviations that may negatively impact the patient outcomes and should be reported to the physician and documented in the clinical record. Figure 15-1 shows an example of a comprehensive pediatric nursing assessment.

The pediatric home care nurse needs to recognize normal infant and child physiology to perform an assessment. The assessment of growth and development is an essential component of understanding an infant or child's care and his or her response to interventions. There are specific, well-accepted growth and development milestones and standards to guide the nurse's assessment.

Pediatric assessments are best compared to baseline data and reassessed with serial measurements of growth. An assessment of physical progression, together with a review of systems, will also provide essential information on the development of the pediatric patient. The pediatric patient's response to interventions can be measured through these assessments and is a significant role for the pediatric home care nurse. The ongoing assessment and evaluation of the pediatric patient in the home is integral in determining outcomes.

The assessment of an infant or child should include measurements of vital signs, weight, height, or length. Head circumference generally should be obtained in the child under the age of 2 years. A review of systems needs to encompass an assessment of the cardiovascular, respiratory, neurological, gastrointestinal, renal, endocrine, musculoskeletal, and hematological systems. Instruments appropriate to the size of the infant or child should be used for the assessment (e.g., a blood pressure cuff of the appropriate size for the child's arm). If a too-large or too-small a cuff is used for a blood pressure, the reading will be inaccurate.

Awareness of the developmental level of the child will assist the home care nurse in approaching the child for a physical assessment. The development level of a child will indicate the strategies the nurse should use to garner the most cooperation from the patient. Developmental assessment is performed through the use of standardized tests, such as the Denver Developmental Screening II, which determines the child's progress towards cognitive, language, and motor activity milestones (Frankenberg and Dodds, 1990). Table 15-1 lists the developmental levels and the methods recommended for the physical examination of a child (Whaley and Wong, 1997).

The physical assessment should begin with the least invasive procedures, such as observation and auscultation. Conclude the assessment with the procedures that are considered invasive or traumatic, such as palpation

Text continued on p. 309.

COMPREHENSIVE PEDIATRIC NURSING ASSESSMENT

DATE OF SERVICE ____/____/____

REFER TO PATIENT/CLIENT DATA MAP FOR DEMOGRAPHICS.

TIME IN ________ OUT ________

PERTINENT BACKGROUND INFORMATION

WELL CHILD CARE FREQUENCY (if applicable) ________

PEDIATRICIAN ________ PHONE ________

CLINIC ________

DATE LAST CONTACTED ____/____/____ DATE LAST VISITED ____/____/____

CHIEF COMPLAINT: ________

PRESENT ILLNESS/NURSING DIAGNOSIS: ________

DISABILITIES: ________

RECENT HOSPITALIZATION? ☐ No ☐ Yes, dates ____/____/____ through ____/____/____

Reason ________

New diagnosis/condition? ☐ No ☐ Yes, specify ________

OTHER PRIOR HOSPITALIZATION(S)? ☐ No ☐ Yes, how many times ________

Reason(s)/Dates ________

VITALS/ALLERGIES

T° ________ ☐ O ☐ R ☐ Ax

Ht. ________ Wt. ________

Resp. ________ ☐ Reg. ☐ Irreg.

Pulse: A ________ R ________ F ________ ☐ Regular ☐ Irregular

B/P	LYING	SITTING	STANDING
Right			
Left			

ALLERGIES: ☐ None known ☐ Aspirin ☐ Penicillin ☐ Sulfa ☐ Pollen ☐ Eggs ☐ Milk products ☐ Insect bites ☐ Other ________

IMMUNIZATIONS (✓ if current.)

☐ DPT ☐ Measles ☐ Polio
☐ DT ☐ Mumps ☐ HBV
☐ MMR ☐ Rubella ☐ Hib
☐ Other (specify) ________

NEWBORN/INFANT (Complete if applicable.)

Newborn screen results ________

Gestational age at birth ________ weeks Birth wt. ________ lb. ________ oz. Length ________ in.

Head circumference ________ Fontanels: ☐ Anterior ☐ Posterior

Umbilicus: ☐ Healed ☐ Hernia ☐ Inverted ☐ Everted

NOTE: Additional newborn/infant related assessment criteria are identified by an asterisk (*) throughout the remainder of this form.

SCREENING/EARLY DETECTION

TB skin test: ☐ No ☐ Yes, if yes, when/results ________

Lead screening: ☐ No ☐ Yes, if yes, when/results ________

Other (specify) ________

CHILDHOOD HISTORY (H-history of; N-negative; P-present problem)

CONDITION	H	N	P	CONDITION	H	N	P
*Thrush				Strep throat			
*Apnea				Sinusitis			
Conjunctivitis				Nosebleeds			
Croup				Fracture(s)			
Pica				Burn(s)			
Rubella				Otitis media			
Rubeola				Frequent ear infection			
Scarlet Fever				Tonsillitis			
Mumps				Frequent sore throat			
Chickenpox				Bleeding problems			
Hepatitis				Rheumatic fever			
Sickle Cell				Headaches			
Lead poisoning				Seizures–grand mal			
HIV				Seizures–petit mal			
Pneumonia				Other (specify)			
Asthma							
Frequent colds							

EYES/EARS

EYES

☐ Glasses ☐ Contacts: (R / L) ☐ Prosthesis: (R / L)
☐ Jaundice ☐ Blurred vision ☐ Legally blind
☐ Infections
☐ Other (specify, incl. hx) ________

☐ NO PROBLEM

EARS

☐ HOH: R / L ☐ Deaf: R / L ☐ Hearing aid: R / L
☐ Vertigo ☐ Tinnitus
☐ Other (specify, incl. hx.) ________

☐ NO PROBLEM

HEAD/NECK

☐ Injuries/Wounds (specify) ________

☐ Masses/Nodes: Site ________ Size ________

☐ Other (specify, incl. hx) ________

☐ NO PROBLEM

NOSE/THROAT/MOUTH

☐ Congestion ☐ Dysphagia ☐ Hoarseness
☐ Lesions ☐ Sore throat ☐ Masses/Tumors
* ☐ Palate intact

General condition of teeth ________

Oral hygiene practices ________

☐ Dentist visits: frequency ________

☐ Other (specify, incl. hx) ________

☐ NO PROBLEM

PATIENT/CLIENT NAME – Last, First, Middle Initial ________ ID# ________

Form 3547HH © 1994 Briggs Corporation, Des Moines, IA 50306 To order, phone 1-800-247-2343 PRINTED IN U.S.A.

Page 1 of 4

COMPREHENSIVE PEDIATRIC NURSING ASSESSMENT

FIGURE 15-1 Comprehensive pediatric nursing assessment form. *(Reprinted with permission of Briggs Health Care Products, Des Moines, Iowa.)*

ENDOCRINE

☐ Fatigue ☐ Intolerance to heat/cold
☐ Diabetes: Onset ___ / ___ / ___
  ☐ Insulin/dose/frequency ___
☐ Other (specify incl. hx) ___

☐ NO PROBLEM

CARDIOVASCULAR

HEART SOUNDS: ☐ Reg. ☐ Irreg. (specify) ___

☐ Palpitations
☐ Pulse deficit (specify) ___
☐ Edema ☐ JVD ☐ Fatigue
☐ Cyanosis (site) ___
☐ Cap refill: <3 sec. / >3 sec.
☐ Pulses: LDP / LPT / RDP / RPT
☐ Other (specify, incl. hx) ___

☐ NO PROBLEM

RESPIRATORY

*Chest circumference ___
☐ Retractions ☐ Dyspnea
BREATH SOUNDS: ☐ Clear ☐ Crackles ☐ Wheeze ☐ Absent
☐ Cough: Dry / Acute / Chronic
  ☐ Productive: Thick / Thin / Difficult
    Color ___
SKIN: ☐ Temp. change ☐ Color change
  Specify: ___
☐ Percussion: Resonant / Tympanic / Dull
☐ Chart lobe: ☐ R ☐ L; ☐ Lat. ☐ Ant. ☐ Post.
☐ O₂ use: ___ L/min. by ☐ Mask ☐ Nasal ☐ Trach.
  ☐ Gas ☐ Liquid ☐ Concentrator
☐ Other (specify, incl. hx) ___

☐ NO PROBLEM

GASTROINTESTINAL

NUTRITIONAL REQUIREMENTS FOR AGE (diet) ___

MEAL PATTERNS ___
EATING BEHAVIORS ___
☐ Eating disorder: ☐ Anorexia ☐ Bulimia
  ☐ Other (specify) ___
APPETITE: ☐ Good ☐ Fair ☐ Poor
☐ Weight change: Gain / Loss ___ lb. x ___ wk./mo./yr.
☐ Increase fluids ___ amt. ☐ Restrict fluids ___ amt.
☐ Nausea/Vomiting: Frequency ___ Amt. ___
LAST BM: ___ / ___ / ___ Usual frequency ___
☐ Diarrhea: ☐ Black ☐ Watery; ☐ <3x/day ☐ >3x/day
  ☐ Mucus ☐ Pain ☐ Foul odor ☐ Frothy
  Amount ___
☐ Abnormal stools; describe ___

GASTROINTESTINAL (continued)

☐ Constipation, describe ___
☐ Flatulence ☐ Abdominal distention
BOWEL SOUNDS: ☐ Active ☐ Hyperactive x ___ quads
  ☐ Absent x ___ quads
  Rebound / Hot / Red / Discolored
☐ Other (specify, incl. hx) ___

☐ NO PROBLEM

GENITOURINARY

☐ Diapers/day ___ ☐ Toilet trained (day / night / both)
Urine: Color ___ Amt. ___ Odor ___
  Frequency ___ ☐ Burning ☐ Itching
☐ Enuresis; bedtime ritual ___
☐ External Catheter; Type/brand ___
☐ Other (specify, incl. hx) ___

☐ NO PROBLEM

GENITALIA

SELF-CONCEPT (describe sexuality, body image, etc.) ___

☐ Puberty
☐ Menarche: If checked, age ___
☐ Discharge/Drainage: Urine / Vag. mucus / Feces
☐ Lesions ___ ☐ Masses ___
☐ Bilaters ___ ☐ Cysts ___
☐ Inflammation ___
☐ Other (specify, incl. hx) ___

☐ NO PROBLEM

HEMATOLOGY

☐ Anemia ☐ Bilirubin, results ___
☐ Other (specify, incl. pertinent hx) ___

☐ NO PROBLEM

NEUROLOGICAL

REFLEXES: Specify N - normal, A - abnormal, NA - not applicable

Rooting ___	Blinking ___	Moro's/Startle ___
Sucking ___	Palmar ___	Tonic neck ___
Orienting ___	Plantar ___	Knee jerk ___
Babinski's ___	Stepping/Dancing ___	

Other (list with results) ___

☐ Oriented x ___ ☐ Disoriented
Cognitive development problems:
  ☐ Concepts ☐ Logic ☐ Impaired decision-making ability
  ☐ Memory loss: Short term / Long term
☐ Stuporous/Hallucinations: Visual / Auditory
☐ Headache: Location ___ Freq.: ___

PATIENT/CLIENT NAME — Last, First, Middle Initial   ID#

COMPREHENSIVE PEDIATRIC NURSING ASSESSMENT   Page 2 of 4

2526 p2 f1 inside hh

FIGURE 15-1, cont'd   For legend see opposite page.

continued

NEUROLOGICAL (continued)	SKIN CONDITIONS/WOUNDS (Check all that apply.)

NEUROLOGICAL (continued)

*INFANT MOTOR SKILLS: ☐ Lifts head ☐ Crawls/creeps
Rolls over: ☐ Stomach to back ☐ Back to stomach
Sits: ☐ With assistance ☐ Without assistance
Stands: ☐ With assistance ☐ Without assistance
MOTOR SKILLS: ☐ Walks ☐ Runs ☐ Jumps
☐ Hops ☐ Skips ☐ Balance
☐ Motor change: Fine / Gross
☐ Tremors: Fine / Gross / Paralysis
☐ Weakness: UE / LE Location ____
HAND GRIPS: Equal / Unequal, specify ____
                      Strong / Weak, specify ____
☐ Sensory loss, specify ____
☐ Numbness, specify ____
COMMUNICATION PATTERNS/ABILITY, describe ____

☐ Unequal pupils: R / L / PERRLA
☐ Psychotropic drug use (specify) ____

Dose/Freq. ____
☐ Other (specify, incl. hx) ____
☐ NO PROBLEM

SKIN CONDITIONS/WOUNDS (Check all that apply.)
* Mongolian spots / Itch / Rash / Dry / Scaling
Incision / Wounds / Lesions / Sutures / Staples
Abrasions / Lacerations / Bruises / Ecchymosis
Edema / Hemangiomas
Pallor: Jaundice / Redness Turgor: Good / Poor
Other (specify, incl. pertinent hx) ____
☐ NO PROBLEM

MUSCULOSKELETAL
POSTURE ____
STRENGTH ____
ENDURANCE ____
☐ Scoliosis, type ____
☐ Swollen/Painful joints, specify ____
☐ Fracture, location ____
☐ Decreased ROM, specify ____
☐ Other (specify, incl. pertinent hx) ____
☐ NO PROBLEM

PSYCHOSOCIAL
☐ Angry ☐ Flat affect ☐ Discouraged
☐ Withdrawn ☐ Difficulty coping ☐ Disorganized
☐ Recent change: ☐ Birth ☐ Death ☐ Moved
☐ Divorce ☐ Other (specify) ____
☐ Suicidal: ☐ Ideation ☐ Verbalized
☐ Depressed: ☐ Recent ☐ Long term
Due to (if known) ____
☐ Substance use: ☐ Drugs ☐ Alcohol ☐ Tobacco
DESCRIBE RELATIONSHIPS WITH THE FOLLOWING:
Parents ____
Siblings ____
Peers ____
BEHAVIOR AT DAY CARE/SCHOOL ____
USUAL SLEEP/REST PATTERN ____
SLEEPING ARRANGEMENTS ____
☐ Other (specify, incl. pertinent hx) ____
☐ NO PROBLEM

APPLIANCES/AIDS/SPECIAL EQUIPMENT
☐ Crutch(es) ☐ Wheelchair ☐ Cane ☐ Walker
☐ Brace/Orthotics (specify) ____
☐ Transfer equipment: Board / Lift
☐ Bedside commode
☐ Prosthesis: RUE / RLE / LUE / LLE / Other ____
☐ Grab bars: Bathroom / Other ____
☐ Hospital bed: Semi-elec. / Crank / Spec. ____
Overlays ____
☐ Oxygen: HME Co. ____
HME Rep. ____ Phone ____
☐ Other (specify, incl. pertinent hx) ____
☐ NONE USED

LIVING SITUATION/CAREGIVER INFORMATION
☐ House ☐ Apartment ☐ New environment
Primary language ____
☐ Language barrier ☐ Needs interpreter
☐ Learning barrier: Mental / Psychosocial / Physical / Functional
Primary caregiver (name) ____
Relationship/Health status ____
☐ Assists with ADLs
☐ Provides physical care
☐ Other (specify) ____
☐ Siblings (specify) ____

PAIN
Location ____
Origin ____ Onset __/__/__
Quality (i.e., burning, dull ache) ____
Intensity level ____
Freq./Duration ____
Relief ____
Other (specify) ____
☐ NO PROBLEM

PATIENT/CLIENT NAME — Last, First, Middle Initial   ID#

Page 3 of 4   **COMPREHENSIVE PEDIATRIC NURSING ASSESSMENT**

FIGURE 15-1, cont'd   Comprehensive pediatric nursing assessment form. *(Reprinted with permission of Briggs Health Care Products, Des Moines, Iowa.)*

SUMMARY OF GROWTH AND DEVELOPMENT FOR AGE

PROGNOSIS/LEARNING POTENTIAL	TEACHING/TRAINING (I-Instruct: R-Reinstruct: D-Demonstrate)		
	SUBJECT	I R D	PATIENT/CLIENT/CAREGIVER RESPONSE
	Diet		
	Medication(s)		
	Disease process		
	Safety		
	S/S to report		
	Well child care		
DISCHARGE PLANS	Activities		
1.	Treatments		
2.	Injury prevention		
3.	Growth and development		
4.	Other (specify)		
Discussed with patient/client/caregiver? ☐ Yes ☐ No			

SKILLED CARE (wound. catheter. administration of meds.. venipuncture. IV. etc.)

PATIENT/CLIENT/CAREGIVER RESPONSE _____

SUMMARY CHECKLIST	SIGNATURES/DATES
MEDICATION STATUS: ☐ No change ☐ Order obtained ☐ PRN order obtained	X ___ / /
BILLABLE SUPPLIES RECORDED? ☐ Yes ☐ No	Caregiver (if applicable) Date
CARE COORDINATION: ☐ Physician ☐ PT ☐ OT ☐ ST ☐ SS	Complete TIME OUT (page 1) prior to signing below.
☐ SN ☐ Aide ☐ Other (specify)___	___ / /
PATIENT/CLIENT NAME – Last, First, Middle Initial	Nurse (signature/title) Date ID#

COMPREHENSIVE PEDIATRIC NURSING ASSESSMENT   Page 4 of 4

2526 p1 f1 outside hh

FIGURE 15-1, cont'd   For legend see opposite page.

TABLE 15-1   AGE-SPECIFIC APPROACHES TO PHYSICAL ASSESSMENT

AGE	DEVELOPMENTAL INDICATORS	POSITIONING	SEQUENCE	PREPARATION
Infant (0-1)	Stranger anxiety begins at 7 mo; peaks at 9 mo Resists being restrained Responds to simple commands by age 9 mo Separation anxiety peaks at 13 mo	Supine or prone before 4-6 mo; can place on examination table After 6 mo sits alone; use this position whenever possible in parent's lap If on table, place with parent in full view	If quiet, auscultate heart, lungs, abdomen Palpate and percuss same areas Proceed in usual head-to-toe manner Perform traumatic procedure last (eyes, ears, mouth, rectal temperature) Elicit reflexes as body part examined	Completely undress if room temperature permits Leave diaper in place Gain cooperation with distraction, bright objects, rattles Smile at infant, use soft, high-pitched voice Pacify with pacifier or feeding

Toddler (1-3)	Autonomy important Egocentric Stranger anxiety increases at 18 mo Speech begins Negativism present Know several external body parts Separation anxiety decreases at 2 yr	Sitting on or standing by parent Prone or supine in parent's lap	Inspect body areas through play: "count fingers," "tickle toes" Minimize physical contact initially Introduce equipment slowly Auscultate, percuss, palpate whenever quiet Perform traumatic procedures last	Have parent remove outer clothing Remove underwear as body part examined Allow to inspect equipment; demonstrating use is usually ineffective If uncooperative, perform procedures quickly Use restraint when appropriate Praise for cooperative behavior Talk about examination if cooperative

continued

Modified from Whaley LF, Wong DL: *Whaley and Wong's nursing care of infants and children*, ed 5, 1995, Mosby.

TABLE 15-1   AGE-SPECIFIC APPROACHES TO PHYSICAL ASSESSMENT—cont'd

AGE	DEVELOPMENTAL INDICATORS	POSITIONING	SEQUENCE	PREPARATION
Preschool child (3-5)	Likes to "help" More cooperative, follows simple instructions Knows most external body parts, three to five parts Fears bodily harm	Prefer standing or sitting Usually cooperative Prefer parent's closeness	If cooperative, proceed in head-to-toe direction If uncooperative, proceed as with toddler	Request self-undressing Allow to wear underpants if shy Offer equipment for inspection, briefly demonstrate use Make up "story" about procedure Use paper doll technique Give choices when possible Expect cooperation; use positive statements

and examination of the eyes, ears, and mouth. This strategy allows for obtaining the most information while the child is most cooperative.

On admission to home care, the nurse should obtain the baseline height or length and weight of the child. Documentation of this data on a growth chart is useful for comparison of the child to established standards for growth by age level. Growth charts are readily available from infant formula manufacturers locally. When a child's height or weight falls below the 10th percentile or the 90th standard, the physician should be notified. Many children may already be below the 10th percentile or 90th standard on admission to home care, so careful serial measurements of anthropometrics are necessary for continual monitoring.

The child's developmental level is a key component of the ongoing assessment. Developmental delays are common in premature infants and children with chronic diseases. Progression in developmental milestones is often an indicator of an improvement in the patient's response to intervention.

The pediatric patient should be assessed for immunization status and whether he or she is current for their age. Table 15-2 lists the recommended immunization schedule for infants and children (American Academy of Pediatrics, 1997). If the immunizations are not up-to-date for the child's age, this information should be discussed with the parent(s) and brought to the physician's attention at the next office or clinic visit.

Some pediatric patients in the home care setting are at extreme risk of cardiopulmonary arrest after hospital discharge. There are occasions when parents will be taught techniques in cardiopulmonary resuscitation (CPR) for their child. These instructions should be clearly written and available in the home. The home care nurse caring for pediatric patients should be aware of CPR techniques for infants and children, including those with a tracheostomy, as recommended by the American Heart Association.

PAIN MANAGEMENT FOR CHILDREN

Pain management is frequently required for the pediatric home care patient. Pain may be classified as acute or chronic, depending on its etiology. Assessing pain in children can include the child's self-report of pain; however, the parent's input concerning the child's previous experience with pain is essential. The pain history is also important when the child is unwilling or unable to report his or her own pain. Knowledge of how the child has handled pain in the past, what measures and medications are most comforting, and what are the child's behaviors and words associated with pain will guide the assessment and intervention.

**TABLE 15-2 RECOMMENDED CHILDHOOD IMMUNIZATION SCHEDULE
UNITED STATES, JANUARY-DECEMBER 1997**

VACCINE	BIRTH	1 MO	2 MOS	4 MOS	6 MOS	12 MOS	15 MOS	18 MOS	4-6 YRS	11-12 YRS	14-16 YRS
Hepatitis B[1,2]	Hep B-1	Hep B-2			Hep B-3					Hep B[2]	
Diphtheria, tetanus, pertussis[3]			DTaP or DTP	DTaP or DTP	DTaP or DTP		DTaP or DTP[4]		DTaP or DTP	Td	
H. influenzae type b[4]			Hib	Hib	Hib[4]	Hib[5]					
Polio[5]			Polio[5]	Polio		Polio[6]			Polio		
Measles, mumps, rubella[6]						MMR			MMR[6] or MMR[6]	MMR[6]	
Varicella[7]							Var			Var	

AGE

(From the American Academy of Pediatrics: Recommended Childhood Immunization Schedule, *AAP News* 13(1):18, 1997.) Approved by the Advisory Committee on Immunization Practices (ACIP), the American Academy of Pediatrics (AAP), and the American Academy of Family Physicians (AAFP).

Infants born to HBsAg-negative mothers should receive 2.5 µg of Merck vaccine (Recombivax HB) or 10 µg of SmithKline Beecham (SB) vaccine (Engerix-B). The 2nd dose should be administered ≥ 1 mo after the 1st dose.

Infants born to HBsAg-positive mothers should receive 0.5 mL hepatitis B immune globulin (HBIG) within 12 hrs of birth, and either 5 µg of Merck vaccine (Recombivax HB) or 10 µg of SB vaccine (Engerix-B) at a separate site. The 2nd dose is recommended at 1-2 mos of age and the 3rd dose at 6 mos of age.

Infants born to mothers whose HBsAg status is unknown should receive either 5 µg of Merck vaccine (Recombivax HB) or 10 µg of SB vaccine (Engerix-B) within 12 hrs of birth. The 2nd dose of vaccine is recommended at 1 mo of age and the 3rd dose at 6 mos of age. Blood should be drawn at the time of delivery to determine the mother's HBsAg status; if it is positive, the infant should receive HBIG as soon as possible (no later than 1 wk of age). The dosage and timing of subsequent vaccine doses should be based upon the mother's HBsAg status.

[2]Children and adolescents who have not been vaccinated against hepatitis B in infancy may begin the series during any childhood visit. Those who have not previously received 3 doses of hepatitis B vaccine should initiate or complete the series during the 11-12 year-old visit. The 2nd dose should be administered at least 1 mo after the 1st dose, and the 3rd dose should be administered at least 4 mos after the 1st dose and at least 2 mos after the 2nd dose.

[3]DTaP (diphtheria and tetanus toxoids and acellular pertussis vaccine) is the preferred vaccine for all doses in the vaccination series, including completion of the series in children who have received ≥1 doses of whole-cell DTP vaccine. Whole-cell DTP is an acceptable alternative to DTaP. The 4th dose of DTaP may be administered as early as 12 months of age, provided 6 months have elapsed since the 3rd dose, and if the child is considered unlikely to return at 15-18 mos of age. Td (tetanus and diphtheria toxoids, ab-

sorbed, for adult use) is recommended at 11-12 years of age if at least 5 years have elapsed since the last dose of DTP, DTaP, or DT. Subsequent routine Td boosters are recommended every 10 years.

[4]Three *H. influenzae* type b (Hib) conjugate vaccines are licensed for infant use. If PRP-OMP (PedvaxHIB [Merck]) is administered at 2 and 4 mos of age, a dose at 6 mos is not required. After completing the primary series, any Hib conjugate vaccine may be used as a booster.

[5]Two poliovirus vaccines are currently licensed in the US: inactivated poliovirus vaccine (IPV) and oral poliovirus vaccine (OPV). The following schedules are all acceptable by the ACIP, the AAP and the AAFP, and parents and providers may choose among them:

1. IPV at 2 and 4 mos; OPV at 12-18 mos and 4-6 yr
2. IPV at 2, 4, 12-18 mos, and 4-6 yr
3. OPV at 2, 4, 6-18 mos, and 4-6 yr

The ACIP routinely recommends schedule 1. IPV is the only poliovirus vaccine recommended for immunocompromised persons and their household contacts.

[6]The 2nd dose of MMR is routinely recommended at 4-6 yrs of age or at 11-12 yrs of age, but may be administered during any visit, provided at least 1 month has elapsed since receipt of the 1st dose and that both doses are administered at or after 12 months of age.

[7]Susceptible children may receive Varicella vaccine (Var) at any visit after the first birthday, and those who lack a reliable history of chickenpox should be immunized during the 11-12 year-old visit. Children ≥ 13 years of age should receive 2 doses, at least 1 mo apart.

[8]This schedule indicates the recommended age for routine administration of currently licensed combination vaccines. Some combination vaccines are available and may be used whenever administration of all components of the vaccine is indicated. Providers should consult the manufacturers' package inserts for detailed recommendations.

Behavioral cues such as crying, grimaces, rubbing the site of pain, and hitting and biting behavior may be the only subjective assessment of pain in infants and toddlers. A pain assessment tool may be used in children age 3 years and older (Figure 15-2). Use of the same pain assessment tool by the health care team and the family will provide consistent feedback on the child's pain and the effectiveness of the interventions. Wong describes the Pain Faces scale, which uses schematic drawings of faces to describe their feelings of pain. The tool rates the pain on a scale of 0 to 5, with 0 being "no pain" and 5 being "the worst pain" (Whaley and Wong, 1995). Using the same pain scale among caregivers will not only help the child describe his or her pain quantitatively to others, but will help others to understand the child's relief from pain.

SAFETY CONSIDERATIONS

The environment and safety issues in the home are another aspect of the home care patient's assessment. The initial visit should determine if there are any risk factors posed to the patient because of his or her condition or disease state and the physical environment of the home. The home should be free of the usual child hazards (e.g., chemical and toxic substances, electrical outlets covered from toddlers). The home should also be assessed for particular risks for mobility hazards (e.g., stairs, loose carpets). An assessment of the availability of utilities (e.g., water, electricity) and emergency services should be included in the initial visit. For some therapies emergency power may be necessary, and the local utility company will need to be notified of the special needs of the child who is ventilator dependent. Environmental/safety issues to be assessed are listed in Figure 15-3.

SAFETY AND INFECTION CONTROL

The home care nurse should use the home visit as an opportunity not only to assess the safety of the home for the child's treatment, but to teach the family safety issues that are hazards for all children. The focus of this teaching should be on prevention and should include measures to prevent falls, choking/strangulation or suffocation, drowning, and burns. Car safety should also be emphasized to the parents and should incorporate teaching on car safety seats and their correct use.

Interventions should be planned to minimize risks the child's condition may pose to others in the home. Patients with AIDS/HIV may require certain infection control precautions to reduce their risk of exposure to infections while also protecting others in the home from the risk of transmission of the disease. These instructions should be based on current universal body fluid precautions. Effective handwashing,

Which Face Shows How Much Hurt You Have Now?

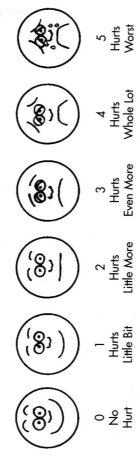

0	1	2	3	4	5
No Hurt	Hurts Little Bit	Hurts Little More	Hurts Even More	Hurts Whole Lot	Hurts Worst

FIGURE 15-2   This face scale is a helpful tool to use to assess the pain of a child who is at least 3 years old. The health care provider should explain each face to the child (e.g., a person feels happy because there is no pain or hurt or sad because there is some or a lot of pain. Face 0 is very happy because there is no pain. Face 1 hurts just a little bit. Face 5 hurts as much as the child can imagine, although a person does not have to cry to feel this bad. The health care provider should ask the child to choose the face that best describes his or her own pain. (From Whaley LF, Wong DL: *Whaley and Wong's nursing care of infants and children*, ed 5, St. Louis, 1995, Mosby.)

HOME SAFETY ASSESSMENT

Patient Name _____ HC # _____ Date: _____

GENERAL HOUSEHOLD SAFETY SCREENING TOOL

Fire Safety	N/A	Yes	No
1. Number of smoke detectors in the home? ____ Are they battery-operated?			
2. Are fire extinguishers present in appropriate locations for use?			
3. Can family members state escape routes and meeting place in the event of a fire?			
4. Can family members state the actions to be taken if a person catches fire?			
Comments:			
Gas/Electric Safety			
1. If a fuse or circuit breaker box is in the home, is it labeled?			
2. For pts with electrical medical equipment is there a back-up power source in case of power outage?			
3. Are flashlights/batteries or candles/matches kept for power outages?			
4. Are electrical outlets two- or three-pronged? two-pronged three-pronged			
5. Are electrical outlets accessible to patient care areas?			
6. Are electrical cords frayed or are wires exposed?			
7. What is the source of heating/cooking fuel? ☐ Electric ☐ Gas ☐ Oil ☐ Other			
8. If gas, does the family know its odor and actions to be taken if a leak is suspected?			
Comments:			

FIGURE 15-3 Home safety assessment form.

General Home Safety	N/A	Yes	No
1. Does the family know emergency phone numbers?			
2. Is the number for poison control posted on or near the phone?			
3. Is there a working telephone in the home?			
4. Are cleansers, drugs and plants out of reach of children or locked in cabinets?			
5. If indicated, do family members wear allergy or medic alert bracelets?			
6. Are fireplaces, radiators, and space heaters screened?			
7. Is the hot water temperature at or below 130 degrees F?			
8. Are hallways and stairs free of clutter, banister present for stairs, and rugs secured?			
9. Is the elevator, hallway, building, or neighborhood safe? (well lit, clean, visible)			
10. Are age specific safety measures followed, per CHHCS protocols followed in the home?			
11. Are rodents, roaches, loose plaster, paint chips, or drugs/alcohol in the home?			
Comments:			

Case Manager Signature _____

FIGURE 15-3, cont'd   For legend see opposite page. *(From Children's Hospital National Medical Center, Preferred Pediatrics Home Care Network, Washington, DC.)*

use of needleless devices for intravenous therapy, wearing gloves, and providing sharps containers for disposal are examples of such interventions.

FAMILY ASSESSMENT

An important aspect of the home care assessment of a pediatric patient is the family assessment. The home care visit is an opportunity to determine the parents'/caregiver's coping abilities, communication patterns, attitudes toward the child's illness, and abilities to carry out the treatment plan. The visit is also a time for reinforcement of teaching and evaluating the effectiveness of the treatment plan.

Pediatric home care nurses may be involved in potential or real cases of child abuse or neglect. These cases of abuse may be the result of violence directed toward the child or neglect. There may be differences of opinion between the nurse and family in the management of specific areas of care to a child. The conflict that may occur could be from care that the nurse would consider ideal for the child as opposed to realistic care according to the family's abilities (Hogue, 1992). The determination of abuse can be subjective, but most codes are based on whether the child is being placed at-risk of harm (i.e., death, disfigurement, or impairment). Not following written medical orders is considered abuse or neglect according to some state codes.

Organizational policies should provide guidelines for nurses in managing care when disagreement exists between the health care team and the family. Policies should also outline the steps to be taken in identifying, documenting, and reporting suspected physical or mental abuse or neglect. The severity and frequency of neglected care should serve as a guide in determining abuse. Differentiation should be made between the family who is unable to manage care because of being overwhelmed and the family who consistently neglects to administer prescribed care.

Documentation of suspected abuse or neglect should be factual. Opinions or subjective statements are not appropriate. Physician statements regarding the necessary medical care and the potential outcome if care is not provided can be used as evidence of neglect or abuse.

Suspected cases of abuse or neglect are to be reported to the appropriate authorities for the community. A Child Protective Services (CPS) worker is assigned to the case to further investigate and identify the educational and psychosocial needs of the family. The home care nurse's role is to encourage the family to cooperate with the investigation. Collaboration of the family, the CPS worker, and the health care team is essential to facilitate appropriate care for the child.

ALTERNATIVE SITES OF CARE: RESPITE FOR CAREGIVERS

Caring for a sick child can be emotionally and physically demanding on parents. When the needs of the child are preventing the caregiver(s) from addressing their own needs, respite care may be needed. Even for a relatively minor or short-term health care problem, a caregiver may need some assistance or relief from the ongoing burden of responsibility. For the chronically ill child with multiple complex therapies, temporary relief of these responsibilities is essential to the emotional well-being of the caregiver and the child.

Respite care may be given by friends or other family members. For the patient receiving complex therapies, the respite caregivers should be trained in care and procedures to safely care for the patient in the primary caregiver's absence. The home care agency may provide respite caregivers at the family's request or at the suggestion of the home care nurse. These caregivers are generally home health aides or licensed nursing staff, depending on the severity and intensity of care needed by the child.

Some pediatric patients may be cared for in daycare centers for the medically fragile. These centers are usually staffed with home health aides and licensed nursing personnel, and care is delivered generally during the business day hours. The centers generally care for patients requiring very complex medical care, including ventilators and infusion therapy. These centers allow the caregivers to resume their jobs during the day and take the pediatric patient home in the evening or are used as a respite from the everyday care of the patient.

PEDIATRIC HOSPICE CARE

The news that a child's prognosis is terminal is always devastating. When a patient has fewer than 6 months to live, the care plan priorities should be focused on the comfort of the patient and reducing or eliminating the pain of the child. Hospice care for the pediatric patient may be available through local hospice programs in the community. The hospice team members should have specialized training programs in the care of the pediatric hospice patient and his or her family. It should also have policies and procedures in place to manage the care of the patient (Sumner, Hurula, 1993; Tobin, 1993).

Hospice services usually include nursing services, social workers, pastoral care counseling, and volunteers. The volunteers play a critical role not only in providing some respite for the primary caregiver to run errands, but also in spending time with siblings of the pediatric patient. With an increased focus on the terminally ill child, the needs of the siblings frequently receive less attention. It is important to remember that siblings have needs that must also be met. For a more in-depth discussion about hospice care in the home, see Chapter 16.

SUMMARY

The range and complexity of children with unique needs will only continue to grow in pediatric home care. Special skills are needed by home care team members with a basis in pediatric care. The pediatric home care nurse must integrate these skills with multifaceted roles to effectively care for this special patient population and their families.

REVIEW EXERCISES

1. Describe some of the therapies and equipment that are prescribed for pediatric home care patients.
2. Discuss the concept of family-centered care and how its focus determines the home care nurse's approach to planning interventions for the pediatric patient in the home setting.
3. Identify the way caring for the pediatric patient in the home setting differs from that in the acute care setting. Describe the way this care differs for the nurse, family, and patient. State interventions that would be appropriate for dealing with these differences.
4. List at least four potential funding sources for pediatric patients receiving home care services. Identify the differences between three managed care product lines, and the way they impact the delivery of home care services to an individual.
5. State three skills needed by the home care nurse caring for pediatric patients that differ from those of the nurse caring for only an adult population.
6. Describe how the assessment of the pediatric patient differs significantly from that of other home care patients.
7. Name at least four areas that should be assessed on every pediatric home care visit.
8. Describe pediatric patients who would be potential candidates for the specialized services of hospice care.
9. Describe the differences in approach to the physical assessment of a pediatric patient based on age and developmental level.
10. Identify areas of documentation that should be included in every nursing visit of the pediatric patient.

RESOURCES

Access to Respite Care Help (ARCH)
800 Eastowne Drive, Suite 105
Chapel Hill, NC 27514
(800)473-1727

American Heart Association
7272 Greenville Avenue
Dallas, TX 75231
(800)242-1793

The Arc (formerly, The Association for Retarded Citizens)
500 East Border Street
Suite 300
Arlington, Texas 76010
(817)261-6003
(800)433-5255

Association for the Care of Children's Health (ACCH)
7910 Woodmont Avenue, Suite 300
Bethesda, MD 20814
(310)654-6549
(800)808-2224

Association of Pediatric Oncology Nursing
4700 W. Lake Avenue
Glenview, IL 60025-1485
(847)375-4724

The Candlelighters Childhood Cancer Foundation
7910 Woodmont Avenue, Suite 460
Bethesda, MD 20814
(301)657-8401
(800)366-2223

Children's Hospice International
2202 Mount Vernon Avenue, Suite 3C
Alexandria, VA 22301
(703)684-0330
(800)24-CHILD

Cystic Fibrosis Foundation
6931 Arlington Road
Bethesda, MD 20814
(800)344-4823

Epilepsy Foundation of America
4351 Garden City Drive
Landover, MD 20785
(301)459-3700
(800)332-1000

Exceptional Parent Magazine
PO Box 3000
Department EP
Denville, NJ 07834
(800)247-8080
(800)562-1973

Friends Network
Funletter TM (Newsletter for Pediatric Cancer Patients)
Kenon Neal, President
P.O. Box 4545
Santa Barbara, CA 93140

Home Care Nurse News
P.O. Box 391
Westerville, OH 43081-9876
(800)993-6397

The Karing Book: Patient's Pal
PO Box 93
Ontario, OR 97914
(800)9KARING

Leukemia Society of America
600 Third Avenue, 4th Floor
New York, NY 10016
(212)573-8484
(800)955-4572

Muscular Dystrophy Association of America
10 East 40th Street, Room 4110
New York, NY 10016
(212)689-9040

National Easter Seal Society
230 West Monroe Street, Suite 1800
Chicago, IL 60606-4802
(312)726-6200
(800)221-6827

National Information Center for Children and Youth with Disabilities
PO Box 1492
Washington, DC 20013-1492, or
1875 Connecticut Avenue, NW
Washington, DC 20009
(202)844-8200
(800)695-0285

The National Parent Network on Disabilities
1727 King Street, Suite 305
Alexandria, Virginia 22314
(703)684-6763

Pediatric Nursing Journal
East Holly Avenue
PO Box 56
Pitman, NJ 08071-9911
(609)256-2300
United Cerebral Palsy Association, Inc.
1660 L Street, NW, Suite 700
Washington, DC 20036
(800)872-5827
(202)776-0406

REFERENCES

Ahmann E: Family-center home care. In Ahmann E, editor: *Home care for the high-risk infant,* Gaithersburg, Md, 1996, Aspen.

American Academy of Pediatrics: Recommended Childhood Immunization Schedule, *AAP News* 13(1):18, 1997.

Cabin B: Cost-effectiveness of pediatric home care, *Caring* 4:45-53, 1985.

Frankenberg WK, Dodds JB: *Denver II,* Denver, 1990, Denver Developmental Materials.

Hack M, et al: School-age outcomes in children with birth weights under 750 g, *N Engl J Med* 331(12):753-759, 1994.

Hill L, Thompson M: Case management of technology-dependent children: a family-centered approach, *J Home Health Care Pract* 6(2),37-41, 1994.

Hogue E: Parental noncompliance in home care, *Pediatr Nurs* 18(6):603-606, 1992.

Lierman C: Failure to thrive. In Ahman E, editor: *Home care for the high-risk infant,* Gaithersburg, Md, 1996, Aspen.

Sumner L, Hurula J: Pediatric hospice nursing: making the most of each moment, *Nursing* 93(8):50-55, 1993.

Tobin C: Holding their own with pediatric hospice, *Caring* pp 56-57, 1993.

Whaley LF, Wong DL: *Whaley and Wong's nursing care of infants and children,* ed 5, St. Louis, 1995, Mosby.

FOR FURTHER READING

Ahmann E: Promoting health maintenance for the high-risk premature infant. In Ahmann E, editor: *Home care for the high-risk infant,* Gaithersburg, Md, 1996, Aspen.

Betz CL, Sowden LA: Growth and development. In *Pediatric nursing reference,* St. Louis, 1996a, Mosby.

Betz CL, Sowden LA: Nursing assessment. In *Pediatric nursing reference,* St. Louis, 1996b, Mosby.

Betz CL, Sowden LA: Taking blood pressure and age-appropriate cuff size, In *Pediatric nursing reference,* St. Louis, 1996c, Mosby.

Brucker JM, Wallin KD: *Manual of pediatric nursing,* Boston, 1996, Little, Brown.

Buzz-Kelley L, Gordin P: Teaching CPR to parents of children with tracheostomies, *MCN* 18:158-163, 1993.

Chandra NC, Hazinski MF: *Textbook of basic life support for healthcare providers,* Dallas, 1994, American Heart Association.

Engvall J, McCarthy A: Innovative approaches for teaching children with chronic conditions, *J Pediatric Health Care* 10:239-242, 1996.

Lonergan JN, et al: *Homecare management of the bone marrow transplant patient,* Sudbury, Mass, 1996, Jones & Bartlett.

Martinson I: Hospice update: home care and children with cancer: grief and the role of the nurse, *Home Care Nurse News* 3(10):5, 1996.

National Association for Home Care: About NAHC: A profile of the National Association for Home Care, Washington, DC, 1994, NAHC.

Shelton TL, Stepanek JS: *Family-centered care for children needing specialized health and developmental services,* Bethesda, Md, 1994, Association for the Care of Children's Health.

Whaley LF, Wong DL: *Essentials of pediatric nursing,* ed 5, St. Louis, 1997, Mosby.

16

HOSPICE CARE IN HOME CARE

Tina M. Marrelli, MSN, MA, RNC

"This is how we should care for all patients."

Tina M. Marrelli

A SPECIAL PROGRAM CHANGING THE FOCUS FROM CURE TO CARE

Hospice is a special kind of care and support that is primarily provided in the privacy and comfort of the patient's home. According to the National Hospice Organization (NHO), 77% of hospice patients died in their own residences (National Hospice Organization, 1995). For this and other reasons, hospice is a special type of home care. Simply put, hospice is an organized method of providing care directed toward comfort and support for patients with a limited life expectancy. Hospice focuses on making every remaining day the best it can be.

Of *all* Medicare costs, 28% goes toward care of people in their last year of life; almost 50% is expended in the final 2 months of life (National Hospice Organization, 1995). Significant savings are seen when terminally ill cancer patients are cared for in the home. Carney and Burns (1991) calculated a savings of 39% to 51% for patients in home hospice care.

The hospice focus, which is very different from the curative-focused rescue medicine mentality of the health care system in the United States, is causing a ground swell of support for palliative care and hospice services. For these reasons, hospice is expected to experience significant growth in patient and financial outlays.

This chapter provides an overview of hospice care and seeks to explain the special aspects of hospice care that contribute to the provision of high-quality care for patients and their families. In addition, the hospice specialty is defined for those wishing to move into this unique and satisfying professional career path.

WHAT IS HOSPICE?

Hospice has strong roots in history. The word hospice is derived from a term used historically to designate a resting place for weary travelers. Today, hospice provides care in a multidimensional package that acts as a rest for the weary patient and the patient's family. Hospice patients have usually been through different treatments for curative purposes and may have been on multiple regimens. These can include chemotherapeutic protocols, radiation therapy, surgeries, and any combination of these modalities. Some patients have been battling cancer, acquired immune deficiency syndrome (AIDS), or other diseases for years. They may come to hospice when the medical model can no longer, in good conscience, continue curative treatment. Hospice then helps assist patients focus their limited time on themselves, their partner, and their loved ones.

WHY THE GROWTH OF HOSPICE?

There are numerous reasons for the growth in hospice, including demographic changes, which includes the growth of the frail and elderly, the population of AIDS patients seeking hospice, cost savings, and the trend toward a quality of life that hospice espouses and actualizes in communities across the country.

The kinds of patients and families cared for through hospice has also grown and changed. Historically hospice provided care primarily to patients with cancer. Alzheimer's patients and their families, patients with amyotrophic lateral sclerosis (ALS), and end-stage heart and other organ failure patients are now finding support and care through hospice.

According to the National Hospice Organization (1993): ". . . hospice provides support and care for persons in the last phases of incurable diseases so that they may live as fully and comfortably as possible. Hospice recognizes dying as part of the normal process of living and focuses on maintaining the quality of remaining life. Hospice affirms life and neither hastens nor postpones death. Hospice exists in the hope and belief that through appropriate care, and the promotion of a caring community sensitive to their needs, patients and families may be free to attain a degree of mental and spiritual preparation for death that is satisfactory to them." These standards then provide the framework for hospices daily as they seek to provide the best care for patients and their families.

PATIENTS SEEN IN HOSPICE

The kinds of patient problems seen in hospice care are in many ways similar to the general home care patient population. Infants, children, and adults are cared for by hospice. Hospices may have a specialty focus, such as a pediatric hospice; they generally have admission policies that state their mission and the patient populations served. Diagnoses cared for by hospices include various cancers, AIDS, end-stage renal disease, cardiac and lung processes, and other diagnoses that have a limited life expectancy.

THE TYPES OF HOSPICE ORGANIZATIONS
Different types or "auspices" of programs provide hospice care. These include the following:

1. An inpatient hospice unit at a facility, such as a hospital, nursing home, or subacute unit
2. A community-based hospice, such as a not-for-profit volunteer organization serving a defined rural geographic area
3. A freestanding inpatient hospice, such as a hospice in a large metropolitan area that cares for patients through death
4. A home health agency (HHA) that provides hospice care with specially trained home care hospice nurses, volunteers and other team members
5. Corporations that provide hospice care
6. Other models, such as health maintenance organizations (HMOs)

As managed care continues to grow, it is expected that other systems, such as alliances or network hospices, may emerge to provide this special care to patients.

HOSPICE TEAM MEMBERS: EFFORTS DIRECTED TOWARD COMFORT AND CARING
The nurse is not alone in creating this special care environment. Rather, an interdisciplinary team is a key component of hospice care.

The following lists the core clinical hospice team members:

- Hospice patient and family
- Hospice nurse
- Home health/hospice aide; also called certified nursing assistants (CNAs) in some parts of the country
- Physician
- Social worker
- Bereavement counselor
- Hospice volunteer
- Dietitian
- Pharmacist
- Occupational or physical therapist

326 part III · Specialty Considerations in Home Care

- Speech-language pathologist
- Spiritual counselor

In addition to the interdisciplinary team, the following administrators and managers may also be found in hospice care:

- Secretaries and office support team members
- Bereavement coordinator
- Volunteer coordinator
- Other team members, as unique as the hospice organization and their mission (e.g., art, music, and massage therapist), are found in hospice care. Depending on the size of the hospice, some team members may carry out more than one role. The team works in collaboration with the patient and family to define and plan care throughout the hospice patient's length of stay.

DEFINING HOSPICE NURSING

Regardless of the organizational structure of the hospice, the hospice nurse plays a key role on the team. Hospice nursing practice is the provision of palliative nursing care for the terminally ill and their families, with emphasis on their physical, psychosocial, emotional, and spiritual needs (Hospice Nurses Association, 1995). Hospice nursing is a synthesis of special skills used to create the environment for the best outcomes for the hospice patient and his or her family.

The hospice nurse's role is often that of case or care manager. Whatever the role defined by the organization, the following paragraphs contain key aspects of the hospice home care specialty that must be learned, nurtured, and improved through continued education and experience. Experienced nurses who are new to hospice may be paired with an experienced hospice nurse as a preceptor through the new hospice nurse's orientation. Like any specialty, home care nurses without additional orientation, education, and experience cannot successfully make the transition to hospice care. *Hospice is very different from home care nursing practice, even though some of the care interventions appear similar.*

HALLMARKS OF EFFECTIVE CARE FOR HOSPICE NURSING

Some areas in which home care hospice nurses must be proficient when caring for hospice patients and their families are as follows:

1. Pain and symptom management
2. Knowledge of concepts related to death and dying

3. Stress management skills
4. Sensitive communication skills
5. Sense of humor
6. Flexibility
7. Hospice knowledge

Pain and Symptom Management Skills

Pain and symptom management is a specialty area in hospice. Because of the teamwork in hospice, often this is a multidisciplinary effort with input from the hospice nurse, the physician, the pharmacist, and other team members such as a massage therapist. Because the focus of care is palliative care and support, it is imperative that hospice nurses be competent in pain assessment, intervention, and evaluation. Pain is emerging as the fifth vital sign and should be assessed during every patient encounter.

Knowledge of Concepts Related to Death and Dying

Hospice integrates the dying process as a part of life. The nurse's philosophy and belief systems should be congruent with the basic tenets of hospice. Dr. Kubler-Ross's research on the stages of dying and other studies may be incorporated into patient care and care planning. These theoretical frameworks provide the strength and rationales for intervention and for identifying resolutions to challenges that individual patients and families may face.

Stress Management Skills

Hospice nurses and colleagues have varied mechanisms for providing support to self and each other. Hospice care may be stressful for nurses and other hospice workers. Most hospices provide staff support to assist in the resolution of problems and for review of care and feelings raised through hospice care. Staff support may be structured, such as scheduled meetings with a trained facilitator, or may be a volunteer initiative with varying models. It is important that all hospice team members take care of themselves and find activities and events that provide emotional well-being, nurturing, and support. Whatever model staff support takes, it is the time for sharing, caring, team building, validating, and processing the work of hospice.

Sensitive Communication Skills

Sensitive communication skills are the key to being an effective hospice team member. There is untold intimacy and poignancy in hospice.

A nurse walks into the home of a patient who may have been battling cancer for years and is now ready to change the focus of the fight from the disease to enjoying the final days as he or she chooses.

Communication skills include active listening, presence as an intervention, and sensitively being cued to what the patient is saying (and sometimes asking for). For example, Sarah is a 39-year-old woman with an aggressive, recurrent breast cancer. At a nursing visit, Sarah said to the hospice nurse, "Anne, I want to renew my vows with my husband before I die." Anne said that she would talk to her later about that because she was doing her dressing change. However, this discussion did not occur, and Sarah later expressed this same sentiment to the home health aide, who reported this statement at the patient care conference. Because of this team effort, Sarah did renew her vows before her death. Especially in hospice, because of the limited time factor, patient needs *must* be addressed in a timely manner and followed up. In addition, this example shows an important component of hospice, psychosocial, and spiritual care.

All patient needs (i.e., needs that are clearly articulated and those that are more veiled) should be developed to ensure that the hospice team is meeting them. These spiritual and other psychosocial needs are a key component in the provision and evaluation of high-quality hospice nursing.

Sense of Humor

It is only in the past few years that the healing power of laughter has been recognized and acknowledged. A kind sense of humor helps the team, patients, and families through particularly rough days or to meet unique challenges.

Flexibility

Patients in hospice control their care and care planning. The days shared with the hospice team are the patient's last months or weeks, and as such the patient calls the shots. This includes scheduling, visit times, length of visits, and other decisions. Respect for and acceptance of these patient choices and decisions is a part of effective daily operations in hospice.

Hospice Knowledge

It is very important that hospice nurses have a strong base of knowledge grounded in hospice. There is body of literature emerging related to hospice, and nurses, as well as other team members, must keep current and have an understanding of hospice's historical roots.

IDENTIFIED DIFFERENCES BETWEEN HOME CARE AND HOSPICE NURSING

It is important to note that many patients may be in a home care or home care oncology program and have been provided home visits. However, the dimensions of scope, depth, and breadth of hospice care extend well beyond that of the standard, medically directed and focused home care program. The following delineates a number of differences between home care and hospice.

1. *Home care:* The patient is the unit or focus of care. Patient care is usually directed toward health and ultimately self-care. Care is the traditional, medical model as Medicare, a medical insurance program, pays for medically necessary care. Care in home care is usually related to illness and therapeutic, curative, interventions.

   Hospice: The patient, partner, family, and/or identified caregivers are the recipients of care. Hospice is what all nurses learned in nursing school; here the patient and family are the unit of care, and the patient is an equal partner in determining that care and making choices related to care and care planning.

2. *Home care:* Much of the care is medically focused on curative interventions and outcomes. Care and programs are structured for reimbursement and regulatory reasons.

   Hospice: The care and outcomes are focused on comfort such as pain and other palliative or symptom-control interventions. Because of this, hospice nurses and their hospice colleagues are often experts in symptom management and care planning. Since hospices have historically grown out of grass roots initiatives to provide special supportive care in a local community, there is a flexibility and creativity unknown to most traditional health care models. This means that there are unique programs to support patients, their families, and surviving loved ones. Creative programs offered by hospices include specialized bereavement camps for children, music therapy programs, art therapy interventions, and others.

3. *Home care:* In the best organizations, home care is a team effort.

   Hospice: Care and care planning are truly team efforts. A standard in all hospice programs is that the patient and family care is planned and provided by an interdisciplinary team.

4. *Home care:* Medicare is a cost-based reimbursement system, sometimes reinforcing unnecessary visits or visits that may be medically unnecessary.

Hospice: The Medicare hospice benefit is a managed-care system of reimbursement. In addition, most hospices have traditionally been not-for-profit entities and admit and care for patients regardless of payment mechanisms or their ability to pay.

5. *Home care:* When needed care cannot be provided under the auspices of regular home care and when the nurse identifies that the patient (and the care team) would have additional support through hospice, it can become frustrating when a patient chooses not to have hospice. Home care may not have the flexibility that supports meeting patient needs, depending on the mission and structure.

Hospice: Volunteer support, staff support mechanisms, and the true team concept all assist and support the nurse and other team members through the patient's death and beyond. Continuity and closure are also offered as bereavement services for the patient's survivors for a period of time.

6. *Home care:* Productivity and other parameters of effectiveness are designated by time frames (e.g., 6 to 7 visits a day average or 25 to 35 visits a week average).

Hospice: Time frames may be more difficult to project in hospice because of lengthy or extended visits. The initial visit to a new hospice patient may take more than one visit and may be more than 2 hours long. There is not only much information to provide, but it must be provided in a sensitive manner with the patient and family sometimes setting the pace. Some hospices have a nurse and social worker admit the patient for the first or initial admitting visit. If the hospice is Medicare-certified and the patient is admitted to the benefit, the rules to be explained, forms to be signed, and clinical and physical assessment data gathering that must occur are labor-intensive. It is only with experience that admission and subsequent visits become more efficient and effective.

MEDICARE HOSPICE 101

Many insurers cover or reimburse hospice programs for hospice services. How hospice services are defined may vary as may the specific coverage and documentation requirements. There is a specific Medicare hospice benefit, and many state Medicaid programs mirror the Medicare hospice benefit. The hospice nurse is often the expert on communicating coverage and other information to patients and families in the advocacy role. It is for this reason that hospice nurses should know about the basis of the Medicare hospice program.

Congress enacted the benefit in 1983 and made it a permanent program in 1986. The following five requirements *must* be met for a patient to be eligible for the hospice Medicare benefit:

1. The patient is eligible for Medicare hospital insurance (Part A).
2. The patient is certified by an attending physician and the hospice medical director to have a limited life expectancy and a poor prognosis.
3. The patient resides in the geographical area where there is a hospice program that is Medicare-certified.
4. A written plan of care is established and regularly reviewed.
5. The patient "elects" the hospice Medicare benefit.

The patient who elects the hospice benefit "gives up" his or her regular Medicare benefits. This is usually not a problem unless the patient wants more care than can be delivered through hospice. Patients who elect the benefit receive palliative and noncurative care and support. In addition, some of the requirements of regular Medicare home care are waived for these patients. For example, the patient neither has to be homebound nor meet skilled care requirements as defined in the traditional home care sense. The strength of the program is that it is a comprehensive managed care program in which all services and care are coordinated through one entity, the hospice organization. Coverage generally includes physician services, nursing care, medical supplies and equipment, short-term inpatient care (including respite care), home health aide, physical therapy, speech-language pathology services, medical social services, and counseling, including dietary counseling. Patients have a limited cost sharing for drugs and inpatient respite care. The hospice program is the expert on the rules related to the Medicare hospice program. Although the Medicare program is a needed and viable program for some Medicare beneficiaries seeking hospice, not all patients may be appropriate for it.

HOSPICE DOCUMENTATION

Whatever the coverage, the hospice nurse plays an important role in supporting coverage of hospice through effective documentation. The nursing documentation should emphasize the patient's prognosis, whatever the diagnoses, as this is the reason for hospice. It is important to note that it is a hallmark of effective and quality hospice care that patients are accepted for service with the understanding that they receive the services in accordance with their unique needs. Identifying and reassessing the patient's unique needs is an ongoing process, and is based on the patient's clinical findings as documented in the clinical record.

The documentation must then reflect that the patient clearly has an illness of a terminal nature, with a limited life expectancy of less than 6 months. For example, if a patient has coronary atherosclerosis, the documentation would need to demonstrate that the patient has a shortened life expectancy. It is known that some patients can live for years with this diagnosis on effective cardiac medications. It is for this reason that the documentation must clearly state the findings and the patient's deteriorating status; this supports that the patient is appropriate for hospice. The nurse can see how sick the patient is and how appropriate hospice care is. The nurse's clinical documentation, including the assessment forms, visit notes, and other tools, must support this covered care. With the increased scrutiny by the government to identify "noncovered" care, the hospice team must document the patient's status that supports appropriate and covered hospice care.

Excellence in hospice documentation is in the details. The nurse must support that the patient and family needs and can benefit from hospice care. The ICD-9 code designation(s) must be correct, the history and physical findings should be complete, assessment information should be detailed, and nursing and other notes should support the terminal prognosis. The documentation should reflect ongoing effects of the terminal condition, the family's difficulty with care or coping skills, and the patient's/family's desire for palliative care.

In summary, the nursing and other documentation must reflect the patient's condition and, in essence, paint a clear picture for any reviewer assessing for coverage or quality (Box 16-1). The reviewer has not seen the patient; express how the patient looks objectively throughout your documentation.

SUMMARY

Special qualities, skills, and characteristics of caring people make up the hospice team. The nurse has the unique role of case manager at many hospices. As such, the nurse coordinates and clarifies the desires of patients and their families or partners. Expertise in symptom control, continued learning related to pain and its relief, flexibility, and a sense of humor are all assets nurses should have if they want to make the transition to a practice setting in which nurses and other hospice workers make an important difference in care and life through the dying process for patients and their families. Whatever the role of the nurse at an individual hospice, the focus is always centered on the patient and caregiver and their unique individualized choices and journey.

BOX 16-1   **EFFECTIVE DOCUMENTATION:**
              A CHECKLIST APPROACH

✔ If handwritten, are notes or other entries legible to team members or others who may require the information?

✔ Are data elements or areas needing completion addressed in an understandable manner? For example, is there a legend or a list of acceptable program abbreviations when abbreviations occur?

✔ Does the care plan reflect the problems identified during the comprehensive assessment?

✔ Are new team members oriented to forms and shown accurately completed examples?

✔ Does the clinical record paint a clear picture of the patient, interventions, responses, and outcomes (or quantifiable goals of care)?

✔ Does the record and documentation pass the test of effective care planning and coordination? Could another colleague, in your absence, review the record and be able to effectively continue with the plan of care?

✔ Are interventions based on the needs as documented in the comprehensive assessment and subsequent entries throughout the patient's care?

✔ Does the documentation emphasize the reason the patient needs hospice services?

✔ Does the documentation support covered care as defined by Medicare, the case manager, or payor?

✔ Are the clinical records reviewed on an ongoing and timely basis for quality, completion, and identification that the patient has either met predetermined goals or needs continued care, with possible changes to the plan based on the ongoing assessment findings and response to interventions? This includes dates, communications, and physician's order follow-procedures.

✔ If a surveyor, payor, patient, or accreditation entity were to review the record, would the clinical documentation reflect the provision of safe, quality, and effective patient care?

REVIEW EXERCISES

1. List six of the core services offered by hospices.
2. Describe the basic tenets of hospice.
3. Identify the reason that documentation is an important component in hospice care.
4. List three reasons for the growth in hospice.
5. Define hospice and hospice nursing.

6. Describe the different kinds of hospice organizations.
7. Identify four of the differences between home care and hospice nursing.
8. What is the focus of hospice?
9. Who is the unit of care in hospice?
10. What kinds of patients and families are cared for through hospice?

RESOURCES

Agency for Health Care Policy and Research (AHCPR). Call for the *free* AHCPR Cancer Pain Guidelines by calling (800)4-CANCER.

Fitchett G: *Spiritual assessment in pastoral care: a guide to selected resources,* The Journal of Pastoral Care Publications, (404) 320-0195.

Hawkins C: *The karing book: patient's pal.* This is a large three-ring notebook to track needed medical information. The book attempts to empower parents of very ill children by encouraging their active participation in their child's care, (800)9-KARING.

The Health Care Financing Administration (HCFA) publishes and distributes a flyer, *Medicare hospice benefits.* There is also a free *Medicare handbook* with detailed information about the Medicare programs, including hospice, and can be ordered by calling (800)638-6833.

Home Care Nurse News is a monthly, clinically focused newsletter for clinicians and managers practicing in home care and hospice. To review an issue, call Marrelli and Associates, Inc. at (800)993-NEWS (6397).

Hospice Nurses Association: *Standards of hospice nursing practice and professional performance,* Pittsburgh, 1995, Hospice Nurses Association. Call (412)361-2470 to obtain information.

Marrelli T, Whittier S: *Home health aide: guidelines for care,* 1996, Marrelli and Associates, Inc., (800)993-6397.

Marrelli T, Friend L: *Home health aide: guidelines for care instructor manual,* 1997, Marrelli and Associates, Inc., (800)993-6397.

National Cancer Institute (NCI): *Fact sheets on anticancer drugs.* These are *free* fact sheets on 55 drugs used to treat cancer. They list the side effects, precautions while taking the drug, and the proper way to use it. They are printed in both English and Spanish. Call the NCI at (800)4-CANCER. Spanish- and English-speaking staff members are available to speak with callers.

National Hospice Organization: *Hospice under Medicare,* 1995, Channing L. Bete Company, Inc., (703)243-5900.

National Hospice Organization (NHO): *The NHO medical guidelines for determining prognoses in selected noncancer diseases.* These guidelines may be obtained be calling the NHO or by writing to: NHO Store, 200 State Rd., S. Deerfield, MA 01373-0200.

Purdue Frederick Company. Write for the Patient Comfort Assessment: The Purdue Frederick Company, 100 Connecticut Ave., Norwalk, CT 06850-3590. Ask for a listing of their free resources available to home care and hospice nurses related to pain and its management.

Ross Labs offers a free videotape entitled *Taking charge: managing the symptoms of HIV.* This videotape addresses interventions for pain and fatigue for patients with

AIDS. Ask your local Ross representative for the tape or call (800)227-5767 if you do not know who the representative in your area is. Ask for tape No. H358V.

Sigrist D: *Journey's end: a guide to understanding the dying process,* Hospice of Rochester Genesee Region Home Care, 49 Stone St., Rochester, NY 14604.

The Roxanne Pain Institute for Cancer and AIDs has a 24-hour toll-free number for services to both professionals and patients. For information and reference materials, such as AHCPR materials, call (800)335-9100.

REFERENCES

Carney K, Burns N: Economics of hospice care, *Oncol Nurs Forum* 18:761-786, 1991.

Hospice Nurses Association: *Standards of hospice nursing practice and professional performance,* Pittsburgh, 1995, Hospice Nurses Association.

National Hospice Organization: *Hospice fact sheet,* Arlington, Va, October 10, 1995, National Hospice Organization.

National Hospice Organization: *Standards of a hospice program of care,* Arlington, 1993, National Hospice Organization.

FOR FURTHER READING

Cody C: Hospice update: documentation in non-cancer diseases, *Home Care Nurse News* 2(10):5, 1995.

Marrelli T: Hospice update: accreditation, *Home Care Nurse News* 3(3):5, 1996.

Marrelli T: *Handbook of home health standards and documentation guidelines for reimbursement,* ed 3, St. Louis, 1998, Mosby.

Marrelli T: *The hospice handbook: assessment, standards, and reimbursement,* St. Louis, 1997, Mosby.

Reese K: Home care 101. Part One: Understanding and assessing pain at home, *Home Care Nurse News* 2(1):1-2, 1995.

Reese K: Home Care 101. Part Two: Understanding and assessing pain at home, *Home Care Nurse News* 2(2):1-3, 1995.

chapter

17

INFUSION CARE IN HOME CARE

Christine A. Pierce, RN, CS, MSN, ANP

"No one's head aches when he is comforting another."

Indian Proverb

The ability to provide intravenous therapy in alternate settings has expanded tremendously throughout the last few decades, driven by an array of factors that include advances in technology and pharmacology, reimbursement changes, patient preference, and nursing versatility. The viable home care organization of today must be prepared to provide high-quality, cost-effective intravenous services as a component of comprehensive care and to commit to the ongoing development of appropriate practitioners in this specialty. This chapter will provide an historical look at the evolution of home infusion, describe the current trends, and explore the methods and resources necessary for preparing competent intravenous nursing practitioners in the home care setting.

HISTORY OF HOME INFUSION THERAPY
Background and Evolution

Throughout history man has experimented with the bloodstream as a route to body systems and possible disease intervention. Discovery of the circulatory system, first accurately described by Sir William Harvey in the late 15th century, prompted work in related fields, eventually leading to the invention of hypodermic needles, development of principles of infection control, and the discovery of a noninvasive means to assess vasculature and vascular access—the radiograph. However, it was many years until all of the needed components would come together as the knowledge base of intravenous therapy.

Initial progress was slow as animal-to-human transfusions were incompatible, patients succumbed to sepsis, and pyrogenic contamination of infusates was unpreventable. By the early 20th century infusion therapy was still considered to be a major procedure, reserved for the most critically ill, and remained solely within the domain of the physician. Treatment and technological advances, stimulated by the needs of war casualties with large-scale fluid losses, human nutrition research, and the invention of synthetic materials, continued. The results were increasingly innovative approaches to fluid and electrolyte resuscitation (e.g., steel needle replacement with flexible catheters, use of plastics, and nonvented delivery containers).

The Beginning of Intravenous Nursing

Intravenous (IV) nursing evolved from the large urban medical setting of Massachusetts General Hospital, Boston, where in 1940 a new nursing specialty was described to include the following responsibilities (Plumer and Consentino, 1987):

1. Administering IV solutions and transfusions
2. Cleaning and sharpening needles
3. Cleaning infusion sets
4. Maintaining patent needles and unobstructed flow

This role, although primarily focused on technical care, represented a milestone in establishing nursing's autonomy from medical practice and also set an important precedent for the infusion nursing specialty.

Today nearly 100% of hospitalized patients receive some form of IV therapy during their stay, and many will continue that therapy after discharge. Whether specialist or generalist, practicing in the community or the institution, a nurse will ultimately be faced with the need to care for patients who require the sophisticated interventions of IV therapy. It is therefore essential that all nurses be prepared with the skills and knowledge that can offset risk and maximize the value of IV treatment, regardless of practice setting.

MODERN INFUSION THERAPY
Infusion Care: A Growing Part of Home Care

Home care is a burgeoning segment of the health care industry, driven by a variety of factors, including economic, technological and social. During 1995 over 17,000 home care providers supplied services to approximately 7 million people, at a cost in excess of $27 billion, representing roughly 3% of national health care spending. These costs reflect the service component of care—mainly that attributable to skilled nursing, rehabilitation, and related home care aide services—and not the additional expenses necessarily associated with home infusion, such as medications, pharmacy services and durable medical equipment (National Association for Home Care, 1996). These latter items, commonly referred to as the product and supply component of the home infusion industry, are accounted for in other health care financial reporting and should not be overlooked when attempting to gain a full cost perspective of this specialty. Conners and Winters, in their 1995 comprehensive report on the home infusion industry, estimate that approximately 850,000 individuals received one or more home infusion therapies during 1994. From this data it is relatively easy to calculate that home IV therapy affects about 12% of all home care recipients and, since it generates nearly $5 billion in annual revenues, that it significantly raises the average cost of caring for this specialty group.

Home infusion is in its infancy as far as specialties are concerned. First introduced in the early 1970s, home infusion programs began as a means to foster independence among patients who required long-term—usually lifelong—administration of total parenteral nutrition (TPN). Affiliated with an acute care hospital, the early home infusion programs provided patient and caregiver training regarding the compounding of TPN components, care of the vascular access, and signs and symptoms for which to return to the hospital. The hospital pharmacy dispensed medications, solutions, and supplies, creating a sort of "miniature pharmacy" within the patient's residence. Although the infusion pumps from that era provided the patient with little mobility, at least the TPN recipient was able to reside in the community and continue some normal socialization.

Antiinfective therapy was soon to follow. In 1979 the Cleveland Clinic was able to demonstrate successful clinical outcomes in 150 patients who participated in the self-administration of antibiotics at home (Portez, 1991). Programs such as this were readily accepted by patients and their families since they facilitated early return to work or school and provided independence in managing chronic diseases such as cystic fibrosis and its recurrent pulmonary infections. Soon many other IV medications began to be considered for administration outside of the hospital setting, offering unprecedented convenience and freedom to those with cancer, hemophilia, acquired immune deficiency syndrome (AIDS), and other diseases.

Factors Contributing to Industry Expansion

Although the seminal notions of home infusion were clearly centered around patient advocacy and enhancement of quality of life, there were additional contributory forces that helped launch this industry into its current state of prevalence (Box 17-1).

BOX 17-1   **FACTORS CONTRIBUTING TO GROWTH OF THE HOME INFUSION INDUSTRY**

1. Acceptance of IV nursing as a specialty—1970s
2. Proliferation of entrepreneurial pharmacy providers—early 1980s
3. Medicare Part B prosthetic device benefit—early 1980s
4. Diagnostic-related groups (DRGs)—1983
5. Pharmaceutical research and development—ongoing
6. Technology development—ongoing
7. Patient quality of life concerns and preference—ongoing

In 1983 Medicare introduced diagnostic-related groups (DRGs) to the hospital setting, marking the first prospective payment reimbursement for in-patient care. Suddenly the hospitals were faced with delivering quality clinical outcomes within the confines of limited, predetermined financial resources. Discharging patients sooner, to a less costly environment, seemed highly desirable. Since it was often the continued need for IV therapy that retained a patient in the hospital, home infusion programs provided one solution. In the home care arena, the Health Care Finance Administration (HCFA) was expanding coverage of TPN through the prosthetic device act. Patients who met specific qualifying criteria could receive their TPN at home, with the expense being covered under Medicare, Part B. Associated professional care, most commonly skilled nursing, was already reimbursable under Part A, fostering comprehensive home care for TPN patients with both cancer and noncancer diagnoses.

Product and supply companies soon caught the momentum and began targeting the mobile, insured, and informed home infusion population and its providers for research and development opportunities. Cumbersome, pole-mounted infusion pumps gave way to lightweight, portable, and even disposable models. Catheter materials were designed for better biocompatibility, translating into longer dwell times with fewer complications. Improved vascular access dressing materials enhanced patient comfort and freedom from infection, whereas advances in needleless systems and other protective technologies fostered increased safety for the caregiver as well as the patient.

Pharmaceutical development made some monumental leaps in the last decade, introducing genetically engineered products such as the biologics that revolutionized the treatment of anemia, neutropenia, and other primary and secondary disorders of the hematopoietic system. The category of antiinfective agents came to include antivirals and antifungals, in addition to an ever-expanding array of antibiotics that have longer half lives, greater stability, and less frequency of administration. Sophisticated antiemetics and other adjunctive medications brought a new comfort and mobility to the administration of chemotherapy and the management of pain. It became increasingly possible to do just about anything, just about anywhere!

Critical to the success of home infusion operations was the provision of skilled, professional nursing. Pharmacists and nurses had begun partnering on both clinical and business issues to collaboratively deliver comprehensive infusion care. IV nursing had evolved from the late 1960s, throughout the 1970s, via the proliferation of hospital-based IV teams. This specialty group of nurses provided vascular access device and site care; started IVs; maintained responsibility for IV quality assurance, including complication rates; selected IV products; and often directly administered the more complicated infusion therapies such as chemotherapy and blood transfusions. Their technical expertise, as well as their ability to oversee and direct a broad range of patient care activities, including education and training, made them a valuable commodity during the 1980s.

Since 1973 the specialty had boasted its own professional nursing organization. The National Intravenous Therapy Association (NITA), which in 1987 became the Intravenous Nurses Society (INS), first published IV recommendations for practice in 1980, just a few years after the American Nurses Association had set forth the initial standards of practice for professional nursing. In 1985 NITA offered the first certification examination for the specialty of IV nursing, adding Certified Registered Nurse, Intravenous (CRNI) to the list of credentials that were increasingly sought by home infusion employers. By the mid 1980s, IV nurses were shaping the face of home infusion care—setting quality standards, introducing new therapies to the home setting, advising companies on new product development—and yes, enjoying some of the profitability in the form of handsome salaries, bonuses, and benefits. It was, by all accounts, an exciting time for IV nurses.

Defining Home Infusion

Home infusion therapy (HIT) is a broad term that has been commonly used to refer to the nonoral administration of pharmaceuticals and the maintenance of vascular access devices outside of the hospital setting. It also generally includes enteral therapy that is delivered through nasogastric, gastrostomy, or jejunostomy tubes. It specifically refers to the delivery of medications, solutions, and/or nutritional products via parenteral (e.g., IV, intraarterial, subcutaneous, intraspinal, and intracavitary) routes, within the patient's place of residence (Table 17-1).

TABLE 17-1 TYPES OF HOME INFUSION THERAPIES

ROUTE	THERAPY
Intravenous—peripheral	Antibiotics
	Hydration fluids and electolytes
	Steroids
	Diuretics
	Blood and blood components
Intravenous—central	Antiinfectives (antibiotics, antifungals, antivirals)
	Total parenteral nutrition
	Analgesics
	Anticoagulants
	Chemotherapy
	Inotropic agents
Subcutaneous	Analgesics
	Tocolytics
	Anticoagulants
	Biologics
Intra-arterial	Chemotherapy
Intraspinal	Analgesics
Intracavitary	Chemotherapy

In the broadest interpretation this means that medications, supplies, and equipment are delivered to the patient's home, which then becomes the core care environment. Administration of the infusion may actually be accomplished outside of the home, such as at school or work, depending on the patient's mobility and independence, but the patient does not return to an institutional setting to receive the doses. This differs from the concept of "ambulatory infusion therapy" that involves clinics or outpatient settings to which patients return at regularly scheduled intervals to receive their dosing from professional caregivers. For purposes of discussion here, HIT will be defined specifically as those therapies originating and controlled from the patient's place of residence.

TABLE 17-2   **HOME INFUSION DISTRIBUTION BY THERAPY TYPE, 1994**

INTRAVENOUS SERVICE	DISTRIBUTION (%)
Total parenteral nutrition	4
Antibiotics	43
Enteral nutrition	6
Chemotherapy	9
Pain management	8
"Other"	30

Data from Conners RB, Winters RW, editors: *Home infusion: current status and future trends,* Chicago, 1995, American Hospital Publishing, p. 12.

Types of Home Infusion Therapy Patients

The home infusion patient of the 1990s may be a neonate with a pulmonary infection, a high-risk pregnancy patient with preterm labor, a geriatric patient with congestive heart failure, or someone of nearly any age and diagnosis that requires any type of infusion services. By far the most frequently administered therapies are the antiinfective agents, followed closely by an ever expanding category of "other" (Table 17-2).

The most common reason for receiving HIT is chronic, resistant infections that are not ameliorated by oral antibiotics (Grace and Tomaselli, 1995), such as osteomyelitis in patients with impaired peripheral circulation. Other common diagnoses are human immunodeficiency virus (HIV)-related infections, cancer, short-gut syndrome, chronic pain and dehydration (Table 17-3).

In 1991 more than 60% of home infusion patients were between the ages of 25 and 64, with only 18% 65 years or older (Winters, Parver, and Sansbury, 1992). Although revenues and profitability in this industry have been negatively impacted by managed care, the clinical demands for home infusion continue to grow.

A home care business today would not be considered complete without some type of infusion pharmacy arrangement. Some home health organizations own and operate their own pharmacy, directly employing pharmacists, technicians, and delivery personnel. Others choose to affiliate with infusion providers, either through partnerships or contracting as preferred providers. Still others remain independent providers of skilled nursing for any infusion pharmacy in their area. There are ad-

TABLE 17-3 COMMON DIAGNOSES IN HOME INFUSION THERAPY

DIAGNOSIS	ICD9 CODE	THERAPY TYPE
Osteomyelitis	730.2	Antibiotic
Anemia	285.9	Blood
		Biologic
Dehydration	276.5	Hydration
Carcinoma	194.3	Chemotherapy
		TPN/enteral nutrition
		Analgesic
		Biologic
		Hydration
		Other
Human immunode-ficiency virus	044.9	Antiinfective
		TPN/enteral nutrition
Malabsorption	579.9	TPN/enteral nutrition
Short bowel syndrome	579.2	TPN
Congestive heart failure	428.9	Inotropic
		Diuretic
Thrombophlebitis	451.9	Anticoagulant
Wound, complicated	879.8	Antibiotic
Hyperemesis gravidarum	643.0	Hydration
		TPN
Labor, premature	644.2	Tocolytic
Hemophilia	286.0	Blood components
Fungal disease	117.9	Antiinfective
Endocarditis, infectious	421.0	Antibiotic
Diabetic ulcer	250.8	Antibiotic
Crohn's disease	555.9	TPN/enteral nutrition
Septicemia	038.9	Antibiotic
Cellulitis	682.9	Antibiotic
Obstruction, intestine	560.9	TPN/enteral nutrition

TPN, Total parenteral nutrition.

vantages and disadvantages to each arrangement. Whatever the nature of the business arrangement, the delivery of IV home care shares some common themes: infusion therapy is a high-technology, high-risk, challenging specialty that demands competent, autonomous, and caring professionals to ensure favorable outcomes.

Insurance Coverage

To deliver comprehensive clinical care in home infusion, it is necessary to have a basic understanding of the way costs are reimbursed (Table 17-4). This seems to be a particular area of confusion for home care nurses who, accustomed to servicing a high percentage of elderly Medicare patients whose home care services have traditionally been covered by Medicare Part A, suddenly are faced with having to explain lack of a payment mechanism for the IV antibiotics, pump, and supplies required by the same patient. This is because HIT is predominantly reimbursed by commercial sources, either primary or secondary, and only under specific conditions, for limited therapies, by Medicare Part B, not Part A. During the last decade the HCFA has considered expansion of benefits for HIT, perhaps most visibly with the Medicare Catastrophic Coverage Act, 1988, which, along with other offerings, proposed coverage for home IV drugs and the services required to administer them (Office of Technology Assessment, 1992). In late 1989 the Medicare Catastrophic Coverage Act was repealed before the benefit was implemented.

To simplify the discussion of HIT reimbursement, it is advisable to separate infusion therapies into two clinical categories: (1) nutrition support, commonly referred to as "home PEN" (parenteral and enteral nutrition), and (2) all others. Home PEN was where home infusion began, and Medicare support was one of the factors fueling its growth. Since 1977 Medicare has provided coverage for this therapy under the Part B Prosthetic Device Benefit. As defined by Medicare, a prosthetic device serves to replace the function of a permanently malfunctioning internal body organ, in this case, the gut. Thus the specific rules that apply to a patient's eligibility for PEN coverage were derived from the following:

- Permanence, defined as long and indefinite duration, minimally 90-day
- Complete, not supplemental, *replacement* for the gut—analysis of protein, calorie, and lipid content in the prescribed infusion must meet Medicare's standard to be eligible for reimbursement
- Certificate of Medical Necessity, adequate physician documentation to permit independent determination that the requirements are met and that TPN is medically necessary

Enteral therapy requires similar qualification and must be ruled unsuccessful before TPN can be considered for coverage. In all instances of PEN it is essential to stay abreast of the Durable Medical Equipment Regional Carrier (DMERC) guidelines because there are occasional minor changes to these fundamental reimbursement criteria. The DMERCs

	MEDICARE	MEDICAID	COMMERCIAL PAYORS
TABLE 17-4	**REIMBURSEMENT FOR HOME INFUSION THERAPY**		
PEN	✔	✔	✔
Antibiotics		✔	✔
Anti-infectives	Limited	✔	✔
Analgesics	Limited	✔	✔
Chemotherapy	Limited	✔	✔
Dobutamine			✔
Hydration		✔	✔
Biologics			✔

are specialty carriers (i.e., payors/insurance companies) who process and adjudicate these specialized claims for HCFA.

Provision of PEN through state Medicaid programs is determined by individual states and generally is subject to stringent qualifying criteria. Coverage for TPN and enteral nutrition (EN) is also available through commercial insurance, either primary or secondary. These sources may demand less rigorous qualifying criteria, but may dictate specific limitations such as equipment type or number of reimbursable nursing visits. It is this latter method of payment that has been the savior of patients with short-term TPN needs such as those with radiation enteritis or pancreatitis. In any case, be prepared for a thorough review of the clinical record and specific discussions with the physician/case manager and detailed documentation when the discharge order to home reads "TPN."

In the broadest sense, there is no HIT coverage beyond PEN under Medicare Part B. In reality, Medicare reimbursement exists for a select few very specific therapies that include: IV morphine; certain chemotherapeutic drugs such as 5-fluorouracil when administered by continuous infusion; and a handful of antiinfectives such as fluconazole, which require a pump for safe administration. Again, your DMERC can provide the most current reimbursement guidelines. That leaves the remaining "other" therapies to generally be supported by commercial insurance or Medicaid. So what about all of those elderly, homebound diabetics with infected ulcers or osteomyelitis? The challenge becomes apparent! Without the luxury of secondary insurance, or the foresight of a visionary managed Medicare plan that includes HIT, these patients are faced with a choice of either personal payment or an extended stay in subacute care.

THE HOME AS PRACTICE SETTING
"There's No Place Like Home. . ."

L. Frank Baum's character, Dorothy, can readily be identified by this famous line from *The Wizard of Oz.* Certainly many home care patients would agree with her, preferring the comfort and familiarity of their own surroundings to the sterile, impersonal environment of the hospital. The home, however, presents unique practice challenges for the nurse who assumes the dual role of guest and caregiver in an unfamiliar setting that varies from patient to patient. What are considered routine elements of institutional care—heat, electricity, running water, food, safety—may be startlingly absent or altered at home and will require specific evaluation in each residence, for each case. The home care nurse can never assume that the living conditions or arrangements of any patient will be compatible with the effective implementation of home care services until thorough evaluation is complete.

Patient Rights and Responsibilities

In return for the provision of care at home, a patient has reciprocal responsibilities, both for his own treatment and that of the visiting staff. These ground rules are required for participation in Medicare and are explained during the initial visit before initiating care (see Figure 4-4). The nurse informs the patient of the services and benefits available through home care, including the scope, any limitations, and source of payment, disclosing any charges for services not covered by Medicare or Medicaid. Because Medicare coverage for home infusion is so limited, it is *imperative* that the nurse have a solid understanding of the other reimbursement mechanisms and the ability to explain them to the patient. In the hospital, billing or admitting personnel may assume this responsibility, but in the home a nurse's role broadens to include the important financial aspects of care. This role also includes developing and maintaining collaborative working relationships with the reimbursement department and putting the patient directly in contact with a representative by phone for more information. In situations of financial hardship, intervention by the organization's social workers is recommended.

Part of the patients' rights is that nurses commit to respectful treatment of patients' environment and property and to providing considerate care that preserves personal dignity, which reflect the dual role of caregiver and guest. Calling ahead to schedule visits and notifying the family when a delay occurs are examples of this courtesy. In return, the patient promises to disclose accurate health history information, to inform the organization when a visit must be canceled or time changed, to participate in designing and following the plan of care, and to treat the visit staff with respect. Violation of the contract by either party may be grounds for termination. Effective introduction of this collaborative contracting model sets the stage for an ongoing, mutually satisfying relationship between the nurse and patient.

Safety Precautions: Risk Management 101

Home infusion practitioners are subject to many of the same risks as their hospital counterparts: infectious and hazardous material exposure, equipment malfunction, accidents, and a host of other possibilities. But nursing practice in the home setting introduces some new challenges to the area of risk management. Within the community environment the nurse must be constantly alert to issues of personal safety.

Home care orientation should effectively address these circumstances and offer opportunities to role play potentially risky situations within the protection of the classroom. Organizational policy and procedure should specifically outline the routine precautions to be taken on all home care visits (Box 17-2) and seasoned home health nurses can be invited to share their experiences (see Chapter 4).

BOX 17-2   HOME CARE VISIT PRECAUTIONS

✔ Carry emergency supplies such as flares and a blanket.
✔ Know exactly where you are going and notify supervisor as to where you will be.
✔ Avoid carrying large sums of money, credit cards, or a purse.
✔ Wear minimal or no jewelry.
✔ Carry appropriate identification.
✔ Have medications and bulk supplies delivered by the pharmacy delivery service.
✔ Carry emergency phone numbers and a cellular phone or change for a pay phone.
✔ If domestic or substance abuse is occurring, leave and call for appropriate help.
✔ Ask that visible weapons be put away during the visit or else leave the home.
✔ Do not consume food or beverages from the patient's home.
✔ Be familiar with agency policy regarding use of security escorts and use as needed.

It is not uncommon to make late-evening/night visits for problems, scheduled antibiotic dosing, or TPN hook-ups; on-call visits for emergencies—often during the night—should be anticipated. A cardinal rule is that safety should *never* be taken for granted. If potentially dangerous situations are identified or there is hesitancy regarding personal safety, organization procedures should be followed for notifying supervisors and involving security escorts. At the first suggestion of proximate personal harm, the nurse should leave the situation *immediately.*

Standards of Care

Infusion therapy, in any practice setting, certainly constitutes a "risky business," but outside the protected environment of the hospital (i.e., in a home where the nurse is alone), it can become positively terrifying. Each patient encounter presents another opportunity for less than ideal outcomes if adequate precautions are not in place. There is so much that can go so wrong so quickly. The patient receiving infusion therapy may be "sicker" and less medically stable than other patients. Infusion equipment is highly technical and can be dangerous in unskilled hands. Invasive procedures involving the bloodstream and the use of needles and sharps places practitioners, patients, and other family members at risk for infectious disease transmission or injury.

Determining a patient's readiness for self care involves a complex set of decisions that requires the nurse to have a high level of critical thinking skills and sound judgment. A wrong decision here could prove fatal. Administering complex medications with attendant adverse reactions demands that the infusion nurse have a solid knowledge of pharmacology and be assertive enough to state when a treatment would be better delivered in a more protected environment. To lessen this risk, it is essential to follow the guidelines and recommendations of experience, better known as standards of practice.

Standards of Practice

Standards of practice are a foundation of the nursing profession and must be applied in the same manner, in all practice settings, to all patients at all times to ensure positive outcomes. Let's take a simple example: in the hospital setting risk of bloodborne pathogen exposure is lessened through the effective use of barriers, proper handwashing, and the use of needleless devices whenever possible. These same principles must be applied in the home setting, even though it means carrying supplies such as liquid or foam soap, paper towels, newspapers, goggles, and gloves on each visit. Inconvenience or planning problems cannot be an excuse for failure to follow standards.

Standards of practice relevant to the infusion specialty have originated from regulatory agencies (The Joint Commission on Accreditation of Health Care Organizations [JCAHO] and the Centers for Disease Control and Prevention [CDC]), as well as from professional organizations (Intravenous Nurses Society, American Society of Parenteral and Enteral Nutrition, American Society of Health System Pharmacists). These resources should be integrated into the practice framework of the home care organization, forming the basis for position descriptions, policies, procedures, and evaluation of clinician competency. The latest revision of global infusion nursing standards was published in 1990 (Intravenous Nurses Society, 1990). Box 17-3 highlights the standards that are essential to the home infusion setting.

HOME INFUSION SUPPLIES AND TECHNOLOGY

Technology has expanded, in some instances to keep pace with the clinical demands of home infusion therapy and, in other instances, to set the pace. The following section provides an overview of current technology in HIT.

Vascular Access Devices

Although enteral, intraspinal, and other parenteral routes of medication administration are included in infusion therapy, the predominant route remains venous. Both peripheral and central catheters have improved considerably in the last decade, favoring lower complication rates and increased biocompatibility and patient mobility and ease and safety of use. Catheter materials have progressed from rigid Teflon and polyurethane to the more flexible silicone and Aquavene, decreasing the incidence of phlebitis and vein perforation. The Groshong valve was developed and added to central catheters, permitting the elimination of heparin dwell solutions and increasing safety from air embolism. Peripherally inserted central catheters (PICCs) made a comeback, becoming a preferred access for patients with contraindications to surgical line placement. The midline catheter was introduced in 1990, bridging the gap between short peripheral catheters and central lines and became a common access for moderate duration (2 to 4 weeks) antibiotic therapy. Table 17-5 provides a brief overview of vascular access devices, uses, advantages and disadvantages.

Infusion Devices

Home infusion therapy has improved because of the abundance of new and improved infusion devices. Once safety, reliability, and portability were king; now devices compete with sophisticated features such as

---

BOX 17-3   ESSENTIAL STANDARDS OF PRACTICE IN HOME INFUSION THERAPY

Disease Transmission and Infection Control

S-24   Implementation of infection control measures minimizes the potential for infectious complications and should encompass handwashing, barrier protection, aseptic technique, disposal of contaminated and/or sharp materials, and a mechanism for tracking and reporting infection complications as a component of quality monitoring.

S-25   Durable medical equipment shall be routinely cleansed with disinfectant.

S-26   Handwashing shall be accomplished before and immediately after all clinical procedures.

Medication Administration

S-30   Intravenous therapy shall be initiated on a physician's order using the nursing process. Consent of the patient or a legally authorized representative and the patient's identity shall be confirmed before initiation of therapy.

S-42   Patients receiving IV therapies shall be monitored at frequent and established intervals based on prescribed therapy, patient's condition and age, and practice setting.

S-46   IV therapy shall be discontinued on the order of a physician.

S-49   Before IV solution/medication administration the nurse shall assess the following: appropriateness of prescribed therapy; patient's age and condition; and dose, route, and rate ordered. The nurse shall have knowledge of the indications, actions, side effects, adverse reactions, and nursing interventions.

S-53   Medications shall not be administered, and products shall not be used beyond their established expiration dates.

S-53   Administration of investigational medications shall be in accordance with state and federal regulations. Signed informed patient consent is required before patient participation in the investigation.

Documentation

S-20   Documentation in the patient's medical record shall contain sufficient information to identify IV procedures, prescribed treatments, complications, and nursing interventions. Docu-

---

Data from Intravenous Nurses Society: *Revised intravenous nursing standards of practice,* Boston, 1990, Intravenous Nurses Society.

BOX 17-3   **ESSENTIAL STANDARDS OF PRACTICE IN HOME INFUSION THERAPY—cont'd**

---

mentation shall be legible and accessible to health care professionals involved in the patient's care.

S-21   Distinctive labeling shall provide pertinent and easily identified information relative to the cannula, dressing, solution, medication, and administration set.

S-21   Statistical data shall be compiled, reviewed, and evaluated to quantify and qualify outcomes of IV care. This data must be easily retrievable.

Patient Education

S-27   Patients shall be informed; when required to participate in their own care, understanding shall be assessed, and a return demonstration performed; continued treatment in the home setting requires that the nurse perform comprehensive education and a written set of instructions; education must include avoidance of and interventions for complications, emergency procedures, accessing the on-call system; all teaching must be documented in the clinical record.

Equipment

S-22   Products are to be assessed for defects.

S-23   Product defects shall be reported to appropriate agencies.

S-58   The nurse's knowledge relative to infusion devices shall include indications for use, mechanical operation, troubleshooting, PSI rating, and safety precautions.

---

remote programming, central venous pressure monitoring, bar coding, and preprogrammed drug compatibility (Jensen, 1995). There is such a variety that keeping track of every new pump has become virtually impossible. Infusion nurses who deliver care to special populations such as those in remote or rural areas, neonates, or bone marrow transplant or AIDS patients may find that they could benefit from some of the special features, especially multichannel delivery and remote programming. For most home infusion nurses, however, their selection of infusion devices is restricted to a common, reliable few, generally selected by a combination of affordability and versatility. Reading the infusion specialty literature and attending the trade shows at professional meetings will raise awareness of features to recommend for a specific patient population.

TABLE 17-5 **VASCULAR ACCESS DEVICES**

TYPE	FEATURES	USES	ADVANTAGES	DISADVANTAGES
Tunnelled	Single/dual lumen Surgical placement	Long-term therapy Extreme pH, osmo-larity Antibiotics Total parenteral nutrition Anti-infectives Chemotherapy Dobutamine Others	Cuff provides infection barrier Location facilitates self-care Wide bore/rapid flow rates Tip placement in superior vena cava Groshong valve ends heparin dwell	Visible exit site May be damaged/dis-lodged Risk of air embolism Requires flush/heparin dwell Requires surgery
Peripherally in-serted central catheters	Groshong valve option Percutaneous insert Median or basilic Single/dual lumen	Same as "tunnelled central"	Eliminates heparin dwell Low-risk air embolism Peripheral insertion Nursing procedure Tip placement in superior vena cava Minimal body image alteration	Valve failure Difficulty with blood draw May be unable to place if peripheral veins are damaged
Ports	Surgical placement	Same as "tunnelled central" May avoid vesicants	Not visible externally	Require needle access Location makes self-care difficult

Pumps in Home Care

Infusion devices, commonly known as "pumps," can be categorized as follows:

1. Power source—mechanical or electronic
2. Portability—ambulatory or stationary
3. Delivery mechanism—volumetric or controller
4. Infusion interval—intermittent, continuous, variable, taper
5. Delivery channels—dual or multi
6. Programmability—absent or present

Furthermore, multiple categories can be combined in an attempt to accurately depict the pump. For instance, a patient receiving a complex antiinfective regimen following bone marrow transplant might be characterized as using a programmable, multichannel, ambulatory, volumetric, electronic infusion pump! What is important to remember is the relevance of these general features and how they can be applied to specific patients (Table 17-6).

Pay close attention to the alarm features and safety options, giving strong consideration to risk management in the uncontrolled environment of home. Another vital feature to assess is complexity or ease of use. Complicated equipment can translate into prolonged or difficult training for staff and patients, as well as increased on-call visits. Speak with someone who is already using the equipment you want to purchase and learn from their experience whenever possible.

HOME INFUSION NURSING: MULTIFACETED ROLE

The goal of home infusion nursing is to holistically manage the highly technical care of a diverse patient population while promoting self-care and the highest possible quality of life within the uniqueness of each home and family. The home infusion nurse serves as a role model to patients and caregivers as she trains them to perform technical, complex, life-threatening tasks. She is a resource for the general home care nursing staff, updating them on industry trends and offering patient care advice in her specialty. Home infusion nursing represents a multifaceted role, requiring a diverse skill set and strong determination.

Critical Success Factors

Before entering the world of home infusion, it is prudent to have received IV experience in the hospital setting. Whether this occurs in critical care or oncology or on an infusion specialty team, the important

TABLE 17-6 INFUSION DEVICE FEATURES AND CLINICAL APPLICABILITY

DEVICE TYPE	FEATURES	CLINICAL APPLICATION
Mechanical	Driven by physics, not electricity Elastomeric balloon or spring types Flow determined by restricted rate tubing Compatible with most drugs Some have PCA option Lightweight, portable, disposable Volumes up to 250 cc	Antibiotics Some chemotherapy Analgesics Small volume parenterals Concentrated drug solutions
Electronic	Powered by battery or wall current Gravity type—controllers Positive-pressure type—volumetric pumps Rate calculated by drop size or volume measure Piston driven syringes—60-cc limit Many alarm features: occlusion, air-in-line, free-flow, low battery, parameter violations, completion, and others	All HIT applications May want to avoid positive pressure with vesicants
Ambulatory	Options: multichannel, ambulatory, programmable Transportable, not stationary Generally lightweight Carrying cases available Electronic or mechanical	Most HIT applications Small-volume parenterals Concentrated drug solutions

Stationary	Pole mounted Electronic	Most HIT applications May be preferred by debilitated TPN patients who find the weight difficult to carry Large-volume parenterals Pole may give unsteady patients some security in ambulating
Controller	Gravity delivery at <5 psi Accuracy relies on drop size Rate and occlusion alarms	Hydration Preferred for vesicants Cannot be used with large-drop sizes such as cyclosporin
Volumetric	Positive pressure delivery at < 12 psi Piston, peristaltic Wide rate range from as low as 0.1 cc High degree of accuracy For features and options, see "electronic" Electronic	All HIT applications
Multichannel	Volumetric Ambulatory or stationary Programmable Intermittent, continuous, variable	Indicated for complex medication regimens such as AIDS, bone marrow transplant

continued

PCA, Patient-controlled analgesia; *HIT,* home infusion therapy; *TPN,* total parenteral nutrition.

TABLE 17-6 INFUSION DEVICE FEATURES AND CLINICAL APPLICABILITY—cont'd

DEVICE TYPE	FEATURES	CLINICAL APPLICATION
Programmable	Electronic Volumetric Ambulatory or stationary Intermittent, continuous, variable Delay start PCA option Taper or "ramp" option For features and options, see "electronic"	Analgesics Antibiotics TPN—taper feature

---

BOX 17-4   **FOUNDATIONS OF IV NURSING PRACTICE**

✔ Autonomy and accountability
✔ Knowledge of anatomy and physiology
✔ Specific knowledge and understanding of the vascular system and its interrelatedness with other body systems and intravenous treatment modalities
✔ Attainment of skills necessary for the administration of IV therapies
✔ Knowledge of state-of-the-art technologies associated with IV therapies
✔ Knowledge of psychosocial aspects, including but not limited to recognition of sensitivity to the patient's wholeness, uniqueness, and significant social relationships, along with the knowledge of community and economic resources
✔ Interaction and collaboration with members of the health care team and participation in the clinical decision making process.

Data from Intravenous Nurses Society: *Revised intravenous nursing standards of practice*, Boston, 1990, Intravenous Nurses Society.

point is familiarity with the principles of care and working knowledge of the skills and technology needed to provide safe and effective patient care. It is then desirable to undertake some general home care experience, learning the uniqueness of nursing in the home environment, the rules of reimbursement and documentation, and the time-management skills that are needed for successful practice. A foundation in the concepts of community health nursing and an understanding of its scope of practice would be ideal. As the specialty's professional organization, the Intravenous Nurses Society has outlined the foundations of IV nursing practice (Box 17-4) and described basic competencies to be attained by the infusion nursing practitioner (Box 17-5). Perhaps most valuable is the willingness to face the unknown with every case that is opened. That flexibility and quest for adventure will sustain the nurse who chooses this specialty, as will a sense of humor, good judgment, and strong critical thinking/problem-solving skills.

Certification

Certification is one form of competency validation, symbolizing a practitioner's ability to meet experience and knowledge requirements and then successfully pass a standardized examination. In the United States

---

BOX 17-5   **COMPETENCIES IN INTRAVENOUS NURSING**

1. Proficiency in all clinical aspects of IV nursing, with validated competency in clinical judgment and practice
2. Verbal and written communication skills
3. Patient education skills, with demonstrated ability to assess level of learning and need for additional instruction learning
4. Familiarity with relevant technology and participation in the evaluation, selection, and implementation of these products in the clinical area
5. Active participation in continuing education
6. Compliance with legal and regulatory standards of the IV specialty
7. Evidence of quality improvement activities and outcomes evaluation
8. Participation in and use of nursing research
9. Familiarity with principles of supervision and fiscal management

---

Data from Intravenous Nurses Society: *Revised intravenous nursing standards of practice,* Boston, 1990, Intravenous Nurses Society.

today there are dozens of nursing specialty certification options (Fickeissen, 1990). Those familiar to the home infusion industry include the following:

- Certified registered nurse, intravenous (CRNI)
- Certified nutritional support nurse (CNSN)
- Oncology certified nurse (OCN)

Certification is generally offered through the independent testing corporations affiliated with specialty professional organizations, such as the Intravenous Nurses Certification Corporation, whose responsibility it is to preserve the quality of nurses displaying the certification credential and protect the public from harm at the hands of the certified nurse (Intravenous Nurses Certification Corporation, 1991). Although certification is voluntary, much like organizational accreditation, the CRNI designation has become highly desirable in competition for home infusion nursing positions.

THE PROCESS OF PATIENT CARE
Assessment
Although the practice of home infusion is classified as a nursing specialty, focus must remain on comprehensive patient care with systematic application of the nursing process. Assessing patient appropriate-

ness for HIT extends far beyond the ability to provide the right drug for the diagnosis and involves thoughtful preplanning. The majority of HIT patients originate from the acute care hospital and require continuing therapy at home for the same diagnosis or related diagnoses. This hospital stay affords the home infusion nurse with an opportunity to interact with the acute care team and begin the discharge planning process very soon after admission. Ideally the infusion nurse can begin predischarge teaching with the patient and caregiver, providing a chance to gain greater insight into the patient's willingness and abilities to sustain care at home.

Every home care provider must design patient acceptance criteria. These guidelines help determine which patients are appropriate for home care services with that agency and who would be better cared for in another environment. The guidelines serve to protect both the agency and the patient. Providers of infusion specialty services should have acceptance criteria that specifically address IV cases, including such requirements as the following (Sheldon and Bender, 1994):

1. Appropriate diagnosis and treatment
2. Medically stable condition
3. Venous accessibility or reasonable plan for initiation and maintenance
4. A safe and appropriate home environment, including physical layout, cleanliness, phone access, and electricity
5. Client and caregiver ability and willingness to be taught and to perform care
6. The financial resources to ensure appropriate scope of services

The admission criteria must then be applied consistently and objectively to each home infusion referral to preserve impartiality and eliminate bias. It is helpful to collect preadmission data on a standardized form that can then be retained as evidence of patient selection processes.

Once the decision is made to accept a patient for HIT, further assessment is required. Visit the patient and evaluate cognitive skills, fine motor skills, and vision. Keep in mind what you will be requiring the patient to learn and do. If the patient requires assisted care and has identified a caregiver, meet and talk with that caregiver. It is not unheard of to have the patient name someone as a caregiver who is completely unaware or unable to provide the patient's needed care. Detail the reality of the patient's care needs as completely as possible, stating the expectations for patient and caregiver training and availability. It is far better to have the potential caregiver decline while the patient is still hospitalized than within the first few days at home.

Look at the big picture. Will the care plan require medical equipment beyond the infusion pump? A home environmental assessment at this point is a rare luxury, so most knowledge about the home will need to be obtained from the patient and family interview. Plan for the hospital bed, wheelchair, infusion pump, and oxygen equipment to be delivered together in advance of the patient's arrival. The first hours at home, especially for a patient with high-tech needs, can be particularly chaotic. It is not unusual for the infusion therapy nurse to be the first intervention required and meet the patient on his or her arrival home.

Meet or talk with the referring physician. Make certain that the physician's understanding of HIT is realistic and that the proposed treatment goals are compatible with the patient's unique home setting. When multiple physicians are involved in caring for the patient in the hospital, clearly establish who is responsible for managing the HIT. Obtain written orders for the home, including the specific IV prescription, using standardized order forms for complex therapies such as TPN (Figure 17-1). Make sure to include requests for related orders such as maintenance of the vascular access with heparin flushing, laboratory work type and frequency, support drugs for therapies with anticipated adverse reactions such as amphotericin B, and any anaphylaxis prevention kits.

Intervention and Evaluation

Once the patient is home, the infusion nurse assumes the predominant role of care or case manager and coordinator, collaborating with the patient, caregiver, physician, and fellow members of the multidisciplinary team to develop a goal-directed plan of care. Depending on the insurance source, there may also be the need to coordinate care with an external case manager or to align goals with external guidelines such as Medicare regulations. If the organization uses standardized care plans or an electronic clinical record, it will be necessary to individualize the care plan according to patient needs that were identified in the assessment phase.

The infusion pharmacy generally assumes responsibility for delivering medications, solutions, and supplies, but it will be the nurse's responsibility to initially ensure proper storage and handling and to verify that the delivery is accurate. Carefully read all prescription labels, verify them against the physician's order, and check the expiration dates before storing. Check that the equipment is working and simulate alarm conditions to test the safety functions. The properly stocked home infusion nursing bag (Figure 17-2) should contain basic items that will promote practice within the standards of care for infection control and safe handling of blood and nee-

Text continued on p. 366.

MERIDIA HOME HEALTH

INFORMATION ON POTENTIAL INFUSION THERAPY REFERRAL

PATIENT _____ DOB _____ HOME PHONE _____
ADDRESS _____
HOSP _____ RM #_____ RM PHONE # _____ MAY CONTACT PT: Y N
Admitting Dx: _____
Dx For Infusion Therapy: _____
Other Dx: _____

TYPE OF INFUSION THERAPY: Antibiotic   TPN   Hydration   Pain Mgmt
THERAPY TO BE ADMINISTERED VIA: Broviac/Hickman   Groshong
  Portacath   Heplock   Landmark   PIC Line   Subq   Other:
  Size: _____   No of lumens _____   Placement date: _____
HOSPITAL INFUSION THERAPY: Date Initiated: _____
  Specific info:_____
  _____
  Hosp. administration times: _____
PROBABLE HOME THERAPY: _____
  Projected length of therapy:_____
M.D.: Primary: _____   For Therapy: _____
OTHER PATIENT INFO: Ht:_____ Wt:_____   Quality of veins: _____
Allergies: _____
Functional Limits: _____
  _____

Mental status/psychosocial info: _____
  _____
  _____

Homecare needs in addition to IV therapy: PT   OT   ST   MSS   Aide
  SN: Wnd. care   Diabetic mgmt.   Foley mgmt.   Other: _____

Pt. ability to participate in IV therapy: _____
  _____
  _____

FIGURE 17-1   Written orders for home IV prescription must be obtained. *(Courtesy Meridia Home Health.)*   continued

Caregiver/Significant other: _____

  Ability/willingness to participate in therapy: _____

_____

_____

Responsibility for patient's care between nursing visits: _____

_____

_____

INSURANCE INFO: Pt's SS #: _____

  PRIMARY INSUR: _____   Policy Holder: _____

  Holder's SS #: _____   Employer: _____

  Policy #: _____   Group #: _____

  SECONDARY INSUR: _____   Policy Holder: _____

  Holder's SS #: _____   Employer: _____

  Policy # : _____   Group #: _____

  Coverage For Infusion Supplies: _____

  Coverage For SN Visits: _____

  Patient Informed Of Coverage: Date: _____   By: _____

  OTHER INFO: _____

_____

DATE OF COORDINATOR'S INITIAL CONTACT WITH:

  Supplier _____   HCM Clin Mgr _____   Other: _____

  Meridia Home Health: IV Suprv _____   DCC _____

Coordinator's Signature: _____

PATIENT'S HOSPITAL DISCHARGE: Date: _____   Time: _____

  Supplier Notified: RX Faxed to Pharmacy: _____

_____

  Meridia Home Health IV Suprv. Notified: _____

  Intake Faxed: _____   Signed MD Orders Faxed: _____

Coordinator's Signature: _____

FIGURE 17-1, cont'd   Written orders for home IV prescription must be obtained.

MERIDIA HOME HEALTH
PHYSICIAN ORDERS FOR HOMECARE SERVICES/TREATMENTS

ADDENDUM FOR TOTAL PARENTERAL NUTRITION

PATIENT: _____   SS#: _____

	BASE SOLUTION:					Daily TPN Bag to Contain:
	Dextrose in water (circle):	10%	20%	50%	70%	ml
	Amino Acid Solution (circle):	5%	8.5%	10%		ml
	Trace Element: 3ml/day is the usual additive (1ml provides Zn-1mg, Cu-0.4mg, Mn-0.1mg, Cr-4mcg)					ml

ADDITIVES: (Indicate ordered additive with a ✓ & enter dosage/bag)

T P N	Supplemental Zinc Sulfate	mg
	Sodium Chloride	mEq
	Sodium Acetate	mEq
F O R M U L A	Potassium Chloride	mEq
	Potassium Phosphate	mEq
	Calcium Gluconate (4.6mEq/10ml)	mEq
	Magnesium Sulfate (8.12mEq/ml)	mEq
	Humulin-R	units
	MVI-12 (10ml/day usual)	ml
	Heparin Sodium	units
	Other:	
	LIPID EMULSION: 10% 20%	ml

TPN TO BE INFUSED OVER: 8 hours   10 hours   12 hours   16 hours   Continuous

	Type	Frequency	Call Results To: (specify Dr.)
L A B	1. CBC/diff	_____	_____
	2. Chem-18	_____	_____
W O R K	3. PT	_____	_____
	4. PTT	_____	_____
	5. Mg	_____	_____
	6. Other	_____	_____

M.D. Signature/Date	M.D. Name (Please Print)

HTPNPO.FRM

FIGURE 17-1, cont'd   For legend see opposite page.

HOME CARE BAG CONTENTS BY DISCIPLINE
SKILLED NURSING

RN/LPN Standard Care	RN IV Therapy	RN Enterostomal Therapy
Newspaper	Newspaper	Newspaper
Agency designated antimicrobial skin cleanser	Agency designated antimicrobial skin cleanser	Agency designated antimicrobial skin cleanser
Cal Stat®	Cal Stat®	Cal Stat®
Paper towels	Paper towels	Paper towels
Plastic aprons	Plastic aprons	Plastic aprons
Disposable gloves	Disposable gloves	Disposable gloves
Disposable gown (2)	Disposable gown (2)	Disposable gown (2)
Disposable masks (2)	Disposable masks (2)	Disposable masks (2)
CPR MicroShield	CPR MicroShield	CPR MicroShield
Protective eyewear	Protective eyewear	Protective eyewear
Stethoscope	Stethoscope	Stethoscope
Sphygmomanometer	Sphygmomanometer	Sphygmomanometer
Thermometer/covers	Thermometer/covers	Thermometer/covers
Plastic Ziploc bags	Plastic Ziploc bags	Plastic Ziploc bags
Plastic Biohazard specimen bags	Plastic Biohazard specimen bags	Plastic Biohazard specimen bags
Sharps container	Sharps container	Sharps container
Blood drawing kit	Blood drawing kit	Blood drawing kit
Syringes and needles: 2-TB 2-10cc 2-3cc 2-20cc 2-5cc	Syringes and needles: 2-TB 2-10cc 2-3cc 2-20cc 2-5cc	Syringes and needles: 2-TB 2-10cc 2-3cc 2-20cc 2-5cc
Insulin syringes (2)	Insulin syringes (2)	Insulin syringes (2)
Dressings:2x2, Kerlix, 4x4, ABD	Dressings:2x2, Kerlix, 4x4, ABD	Dressings:2x2, Kerlix, 4x4, ABD
Culture tube	Culture tubes	Culture tubes
Sterile urine spec. cup	Sterile urine spec. cup	Sterile urine spec. cup
Sterile gloves (1)	Sterile gloves (2)	Sterile gloves (2)
Sterile instrument set (1)	Sterile instrument set (1)	Sterile instrument set (1)
Tape (1)	Tape (1)	Tape (1)
Betadine wipes (4)	Betadine wipes (4)	Betadine wipes (4)
Accu-Chek Advantage and supplies	Accu-Chek Advantage and supplies	Accu-Chek Advantage and supplies
Sterile applicators (3)	Sterile applicators (3)	Sterile applicators (3)
Sterile tongue blades (3)	Sterile tongue blades (3)	Sterile tongue blades (3)
Moni-Chlor™ towelettes (4)	Moni-Chlor™ towelettes (4)	Moni-Chlor™ towelettes (4)
Asepti-Chlor™ towelette (1)	Asepti-Chlor™ towelette (1)	Asepti-Chlor™ towelette (1)
Staple removal kit (1)	Staple removal kit (1)	Staple removal kit (1)
Paper tape measure	Paper tape measure	Paper tape measure
Surgi lube	Surgi lube	Surgi lube
Skin prep	Skin prep	Skin prep
Telfa pad	Telfa pad	Telfa pad
Steri-strips	Steri-strips	Steri-strips
Shoe covers (1 pr)	IV start kit (1)	S/H powder
Flashlight	Central dressing kit (1)	S/H paste
	IV angio caths (2)	Curved scissors
	Needleless connectors (2)	Duoderm (1)
	Shoe covers (1 pr)	Stoma measuring guide
	Flashlight	Shoe covers (1 pr)
		Flashlight

FIGURE 17-2   List of a properly stocked nursing bag, based on nurse specialty. (*Courtesy Meridia Home Health.*)

HOME CARE BAG CONTENTS BY DISCIPLINE
SKILLED NURSING (Cont'd)

hcbcbdsn.frm

RN Diabetes Education	RN Maternity Services	RN Mental Health Services
Newspaper	Newspaper	Newspaper
Agency designated antimicrobial skin cleanser	Agency designated antimicrobial skin cleanser	Agency designated antimicrobial skin cleanser
Cal Stat®	Cal Stat®	Cal Stat®
Paper towels	Paper towels	Paper towels
Plastic aprons	Plastic aprons	Plastic aprons
Disposable gloves	Disposable gloves (2)	Disposable gloves (2)
Disposable gown (2)	Disposable gown (2)	Disposable gown (2)
Disposable masks (2)	Disposable masks (2)	Disposable masks (2)
CPR MicroShield	RESUSCI® patient face shield	CPR MicroShield
Protective eyewear	Protective eyewear	Protective eyewear
Stethoscope	Stethoscope - Adult/Infant	Stethoscope
Sphygmomanometer	Sphygmomanometer	Sphygmomanometer
Thermometer/covers	Thermometer/covers	Thermometer/covers
Plastic Ziploc bags	Plastic Biohazard specimen bags	Plastic Biohazard specimen bags
Plastic Biohazard specimen bags	Sharps container	Plastic Ziploc bags
Sharps container	Blood drawing kit	Sharps container
Blood drawing kit	Syringes: 10cc	Blood drawing kit
Syringes and needles: 2-TB 2-10cc 2-3cc 2-20cc 2-5cc	Dressings: 2x2 4x4 ABD	Syringes and needles: 2-3cc
Insulin syringes (2)	Culture tube	Insulin syringes (2)
Dressings:2x2, Kerlix, 4x4, ABD	Sterile urine spec. cup	Dressings:2x2, Kerlix, 4x4, ABD
Culture tubes	Sterile gloves	Culture tubes
Sterile urine spec. cup	Sterile instrument set	Sterile instrument set
Sterile gloves (2)	Tape	Moni-Chlor™ towelettes (4)
Sterile instrument set (1)	Urine specimen bags (Infant)	Asepti-Chlor™ towelette (1)
Tape (1)	Cord clamps	Staple removal kit (1)
Betadine wipes (4)	Clamp remover	Paper tape measure
Accu-Chek Advantage and supplies	Pen light	Surgi lube
Sterile applicators (3)	Asepti-Chlor™ towelette	Skin prep
Sterile tongue blades (3)	Steri-strips	Telfa pad
Moni-Chlor™ towelettes (4)	Biowipes	Steri-strips
Asepti-Chlor™ towelette (1)	Paper tape measures	Flashlight
Staple removal kit (1)	Surgi lube	Accu-Chek Advantage and supplies
Paper tape measure	Staple removal kit (1)	Sterile applicators (3)
Surgi lube	Shoe covers (1 pr)	Sterile tongue blades (3)
Skin prep		Shoe covers (1 pr)
Telfa pad		
Steri-strips		
Glucose tablets		
Shoe covers (1 pr)		
Flashlight		

FIGURE 17-2, cont'd   For legend see opposite page.

dles. Special items that may be required, such as a chemotherapy spill kit, should be included with the pharmacy delivery.

The role of teacher begins the moment the nurse enters the patient's home. *Every action performed, every direction given is a model for the patient learning self care.* It is helpful in HIT training to use both printed materials and demonstration/return demonstration. A modular teaching manual, enabling customization for various access devices, therapies, and infusion pumps, is convenient. All teaching materials should include a review of the purpose of therapy and principles of infection control. Remember to use sound principles of adult education, including assessment of learning readiness and previous knowledge. Other success factors can include minimizing environmental distractions and planning teaching sessions for periods of maximum comfort and energy; setting realistic goals; and holding shorter, more frequent classes.

Evaluation of learning is an essential part of the teaching/learning process. Assessing a patient or caregiver's competency to perform HIT independently is a major responsibility of the nurse and requires sound judgment. Documentation of the teaching process should include content provided and correlate knowledge demonstrated. This is best accomplished by a standardized education evaluation tool (Figure 17-3) that lists all important components to be taught, allows for individualization, and provides an area in which to record level of performance from the learner. Ultimately this form is signed by both the teacher and learner, signifying their agreement with the recorded level of achievement. This level of documentation is a valuable addition to good risk management.

SUMMARY

Infusion therapy is an essential component of home care. Having evolved over the last two decades, it has arrived at a point of common acceptance despite the inherently risky nature of high-technology care. Ongoing development of pharmaceuticals and technology, as well as newly identified clinical needs, continue to drive growth in this industry. Medicare, the largest payor in home care, still does not pay for the most commonly prescribed HIT—antibiotics—in spite of repeated consideration and analysis, leaving a gap in the provision of comprehensive home care for seniors. Nursing has responded to the demand for specialty practitioners with increasing levels of skill and experience by evolving the role of the home infusion nurse. Ongoing development of that role through competency-based job descriptions and performance evaluations, coupled with research in the infusion practice area, will set the stage for the continued growth of the specialty of infusion nursing into the next century.

MERIDIA HOME HEALTH
THERAPY EDUCATION/EVALUATION

☐ Initial   ☐ Subsequent

PATIENT NAME		THERAPY		SOCIAL SECURITY #		
	TOPIC Complete each category with appropriate dates and instructor initials.	ASSESSMENT/ DISCUSSION/ DEMONSTRATION	RETURN DEMONSTRATION WITH ASSISTANCE	RETURN DEMONSTRATION WITHOUT ASSISTANCE	ADDITIONAL COMMENTS	
INTRO	Purpose/Principle of Therapy					
INFECTION CONTROL	Handwashing					
	Work Area					
	Maintaining Asepsis					
	Blood/Body Fluid Precautions					
SOLUTION/ MEDS/ FORMULA	Storage					
	Inspection					
	Additives					
	Preparation					
	Dosage/Concentration					
ADMINISTRATION PROCEDURES	Administration Set					
	Gravity/Bolus					
	Pump: Operation					
	Maintenance					
	Alarm System					
	Catheter/Tube Placement					
	Connection Procedure					
	Disconnection Procedure					
	Rate of Administration					
	Fat Administration					
CATH/ TUBE CARE	Heparinization/Irrigation					
	Site Care/Dressing Change					
HOME MONITORING/ CONDITIONS	Weight					
	Temperature					
	Intake/Output					
	Urine Testing					
	Environmental Safeguards					
SUPPLY MGMT.	Equipment/Supplies					
	Inventory Control					

COMPLICATIONS EMERGENCY INTERVENTIONS				
____ Administration Set Malfunction	____ Catheter Blockage	____ Electrolyte Imbalance	____ Nausea/Vomiting
____ Air Embolism	____ Catheter Damage	____ Hypo/Hyperglycemia	____ Phlebitis
____ Air In Line	____ Catheter Disconnection	____ Infection	____ Pump Malfunction
____ Allergic Reaction	____ Catheter Displacement	____ Infiltration	____ 24 Hour Emergency Number
____ Blood Back-up	____ Drug Specific Complication		

SPECIAL INSTRUCTIONS/ COMMENTS

SIGNATURES	Instructor/Title	I/we, _____ , (patient and/or caregiver) have received educational materials, have been instructed and feel competent to safely and effectively perform some/all of the functions associated with the prescribed therapy with the assistance of Meridia Home Health staff/services. I/we understand these functions will be routinely performed in a facility other than a hospital or medical institution.
		Patient/Spouse/Guardian Date

DISTRIBUTION: WHITE-Meridia Home Health Clinical Record CANARY-CareMark PINK-LifeFocus GOLDENROD-Hospital Copy
CC 732G 2/90 1M

FIGURE 17-3 Example of an education/evaluation form. *(Courtesy Meridia Home Health.)*

REVIEW EXERCISES

1. Which of the following factors have contributed to the growth of home infusion:
   a. New technology
   b. Consumer preference
   c. Pharmaceutical development
   d. All of the above
2. IV nursing was first recognized as a specialty in 1940. (True or False)
3. The first IV therapy to be successfully administered at home was antibiotics. (True or False)
4. All of the following are responsibilities of the home infusion nurse, *except:*
   a. Patient education
   b. Pump evaluation
   c. Drug administration
   d. Implanted port insertion
5. The most common reason for receiving HIT is chronic, resistant infections that are not eliminated by oral antibiotics. (True or False)
6. For what do the letters "PICC" stand?
7. Explain the fundamental difference between a "pump" and a "controller."
8. Describe the proper catheter tip placement for each of the following devices:
   a. Midline catheter
   b. Tunnelled Groshong
   c. Implanted port

RESOURCES
Abbott Laboratories
1 Abbott Park Rd.
Abbott Park, IL 60064-3502
(800)222-6883
Bard Access Systems
5425 West Amelia Earhart Dr.
Salt Lake City, UT 84116
(801)595-973
Baxter Healthcare Corporation
IV Systems Division/Ambulatory Infusion Business
Route 120 and Wilson Rd.
Round Lake, IL 60073-090
(708)546-6311

Becton Dickinson Infusion Systems
Division of Becton Dickinson and Co.
2 Bridgewater Lane
Lincoln Park, NJ 07035-139
(800)232-8666
Infusion
P.O. Box 3066
Langhorne, PA 19047-9396
Intravenous Nurses Certification Corporation (INCC)
Fresh Pond Square
10 Fawcett St.
Cambridge, MA 02138
(617)441-3008
Intravenous Nurses Society (INS)
Fresh Pond Square
10 Fawcett St.
Cambridge, MA 02138
(617)441-3008
National Home Infusion Association
205 Daingerfield Rd.
Alexandria, VA 22314
(703)59-3740
SIMS-Deltec, Inc.
1265 Grey Fox Rd.
St. Paul, MN 55112-6967
(800)433-5832

REFERENCES

Conners RB, Winters RW, editors: *Home infusion: current status and future trends,* Chicago, 1995, American Hospital Publishing.

Fickeissen J: 56 ways to get certified, *Am J Nurs* 90(3):50, March, 1990.

Grace LA, Tomaselli BJ: Intravenous therapy in the home. In Terry J, et al, editors: *Intravenous therapy: clinical principles and practice,* Philadelphia, WB Saunders, 1995.

Intravenous Nurses Certification Corporation: *Mission statement,* Boston, 1991, Intravenous Nurses Certification Corp.

Intravenous Nurses Society: *Revised intravenous nursing standards or practice,* Boston, 1990, Intravenous Nurses Society.

Jensen BL: Types of intravenous therapy equipment. In Terry J, et al, editors: *Intravenous therapy: clinical principles and practice,* Philadelphia, 1995, WB Saunders.

National Association for Home Care: *Basic statistics about home care 1995,* Washington, DC, 1996, National Association for Home Care.

Office of Technology Assessment: *Home drug infusion therapy under Medicare,* Washington, DC, 1992, Government Printing Office.

Plumer AL, Consentino F: *Principles and practice of intravenous therapy,* ed 4, Boston, 1987, Little, Brown.

Poretz DM: High tech comes home, *Am J Med* 91:453-454, 1991.

Sheldon P, Bender M: High-technology in home care, *Nurs Clin North Am* 29:507-519, 1994.

Winters RW, Parver AK, Sansbury AJ: *Home infusion therapy: a service and demographic profile,* Washington, DC, 1992, National Alliance for Infusion Therapy.

FOR FURTHER READING

Humphrey CJ, Milone-Nuzzo P: *Orientation to home care nursing,* Gaithersburg, Md, 1996, Aspen.

LaRocca JC: *Handbook of home care IV therapy,* St. Louis, 1994, Mosby.

Phillips LD: *Manual of IV therapeutics,* Philadelphia, 1993, FA Davis.

Terry J, et al, editors: *Intravenous therapy clinical principles and practice,* Philadelphia, 1995, WB Saunders.

Winters RW: The home infusion industry: an overview. In Conners RB, Winters RW, editors: *Home infusion therapy: current status and future trends,* Chicago, 1995, American Hospital Publishing.

part
IV

OTHER CONSIDERATIONS

chapter

18

WHERE TO FROM HERE: PROFESSIONAL GROWTH IN HOME CARE

Tina M. Marrelli, MSN, MA, RNC

> *"A new idea is first condemned as ridiculous and then dismissed as trivial, until it becomes what everyone knows."*
>
> William James

Many new ideas will come to be norms in practice and operations over the coming years in home care. This quote points out the need that there is still much to know and continue to learn as you pursue goals throughout your career. Learning truly must be lifelong in health care, and nowhere is this more true than in home care. This final chapter addresses methods for self-development, goals and planning, and career strategies that make prospective employers value your skills and expertise. Essential skills such as time management are also addressed as the need to be more effective with limited resources will only continue in the coming years. Information has been provided about the norms and best practices related to the rules in home care in previous chapters. The information in Box 18-1 summarizes the important activities from a humorous and regulatory perspective.

"THE BEST" HOME CARE NURSES

The following lists some of the hallmarks of the best nurses who practice in home care. The assumption is made that they perform these activities or demonstrate these behaviors while providing skillful, caring, and competent patient care.

1. Follows the organization's defined clinical protocols
2. Individualizes standardized care plans

BOX 18-1   THE HOME HEALTH CARE NURSE'S COMMANDMENTS

I. Thou shalt be sure the patient meets admission criteria.

II. Thou shalt read thy documentation objectively. (Does it reflect homebound status and/or why skilled nursing or therapy is required?)

III. Thou shalt emphasize:
   a. Why care was initiated.
   b. What skilled nursing interventions were performed.
   c. Where the patient's plan is going (patient-centered goals).
   d. What the rehabilitation potential of the patient is (plan for discharge).

IV. Thou shalt complete thy documentation in a timely manner.

V. Remember the plan of care (POC), keep it current, that your days may be long in home health.

VI. Thou shalt focus on the patient's problems in thy documentation.

VII. Demonstrate through thy documentation that the care provided is patient-centered so reimbursement shall be thy reward.

VIII. Have pity on the soul who reads thy flowsheets, that he or she may see the patient's problems and needs, as well as thy focus toward achievement of goals.

IX. Keep thy documentation concise.

X. Document all communication thee has with thy associates and physicians, that light may dawn on those confined to the office regarding patient charges.

XI. Remember the nursing process, to keep it visible in your charting.

XII. Thou shalt document goal achievement and/or progress toward goals and outcomes.

XIII. Thou shalt document reasons goals are unattainable.

XIV. Thou shalt document the patient's response to interventions and nursing actions.

XV. Remember to comply with regulatory, licensure, and quality standards, that thee may avoid the bottomless pit of overwhelming expectations of state, agency, and patient.

3. Adheres to the organization's administrative policies related to paperwork completion, timelines, and other systems
4. Are customer-service oriented
5. Meets productivity and other standards
6. Identifies solutions to identified challenges to improve patient care, as well as the organization
7. Demonstrates lifelong learning by attending in-services, taking courses, or other self-directed education endeavors
8. Documents effectively to meet state, federal, and accreditation standards
9. Others, based on the organization's unique requirements

EFFECTIVE TIME MANAGEMENT: A MUST FOR SUCCESS IN HOME CARE

Clinicians must be excellent planners and improvisers in the home care. There is a saying that, if you want to have something done, delegate it to a busy person. Although some people seem to be born with these skills, they are not. Effective personal and professional time management skills are learned, a wealth of books and tapes are available on this topic. Although an in-depth discussion of these important skills is beyond the scope of this text, the following are some key tips to improve your skills.

- Organize and update your list of needed phone numbers. This includes the office, your supervisor's pager number, drug stores and their hours of operation, and other details that facilitate great patient care and effective office operations.
- Remember that becoming and staying organized is a learned skill and that, like any skill, increased performance comes only with improvement.
- Observe and model skills of others at your organization who are organized and enjoy their work in home care.
- Plan, plan, plan for scheduled patient visits and learn to anticipate patient needs.
- Make and use "to do" lists; once the task is checked off, the feeling of accomplishment is well worth it!
- Remember that successful home care clinicians and managers usually have effective personal organizational and time management skills!
- Touch paper (or the keyboard) once; finish the task at hand, particularly when it comes to timely and accurate completion of clinical documentation.

STAYING COMPETITIVE IN THE MARKETPLACE

The skills listed in the previous section also assist in making you a marketable and flexible team member—valued assets in any organization. Unfortunately, some parts of the county have a glut of nurses who cannot find work in their area of choice. This dilemma speaks to the need for further education and training to meet the needs of the community at large. There is no question that, as the nursing and home care markets continue to expand, the nurses and other clinicians and managers with the most education, experience, credentials, and demonstrated flexibility will be most valued in the job market. Nurses will continue to see many of the hallmarks of managed care continue in the coming years, including expansion of cross-training and patient-centered care.

THE ROLE OF NURSING IN THE FUTURE: CASE MANAGER

There are many and varied titles for nurses in home care and hospice who care for patients in the home. Whatever the title, there will be an increase in nurse career diversity unlike any nurses have seen in the past. Expanded roles of nurses as case managers in all kinds of emerging site settings will occur as inpatient hospitals continue to rachet down their length of stay. Nurses will need to be interested in research findings and processes and many will need to develop as researchers as the need for outcome- and research-based practice only increase. Nursing and other scientific-based professions must determine ways to prove or identify the effectiveness of care interventions on patient outcomes.

Simply put, nurses can be a part of the future and solution of health care or tacitly let it be "above us" and our daily professional lives. Assume the power and act in the patient's and your organization's best interest. Nurses or other health care professionals must have input into the process; this patient advocacy role has strong roots in history and must be clearly articulated to policy makers. Outcomes are one way to speak articulately as they are quantifiable or measurable.

The expectation in all health care settings is that the emphasis on increased productivity and efficiencies will only increase. For many years, Medicare paid claims in home care, sometimes whether they were appropriate or not. Home care and hospice organizations have the threat of Operation Restore Trust (ORT) and other initiatives as the government seeks to limit overuse, fraud, and abuse in the Medicare systems. Nurses have a moral and ethical obligation to identify, report, and speak out against such unlawful and costly practices.

BOX 18-2   **STRESS MANAGEMENT: WHEN YOU NEED A CHANGE OF ACTIVITIES**

Call a friend and go to a spa for a day or the movies for an afternoon.

Spend some time with a trusted friend hashing out the pros and cons.

Sign up for some continuing education credits in an area of interest.

Start working on your BSN or Master's (again) and pick a timeline for completion.

Exercise, eat healthy, and sleep— naps are a forgotten art!

Take a public-speaking course (health education will only grow).

Register for a typing or word processing class (these skills are invaluable when your organization goes to computerized documentation or scheduling).

Call about certification in the specialty area of your choice and work toward meeting the defined requirements. Know that there is home care certification by the American Nurses Credentialing Center (ANCC) for both BSN and Master's prepared nurses. Other certifications include intravenous, oncology, hospice, pediatric, and community health.

Start a journal club for your team members.

There will be times when you will be frustrated, particularly on difficult days (e.g., when your entire caseload needs to be seen on the same day, all for very good reasons). This is where having effective stress management skills and a sense of humor can help (Box 18-2)!

SUMMARY

There is much to learn but, as you practice in home care, the information and responsibilities start to become a seamless whole that begins with patient admission and continues through discharge. Home care clinicians have important roles in assisting patients to meet their desired outcomes. In this specialty there are many opportunities for growth and learning. The learning in home care must truly be lifelong to safely care for patients. Seeking certification, pursuing a degree, and ongoing attendance at organizational and external offerings contributes to both continuing competence as well as personal professional fulfillment. Welcome to home care, the health care setting of the future!

REVIEW EXERCISES

1. Identify one or two professional goals to be accomplished and define a time frame for implementation and achievement of the goals.

2. Determine an area of specialization of home care (e.g., call schools, read information) and seriously consider pursuing additional education or training.
3. List three educational endeavors (e.g., literature search, benchmarking) that you have initiated or accomplished in the last year and identify areas to improve on this year.

RESOURCE

Michigan Foundation for Home Care: Home care: a research guide, Michigan Foundation for Home Care, 1996, (517)349-8089.

FOR FURTHER READING

Bailey C: Education for home-care providers, *J Obstet Gynecol Nurs* 23(8):714-719, 1994.

Bennis S, Davis S: Empowering home care nurses through education, *Caring,* September 1992, pp 65-66.

Green P: Meeting the learning needs of home health nurses, *J Home Health Care Pract* 6(4):25-32, 1994.

Zabkar F: Getting organized to practice home health nursing, *Home Care Provider* 1(4):195-197, 218, 1996.

OASIS-B*

**Medicare Home Health Care Quality Assurance and Improvement Demonstration
Outcome and Assessment Information Set (OASIS-B)**

> This data set should not be reviewed or used without first reading the accompanying
> narrative prologue that explains the purpose of the OASIS and its past and planned
> evolution.

Items to be Used at Specific Time Points

Start of Care (or Resumption of Care Following Inpatient Facility Stay):   1-79

Follow-Up: 1-11, 14, 19-21, 23, 26-36, 39-81

Discharge (not to inpatient facility):   1-11, 14, 19-21, 23, 26-36, 39-84, 88-89

Transfer to Inpatient Facility (with or without agency discharge): 1-11, 80-82, 85-89

Death at Home: 1-11, 89

Note: For items 61-77, please note special instructions at the beginning of the section.

DEMOGRAPHICS AND PATIENT HISTORY

1.   **(M0010) Agency ID:** __ __ __ __ __ __ __ __

2.   **(M0020) Patient ID Number:** _____

3.   **(M0030) Start of Care Date:** __ __ / __ __ / __ __ __ __
     month   day   year

4.   **(M0040) Patient's Last Name:** __ __ __ __ __ __ __ __ __ __ __ __ __ __

5.   **(M0050) Patient State of Residence:** __ __

6.   **(M0060) Patient Zip Code:** __ __ __ __ __

7.   **(M0063) Medicare Number:** __ __ __ __ __ __ __ __ __ __ __
     (including suffix if any)

     ☐ NA   No Medicare

8.   **(M0066) Birth Date:** __ __ / __ __ / __ __ __ __
     month   day   year

9.   **(M0080) Discipline of Person Completing Assessment:**
     ☐ 1-RN ☐ 2-LPN ☐ 3-PT ☐ 4-SLP/ST ☐ 5-OT ☐ 6-MSW

10. **(M0090) Date Assessment Information Recorded:** __ __ / __ __ / __ __ __ __
     month   day   year

11. **(M0100) This Assessment is Currently Being Completed for the Following Reason:**

☐ 1 - Start of care
☐ 2 - Resumption of care (after inpatient stay)
☐ 3 - Discharge from agency - not to an inpatient facility [Go to *M0150*]
☐ 4 - Transferred to an inpatient facility - discharged from agency [Go to *M0830*]
☐ 5 - Transferred to an inpatient facility - not discharged from agency [Go to *M0830*]
☐ 6 - Died at home [Go to *M0906*]
☐ 7 - Recertification reassessment (follow-up) [Go to *M0150*]
☐ 8 - Other follow-up [Go to *M0150*]

12. **(M0130) Gender:**

☐ 1 - Male
☐ 2 - Female

13. **(M0140) Race/Ethnicity** (as identified by patient):

☐ 1 - White, non-Hispanic
☐ 2 - Black, African-American
☐ 3 - Hispanic
☐ 4 - Asian, Pacific Islander
☐ 5 - American Indian, Eskimo, Aleut
☐ 6 - Other
☐ UK - Unknown

14. **(M0150) Current Payment Sources for Home Care: (Mark all that apply.)**

☐ 0 - None; no charge for current services
☐ 1 - Medicare (traditional fee-for-service)
☐ 2 - Medicare (HMO/managed care)
☐ 3 - Medicaid (traditional fee-for-service)
☐ 4 - Medicaid (HMO/managed care)
☐ 5 - Workers' compensation
☐ 6 - Title programs (e.g., Title III, V, or XX)
☐ 7 - Other government (e.g., CHAMPUS, VA, etc.)
☐ 8 - Private insurance
☐ 9 - Private HMO/managed care
☐ 10 - Self-pay
☐ 11 - Other (specify) _____
☐ UK - Unknown

15. **(M0160) Financial Factors** limiting the ability of the patient/family to meet basic health needs: **(Mark all that apply.)**

☐ 0 - None
☐ 1 - Unable to afford medicine or medical supplies
☐ 2 - Unable to afford medical expenses that are not covered by insurance/Medicare (e.g., copayments)
☐ 3 - Unable to afford rent/utility bills
☐ 4 - Unable to afford food
☐ 5 - Other (specify) _____

16. **(M0170) From which of the following Inpatient Facilities was the patient discharged <u>during the past 14 days</u>? (Mark all that apply.)**

☐ 1 - Hospital
☐ 2 - Rehabilitation facility
☐ 3 - Nursing home
☐ 4 - Other (specify) _____
☐ NA - Patient was not discharged from an inpatient facility   [If NA, go to *M0200*]

17. **(M0180) Inpatient Discharge Date** (most recent):

__ __/__ __/__ __ __ __
month day   year

☐ UK - Unknown

18. **(M0190) Inpatient Diagnoses** and three-digit ICD code categories <u>for only those conditions treated during an inpatient facility stay within the last 14 days</u> (no surgical or V-codes):

Inpatient Facility Diagnosis   ICD

a. _____   (__ __ __)

b. _____   (__ __ __)

19. **(M0200) Medical or Treatment Regimen Change Within Past 14 Days:** Has this patient experienced a change in medical or treatment regimen (e.g., medication, treatment, or service change due to new or additional diagnosis, etc.) within the last 14 days?

  ☐ 0 - No [If No, go to *M0220*]
  ☐ 1 - Yes

20. **(M0210)** List the patient's **Medical Diagnoses** and three-digit ICD code categories <u>for those conditions requiring changed medical or treatment regimen</u> (no surgical or V-codes):

  Changed Medical Regimen Diagnosis   ICD

  a. _____   (__ __ __)
  b. _____   (__ __ __)
  c. _____   (__ __ __)
  d. _____   (__ __ __)

21. **(M0220) Conditions Prior to Medical or Treatment Regimen Change or Inpatient Stay Within Past 14 Days:** If this patient experienced an inpatient facility discharge or change in medical or treatment regimen within the past 14 days, indicate any conditions which existed <u>prior to</u> the inpatient stay or change in medical or treatment regimen. **(Mark all that apply.)**

  ☐ 1 - Urinary incontinence
  ☐ 2 - Indwelling/suprapubic catheter
  ☐ 3 - Intractable pain
  ☐ 4 - Impaired decision-making
  ☐ 5 - Disruptive or socially inappropriate behavior
  ☐ 6 - Memory loss to the extent that supervision required
  ☐ 7 - None of the above
  ☐ NA - No inpatient facility discharge <u>and</u> no change in medical or treatment regimen in past 14 days
  ☐ UK - Unknown

22. **(M0230/M0240) Diagnoses and Severity Index:** List each medical diagnosis or problem for which the patient is receiving home care and ICD code category (no surgical or V-codes) and rate them using the following severity index. (Choose one value that represents the most severe rating appropriate for each diagnosis.)

  0 - Asymptomatic, no treatment needed at this time
  1 - Symptoms well controlled with current therapy
  2 - Symptoms controlled with difficulty, affecting daily functioning; patient needs ongoing monitoring
  3 - Symptoms poorly controlled, patient needs frequent adjustment in treatment and dose monitoring
  4 - Symptoms poorly controlled, history of rehospitalizations

(M0230) Primary Diagnosis	ICD		Severity Rating			
a. _____	(__ __ __)	☐ 0	☐ 1	☐ 2	☐ 3	☐ 4

(M0240) Other Diagnoses	ICD		Severity Rating			
b. _____	(__ __ __)	☐ 0	☐ 1	☐ 2	☐ 3	☐ 4
c. _____	(__ __ __)	☐ 0	☐ 1	☐ 2	☐ 3	☐ 4
d. _____	(__ __ __)	☐ 0	☐ 1	☐ 2	☐ 3	☐ 4
e. _____	(__ __ __)	☐ 0	☐ 1	☐ 2	☐ 3	☐ 4
f. _____	(__ __ __)	☐ 0	☐ 1	☐ 2	☐ 3	☐ 4

23. **(M0250) Therapies** the patient receives <u>at home</u>: **(Mark all that apply.)**

  ☐ 1 - Intravenous or infusion therapy (excludes TPN)
  ☐ 2 - Parenteral nutrition (TPN or lipids)
  ☐ 3 - Enteral nutrition (nasogastric, gastrostomy, jejunostomy, or any other artificial entry into the alimentary canal)
  ☐ 4 - None of the above

24. **(M0260) Overall Prognosis:** BEST description of patient's overall prognosis for <u>recovery from this episode of illness</u>.

  ☐ 0 - Poor: little or no recovery is expected and/or further decline is imminent
  ☐ 1 - Good/Fair: partial to full recovery is expected
  ☐ UK - Unknown

25. **(M0270) Rehabilitative Prognosis:** BEST description of patient's prognosis for <u>functional status</u>.

  ☐ 0 - Guarded: minimal improvement in functional status is expected; decline is possible
  ☐ 1 - Good: marked improvement in functional status is expected
  ☐ UK - Unknown

26. **(M0280) Life Expectancy:** (Physician documentation is not required.)

☐ 0 - Life expectancy is greater than 6 months
☐ 1 - Life expectancy is 6 months or fewer

27. **(M0290) High Risk Factors** characterizing this patient: **(Mark all that apply.)**

☐ 1 - Heavy smoking
☐ 2 - Obesity
☐ 3 - Alcohol dependency
☐ 4 - Drug dependency
☐ 5 - None of the above
☐ UK - Unknown

LIVING ARRANGEMENTS

28. **(M0300) Current Residence:**

☐ 1 - Patient's owned or rented residence (house, apartment, or mobile home owned or rented by patient/couple/significant other)
☐ 2 - Family member's residence
☐ 3 - Boarding home or rented room
☐ 4 - Board and care or assisted living facility
☐ 5 - Other (specify) _____

29. **(M0310) Structural Barriers** in the patient's environment limiting independent mobility: **(Mark all that apply.)**

☐ 0 - None
☐ 1 - Stairs inside home which <u>must</u> be used by the patient (e.g., to get to toileting, sleeping, eating areas)
☐ 2 - Stairs inside home which are used optionally (e.g., to get to laundry facilities)
☐ 3 - Stairs leading from inside house to outside
☐ 4 - Narrow or obstructed doorways

30. **(M0320) Safety Hazards** found in the patient's current place of residence: **(Mark all that apply.)**

☐ 0 - None
☐ 1 - Inadequate floor, roof, or windows
☐ 2 - Inadequate lighting
☐ 3 - Unsafe gas/electric appliance
☐ 4 - Inadequate heating
☐ 5 - Inadequate cooling
☐ 6 - Lack of fire safety devices
☐ 7 - Unsafe floor coverings
☐ 8 - Inadequate stair railings
☐ 9 - Improperly stored hazardous materials
☐ 10 - Lead-based paint
☐ 11 - Other (specify) _____

31. **(M0330) Sanitation Hazards** found in the patient's current place of residence: **(Mark all that apply.)**

☐ 0 - None
☐ 1 - No running water
☐ 2 - Contaminated water
☐ 3 - No toileting facilities
☐ 4 - Outdoor toileting facilities only
☐ 5 - Inadequate sewage disposal
☐ 6 - Inadequate/improper food storage
☐ 7 - No food refrigeration
☐ 8 - No cooking facilities
☐ 9 - Insects/rodents present
☐ 10 - No scheduled trash pickup
☐ 11 - Cluttered/soiled living area
☐ 12 - Other (specify) _____

32. **(M0340) Patient Lives With:** **(Mark all that apply.)**

☐ 1 - Lives alone
☐ 2 - With spouse or significant other
☐ 3 - With other family member
☐ 4 - With a friend
☐ 5 - With paid help (other than home care agency staff)
☐ 6 - With other than above

SUPPORTIVE ASSISTANCE

33. **(M0350) Assisting Person(s) Other than Home Care Agency Staff:** (Mark all that apply.)

    ☐ 1 - Relatives, friends, or neighbors living outside the home
    ☐ 2 - Person residing in the home (EXCLUDING paid help)
    ☐ 3 - Paid help
    ☐ 4 - None of the above [If None of the above, go to *M0390*]
    ☐ UK - Unknown [If Unknown, go to *M0390*]

34. **(M0360) Primary Caregiver** taking <u>lead</u> responsibility for providing or managing the patient's care, providing the most frequent assistance, etc. (other than home care agency staff):

    ☐ 0 - No one person [If No one person, go to *M0390*]
    ☐ 1 - Spouse or significant other
    ☐ 2 - Daughter or son
    ☐ 3 - Other family member
    ☐ 4 - Friend or neighbor or community or church member
    ☐ 5 - Paid help
    ☐ UK - Unknown [If Unknown, go to *M0390*]

35. **(M0370) How Often** does the patient receive assistance from the primary caregiver?

    ☐ 1 - Several times during day and night
    ☐ 2 - Several times during day
    ☐ 3 - Once daily
    ☐ 4 - Three or more times per week
    ☐ 5 - One to two times per week
    ☐ 6 - Less often than weekly
    ☐ UK - Unknown

36. **(M0380) Type of Primary Caregiver Assistance:** (Mark all that apply.)

    ☐ 1 - ADL assistance (e.g., bathing, dressing, toileting, bowel/bladder, eating/feeding)
    ☐ 2 - IADL assistance (e.g., meds, meals, housekeeping, laundry, telephone, shopping, finances)
    ☐ 3 - Environmental support (housing, home maintenance)
    ☐ 4 - Psychosocial support (socialization, companionship, recreation)
    ☐ 5 - Advocates or facilitates patient's participation in appropriate medical care
    ☐ 6 - Financial agent, power of attorney, or conservator of finance
    ☐ 7 - Health care agent, conservator of person, or medical power of attorney
    ☐ UK - Unknown

SENSORY STATUS

37. **(M0390) Vision** with corrective lenses if the patient usually wears them:

    ☐ 0 - Normal vision: sees adequately in most situations; can see medication labels, newsprint.
    ☐ 1 - Partially impaired: cannot see medication labels or newsprint, but <u>can</u> see obstacles in path, and the surrounding layout; can count fingers at arm's length.
    ☐ 2 - Severely impaired: cannot locate objects without hearing or touching them <u>or</u> patient nonresponsive.

38. **(M0400) Hearing and Ability to Understand Spoken Language** in patient's own language (with hearing aids if the patient usually uses them):

    ☐ 0 - No observable impairment. Able to hear and understand complex or detailed instructions and extended or abstract conversation.
    ☐ 1 - With minimal difficulty, able to hear and understand most multi-step instructions and ordinary conversation. May need occasional repetition, extra time, or louder voice.
    ☐ 2 - Has moderate difficulty hearing and understanding simple, one-step instructions and brief conversation; needs frequent prompting or assistance.
    ☐ 3 - Has severe difficulty hearing and understanding simple greetings and short comments. Requires multiple repetitions, restatements, demonstrations, additional time.
    ☐ 4 - <u>Unable</u> to hear and understand familiar words or common expressions consistently, <u>or</u> patient nonresponsive.

39. **(M0410) Speech and Oral (Verbal) Expression of Language** (in patient's own language):

    ☐ 0 - Expresses complex ideas, feelings, and needs clearly, completely, and easily in all situations with no observable impairment.
    ☐ 1 - Minimal difficulty in expressing ideas and needs (may take extra time; makes occasional errors in word choice, grammar or speech intelligibility; needs minimal prompting or assistance).
    ☐ 2 - Expresses simple ideas or needs with moderate difficulty (needs prompting or assistance, errors in word choice, organization, or speech intelligibility). Speaks in phrases or short sentences.
    ☐ 3 - Has severe difficulty expressing basic ideas or needs and requires maximal assistance or guessing by listener. Speech limited to single words or short phrases.
    ☐ 4 - <u>Unable</u> to express basic needs even with maximal prompting or assistance but is not comatose or unresponsive (e.g., speech is nonsensical or unintelligible).
    ☐ 5 - Patient nonresponsive or unable to speak.

40. **(M0420) Frequency of Pain** interfering with patient's activity or movement:

    ☐ 0 - Patient has no pain or pain does not interfere with activity or movement
    ☐ 1 - Less often than daily
    ☐ 2 - Daily, but not constantly
    ☐ 3 - All of the time

41. **(M0430) Intractable Pain:** Is the patient experiencing pain that is <u>not easily relieved</u>, occurs at least daily, and affects the patient's sleep, appetite, physical or emotional energy, concentration, personal relationships, emotions, or ability or desire to perform physical activity?

    ☐ 0 - No
    ☐ 1 - Yes

INTEGUMENTARY STATUS

42. **(M0440) Does this patient have a Skin Lesion** or an Open Wound? This excludes "OSTOMIES."

    ☐ 0 - No [If No, go to *M0490*]
    ☐ 1 - Yes

43. **(M0445) Does this patient have a Pressure Ulcer?**

    ☐ 0 - No [If No, go to *M0468*]
    ☐ 1 - Yes

   43a. **(M0450) Current Number of Pressure Ulcers at Each Stage:** (Circle one response for each stage.)

Pressure Ulcer Stages	Number of Pressure Ulcers				
a) Stage 1: Nonblanchable erythema of intact skin; the heralding of skin ulceration. In darker-pigmented skin, warmth, edema, hardness, or discolored skin may be indicators.	0	1	2	3	4 or more
b) Stage 2: Partial thickness skin loss involving epidermis and/or dermis. The ulcer is superficial and presents clinically as an abrasion, blister, or shallow crater.	0	1	2	3	4 or more
c) Stage 3: Full-thickness skin loss involving damage or necrosis of subcutaneous tissue which may extend down to, but not through, underlying fascia. The ulcer presents clinically as a deep crater with or without undermining of adjacent tissue.	0	1	2	3	4 or more
d) Stage 4: Full-thickness skin loss with extensive destruction, tissue necrosis, or damage to muscle, bone, or supporting structures (e.g., tendon, joint capsule, etc.).	0	1	2	3	4 or more
e) In addition to the above, is there at least one pressure ulcer that cannot be observed due to the presence of eschar or a nonremovable dressing, including casts? ☐ 0 - No ☐ 1 - Yes					

   43b. **(M0460) Stage of Most Problematic (Observable) Pressure Ulcer:**

   ☐ 1 - Stage 1
   ☐ 2 - Stage 2
   ☐ 3 - Stage 3
   ☐ 4 - Stage 4
   ☐ NA - No observable pressure ulcer

43c. (M0464) Status of Most Problematic (Observable) Pressure Ulcer:

☐ 1 - Fully granulating
☐ 2 - Early/partial granulation
☐ 3 - Not healing
☐ NA - No observable pressure ulcer

44. (M0468) Does this patient have a Stasis Ulcer?

☐ 0 - No [If No, go to *M0482*]
☐ 1 - Yes

44a. (M0470) Current Number of Observable Stasis Ulcer(s):

☐ 0 - Zero
☐ 1 - One
☐ 2 - Two
☐ 3 - Three
☐ 4 - Four or more

44b. (M0474) Does this patient have at least one Stasis Ulcer that Cannot be Observed due to the presence of a nonremovable dressing?

☐ 0 - No
☐ 1 - Yes

44c. (M0476) Status of Most Problematic (Observable) Stasis Ulcer:

☐ 1 - Fully granulating
☐ 2 - Early/partial granulation
☐ 3 - Not healing
☐ NA - No observable stasis ulcer

45. (M0482) Does this patient have a Surgical Wound?

☐ 0 - No [If No, go to *M0490*]
☐ 1 - Yes

45a. (M0484) Current Number of (Observable) Surgical Wounds: (If a wound is partially closed but has <u>more</u> than one opening, consider each opening as a separate wound.)

☐ 0 - Zero
☐ 1 - One
☐ 2 - Two
☐ 3 - Three
☐ 4 - Four or more

45b. (M0486) Does this patient have at least one Surgical Wound that Cannot be Observed due to the presence of a nonremovable dressing?

☐ 0 - No
☐ 1 - Yes

45c. (M0488) Status of Most Problematic (Observable) Surgical Wound:

☐ 1 - Fully granulating
☐ 2 - Early/partial granulation
☐ 3 - Not healing
☐ NA - No observable surgical wound

RESPIRATORY STATUS

46. (M0490) When is the patient dyspneic or noticeably Short of Breath?

☐ 0 - Never, patient is not short of breath
☐ 1 - When walking more than 20 feet, climbing stairs
☐ 2 - With moderate exertion (e.g., while dressing, using commode or bedpan, walking distances less than 20 feet)
☐ 3 - With minimal exertion (e.g., while eating, talking, or performing other ADLs) or with agitation
☐ 4 - At rest (during day or night)

47. **(M0500) Respiratory Treatments utilized at home: (Mark all that apply.)**

    ☐ 1 - Oxygen (intermittent or continuous)
    ☐ 2 - Ventilator (continually or at night)
    ☐ 3 - Continuous positive airway pressure
    ☐ 4 - None of the above

ELIMINATION STATUS

48. **(M0510)** Has this patient been treated for a **Urinary Tract Infection** in the past 14 days?

    ☐ 0 - No
    ☐ 1 - Yes
    ☐ NA - Patient on prophylactic treatment
    ☐ UK - Unknown

49. **(M0520) Urinary Incontinence or Urinary Catheter Presence:**

    ☐ 0 - No incontinence or catheter (includes anuria or ostomy for urinary drainage) [**If No, go to** **M0540**]
    ☐ 1 - Patient is incontinent
    ☐ 2 - Patient requires a urinary catheter (i.e., external, indwelling, intermittent, suprapubic) [**Go to** **M0540**]

50. **(M0530) When does Urinary Incontinence occur?**

    ☐ 0 - Timed-voiding defers incontinence
    ☐ 1 - During the night only
    ☐ 2 - During the day and night

51. **(M0540) Bowel Incontinence Frequency:**

    ☐ 0 - Very rarely or never has bowel incontinence
    ☐ 1 - Less than once weekly
    ☐ 2 - One to three times weekly
    ☐ 3 - Four to six times weekly
    ☐ 4 - On a daily basis
    ☐ 5 - More often than once daily
    ☐ NA - Patient has ostomy for bowel elimination
    ☐ UK - Unknown

52. **(M0550) Ostomy for Bowel Elimination:** Does this patient have an ostomy for bowel elimination that (within the last 14 days): a) was related to an inpatient facility stay, <u>or</u> b) necessitated a change in medical or treatment regimen?

    ☐ 0 - Patient does <u>not</u> have an ostomy for bowel elimination.
    ☐ 1 - Patient's ostomy was <u>not</u> related to an inpatient stay and did <u>not</u> necessitate change in medical or treatment regimen.
    ☐ 2 - The ostomy <u>was</u> related to an inpatient stay or <u>did</u> necessitate change in medical or treatment regimen.

NEURO/EMOTIONAL/BEHAVIORAL STATUS

53. **(M0560) Cognitive Functioning:** (Patient's current level of alertness, orientation, comprehension, concentration, and immediate memory for simple commands.)

    ☐ 0 - Alert/oriented, able to focus and shift attention, comprehends and recalls task directions independently.
    ☐ 1 - Requires prompting (cueing, repetition, reminders) only under stressful or unfamiliar conditions.
    ☐ 2 - Requires assistance and some direction in specific situations (e.g., on all tasks involving shifting of attention), or consistently requires low stimulus environment due to distractibility.
    ☐ 3 - Requires considerable assistance in routine situations. Is not alert and oriented or is unable to shift attention and recall directions more than half the time.
    ☐ 4 - Totally dependent due to disturbances such as constant disorientation, coma, persistent vegetative state, or delirium.

54. **(M0570) When Confused (Reported or Observed):**

    ☐ 0 - Never
    ☐ 1 - In new or complex situations only
    ☐ 2 - On awakening or at night only
    ☐ 3 - During the day and evening, but not constantly
    ☐ 4 - Constantly
    ☐ NA - Patient nonresponsive

55. (M0580) When Anxious (Reported or Observed):

- ☐ 0 - None of the time
- ☐ 1 - Less often than daily
- ☐ 2 - Daily, but not constantly
- ☐ 3 - All of the time
- ☐ NA - Patient nonresponsive

56. (M0590) Depressive Feelings Reported or Observed in Patient: (Mark all that apply.)

- ☐ 1 - Depressed mood (e.g., feeling sad, tearful)
- ☐ 2 - Sense of failure or self reproach
- ☐ 3 - Hopelessness
- ☐ 4 - Recurrent thoughts of death
- ☐ 5 - Thoughts of suicide
- ☐ 6 - None of the above feelings observed or reported

57. (M0600) Patient Behaviors (Reported or Observed): (Mark all that apply.)

- ☐ 1 - Indecisiveness, lack of concentration
- ☐ 2 - Diminished interest in most activities
- ☐ 3 - Sleep disturbances
- ☐ 4 - Recent change in appetite or weight
- ☐ 5 - Agitation
- ☐ 6 - A suicide attempt
- ☐ 7 - None of the above behaviors observed or reported

58. (M0610) Behaviors Demonstrated <u>at Least Once a Week</u> (Reported or Observed): (Mark all that apply.)

- ☐ 1 - Memory deficit: failure to recognize familiar persons/places, inability to recall events of past 24 hours, significant memory loss so that supervision is required
- ☐ 2 - Impaired decision-making: failure to perform usual ADLs or IADLs, inability to appropriately stop activities, jeopardizes safety through actions
- ☐ 3 - Verbal disruption: yelling, threatening, excessive profanity, sexual references, etc.
- ☐ 4 - Physical aggression: aggressive or combative to self and others (e.g., hits self, throws objects, punches, dangerous maneuvers with wheelchair or other objects)
- ☐ 5 - Disruptive, infantile, or socially inappropriate behavior (**excludes** verbal actions)
- ☐ 6 - Delusional, hallucinatory, or paranoid behavior
- ☐ 7 - None of the above behaviors demonstrated

59. (M0620) Frequency of Behavior Problems (Reported or Observed) (e.g., wandering episodes, self abuse, verbal disruption, physical aggression, etc.):

- ☐ 0 - Never
- ☐ 1 - Less than once a month
- ☐ 2 - Once a month
- ☐ 3 - Several times each month
- ☐ 4 - Several times a week
- ☐ 5 - At least daily

60. (M0630) Is this patient receiving Psychiatric Nursing Services at home provided by a qualified psychiatric nurse?

- ☐ 0 - No
- ☐ 1 - Yes

ADL/IADLs

> For M0640-M0800, complete the "current" column for all patients. For these same items, complete the "prior" column only at start of care; mark the level that corresponds to the patient's condition 14 days prior to start of care. In all cases, record what the patient is *able to do.*

61. (M0640) Grooming: Ability to tend to personal hygiene needs (i.e., washing face and hands, hair care, shaving or make up, teeth or denture care, fingernail care).

Prior Current
- ☐ ☐ 0 - Able to groom self unaided, with or without the use of assistive devices or adapted methods.
- ☐ ☐ 1 - Grooming utensils must be placed within reach before able to complete grooming activities.
- ☐ ☐ 2 - Someone must assist the patient to groom self.
- ☐ ☐ 3 - Patient depends entirely upon someone else for grooming needs.
- ☐   UK - Unknown

62. (M0650) Ability to Dress Upper Body (with or without dressing aids) including undergarments, pullovers, front-opening shirts and blouses, managing zippers, buttons, and snaps:

Prior Current

☐ ☐ 0 - Able to get clothes out of closets and drawers, put them on and remove them from the upper body without assistance.

☐ ☐ 1 - Able to dress upper body without assistance if clothing is laid out or handed to the patient.

☐ ☐ 2 - Someone must help the patient put on upper body clothing.

☐ ☐ 3 - Patient depends entirely upon another person to dress the upper body.

☐ UK - Unknown

63. (M0660) Ability to Dress Lower Body (with or without dressing aids) including undergarments, slacks, socks or nylons, shoes:

Prior Current

☐ ☐ 0 - Able to obtain, put on, and remove clothing and shoes without assistance.

☐ ☐ 1 - Able to dress lower body without assistance if clothing and shoes are laid out or handed to the patient.

☐ ☐ 2 - Someone must help the patient put on undergarments, slacks, socks or nylons, and shoes.

☐ ☐ 3 - Patient depends entirely upon another person to dress lower body.

☐ UK - Unknown

64. (M0670) Bathing: Ability to wash entire body. **Excludes grooming (washing face and hands only).**

Prior Current

☐ ☐ 0 - Able to bathe self in shower or tub independently.

☐ ☐ 1 - With the use of devices, is able to bathe self in shower or tub independently.

☐ ☐ 2 - Able to bathe in shower or tub with the assistance of another person:
(a) for intermittent supervision or encouragement or reminders, OR
(b) to get in and out of the shower or tub, OR
(c) for washing difficult to reach areas.

☐ ☐ 3 - Participates in bathing self in shower or tub, but requires presence of another person throughout the bath for assistance or supervision.

☐ ☐ 4 - Unable to use the shower or tub and is bathed in bed or bedside chair.

☐ ☐ 5 - Unable to effectively participate in bathing and is totally bathed by another person.

☐ UK - Unknown

65. (M0680) Toileting: Ability to get to and from the toilet or bedside commode.

Prior Current

☐ ☐ 0 - Able to get to and from the toilet independently with or without a device.

☐ ☐ 1 - When reminded, assisted, or supervised by another person, able to get to and from the toilet.

☐ ☐ 2 - Unable to get to and from the toilet but is able to use a bedside commode (with or without assistance).

☐ ☐ 3 - Unable to get to and from the toilet or bedside commode but is able to use a bedpan/urinal independently.

☐ ☐ 4 - Is totally dependent in toileting.

☐ UK - Unknown

66. (M0690) Transferring: Ability to move from bed to chair, on and off toilet or commode, into and out of tub or shower, and ability to turn and position self in bed if patient is bedfast.

Prior Current

☐ ☐ 0 - Able to independently transfer.

☐ ☐ 1 - Transfers with minimal human assistance or with use of an assistive device.

☐ ☐ 2 - Unable to transfer self but is able to bear weight and pivot during the transfer process.

☐ ☐ 3 - Unable to transfer self and is unable to bear weight or pivot when transferred by another person.

☐ ☐ 4 - Bedfast, unable to transfer but is able to turn and position self in bed.

☐ ☐ 5 - Bedfast, unable to transfer and is unable to turn and position self.

☐ UK - Unknown

67. (M0700) Ambulation/Locomotion: Ability to SAFELY walk, once in a standing position, or use a wheelchair, once in a seated position, on a variety of surfaces.

Prior Current

☐ ☐ 0 - Able to independently walk on even and uneven surfaces and climb stairs with or without railings (i.e., needs no human assistance or assistive device).

☐ ☐ 1 - Requires use of a device (e.g., cane, walker) to walk alone or requires human supervision or assistance to negotiate stairs or steps or uneven surfaces.

☐ ☐ 2 - Able to walk only with the supervision or assistance of another person at all times.

☐ ☐ 3 - Chairfast, unable to ambulate but is able to wheel self independently.

☐ ☐ 4 - Chairfast, unable to ambulate and is unable to wheel self.

☐ ☐ 5 - Bedfast, unable to ambulate or be up in a chair.

☐ UK - Unknown

68. (M0710) Feeding or Eating: Ability to feed self meals and snacks. **Note: This refers only to the process of <u>eating</u>, <u>chewing</u>, and <u>swallowing</u>, not preparing the food to be eaten.**

Prior	Current			
☐	☐	0	-	Able to independently feed self.
☐	☐	1	-	Able to feed self independently but requires:
				(a) meal set-up; <u>OR</u>
				(b) intermittent assistance or supervision from another person; <u>OR</u>
				(c) a liquid, pureed or ground meat diet.
☐	☐	2	-	<u>Unable</u> to feed self and must be assisted or supervised throughout the meal/snack.
☐	☐	3	-	Able to take in nutrients orally <u>and</u> receives supplemental nutrients through a nasogastric tube or gastrostomy.
☐	☐	4	-	<u>Unable</u> to take in nutrients orally and is fed nutrients through a nasogastric tube or gastrostomy
☐	☐	5	-	<u>Unable</u> to take in nutrients orally or by tube feeding.
☐		UK	-	Unknown

69. (M0720) Planning and Preparing Light Meals (e.g., cereal, sandwich) or reheat delivered meals:

Prior	Current			
☐	☐	0	-	(a) Able to independently plan and prepare all light meals for self or reheat delivered meals; <u>OR</u>
				(b) Is physically, cognitively, and mentally able to prepare light meals on a regular basis but has not routinely performed light meal preparation in the past (i.e., prior to this home care admission).
☐	☐	1	-	<u>Unable</u> to prepare light meals on a regular basis due to physical, cognitive, or mental limitations.
☐	☐	2	-	Unable to prepare any light meals or reheat any delivered meals.
☐		UK	-	Unknown

70. (M0730) Transportation: Physical and mental ability to <u>safely</u> use a car, taxi, or public transportation (bus, train, subway).

Prior	Current			
☐	☐	0	-	Able to independently drive a regular or adapted car; <u>OR</u> uses a regular or handicap-accessible public bus.
☐	☐	1	-	Able to ride in a car only when driven by another person; <u>OR</u> able to use a bus or handicap van only when assisted or accompanied by another person.
☐	☐	2	-	<u>Unable</u> to ride in a car, taxi, bus, or van, and requires transportation by ambulance.
☐		UK	-	Unknown

71. (M0740) Laundry: Ability to do own laundry -- to carry laundry to and from washing machine, to use washer and dryer, to wash small items by hand.

Prior	Current			
☐	☐	0	-	(a) Able to independently take care of all laundry tasks; <u>OR</u>
				(b) Physically, cognitively, and mentally able to do laundry and access facilities, <u>but</u> has not routinely performed laundry tasks in the past (i.e., prior to this home care admission).
☐	☐	1	-	Able to do only light laundry, such as minor hand wash or light washer loads. Due to physical, cognitive, or mental limitations, needs assistance with heavy laundry such as carrying large loads of laundry.
☐	☐	2	-	<u>Unable</u> to do any laundry due to physical limitation or needs continual supervision and assistance due to cognitive or mental limitation.
☐		UK	-	Unknown

72. (M0750) Housekeeping: Ability to safely and effectively perform light housekeeping and heavier cleaning tasks.

Prior	Current			
☐	☐	0	-	(a) Able to independently perform all housekeeping tasks; <u>OR</u>
				(b) Physically, cognitively, and mentally able to perform <u>all</u> housekeeping tasks but has not routinely participated in housekeeping tasks in the past (i.e., prior to this home care admission).
☐	☐	1	-	Able to perform only <u>light</u> housekeeping (e.g., dusting, wiping kitchen counters) tasks independently.
☐	☐	2	-	Able to perform housekeeping tasks with intermittent assistance or supervision from another person.
☐	☐	3	-	<u>Unable</u> to consistently perform any housekeeping tasks unless assisted by another person throughout the process.
☐	☐	4	-	Unable to effectively participate in any housekeeping tasks.
☐		UK	-	Unknown

73. **(M0760) Shopping:** Ability to plan for, select, and purchase items in a store and to carry them home or arrange delivery.

Prior Current
- ☐ ☐ 0 - (a) Able to plan for shopping needs and independently perform shopping tasks, including carrying packages; OR
  (b) Physically, cognitively, and mentally able to take care of shopping, but has not done shopping in the past (i.e., prior to this home care admission).
- ☐ ☐ 1 - Able to go shopping, but needs some assistance:
  (a) By self is able to do only light shopping and carry small packages, but needs someone to do occasional major shopping; OR
  (b) Unable to go shopping alone, but can go with someone to assist.
- ☐ ☐ 2 - Unable to go shopping, but is able to identify items needed, place orders, and arrange home delivery.
- ☐ ☐ 3 - Needs someone to do all shopping and errands.
- ☐   UK - Unknown

74. **(M0770) Ability to Use Telephone:** Ability to answer the phone, dial numbers, and <u>effectively</u> use the telephone to communicate.

Prior Current
- ☐ ☐ 0 - Able to dial numbers and answer calls appropriately and as desired.
- ☐ ☐ 1 - Able to use a specially adapted telephone (i.e., large numbers on the dial, teletype phone for the deaf) and call essential numbers.
- ☐ ☐ 2 - Able to answer the telephone and carry on a normal conversation but has difficulty with placing calls.
- ☐ ☐ 3 - Able to answer the telephone only some of the time or is able to carry on only a limited conversation.
- ☐ ☐ 4 - Unable to answer the telephone at all but can listen if assisted with equipment.
- ☐ ☐ 5 - Totally unable to use the telephone.
- ☐ ☐ NA - Patient does not have a telephone.
- ☐   UK - Unknown

MEDICATIONS

75. **(M0780) Management of Oral Medications:** <u>Patient's ability</u> to prepare and take <u>all</u> prescribed oral medications reliably and safely, including administration of the correct dosage at the appropriate times/intervals. <u>Excludes</u> injectable and IV medications. **(NOTE: This refers to ability, not compliance or willingness.)**

Prior Current
- ☐ ☐ 0 - Able to independently take the correct oral medication(s) and proper dosage(s) at the correct times.
- ☐ ☐ 1 - Able to take medication(s) at the correct times if:
  (a) individual dosages are prepared in advance by another person; OR
  (b) given daily reminders; OR
  (c) someone develops a drug diary or chart.
- ☐ ☐ 2 - Unable to take medication unless administered by someone else.
- ☐ ☐ NA - No oral medications prescribed.
- ☐   UK - Unknown

76. **(M0790) Management of Inhalant/Mist Medications:** <u>Patient's ability</u> to prepare and take <u>all</u> prescribed inhalant/mist medications (nebulizers, metered dose devices) reliably and safely, including administration of the correct dosage at the appropriate times/intervals. **Excludes all other forms of medication (oral tablets, injectable and IV medications).**

Prior Current
- ☐ ☐ 0 - Able to independently take the correct medication and proper dosage at the correct times.
- ☐ ☐ 1 - Able to take medication at the correct times if:
  (a) individual dosages are prepared in advance by another person, OR
  (b) given daily reminders.
- ☐ ☐ 2 - Unable to take medication unless administered by someone else.
- ☐ ☐ NA - No inhalant/mist medications prescribed.
- ☐   UK - Unknown

77. **(M0800) Management of Injectable Medications:** <u>Patient's ability</u> to prepare and take <u>all</u> prescribed injectable medications reliably and safely, including administration of correct dosage at the appropriate times/intervals. <u>Excludes</u> IV medications.

Prior	Current		
☐	☐	0 -	Able to independently take the correct medication and proper dosage at the correct times.
☐	☐	1 -	Able to take injectable medication at correct times if: (a) individual syringes are prepared in advance by another person, <u>OR</u> (b) given daily reminders.
☐	☐	2 -	<u>Unable</u> to take injectable medications unless administered by someone else.
☐	☐	NA -	No injectable medications prescribed.
☐		UK -	Unknown

EQUIPMENT MANAGEMENT

78. **(M0810) Patient Management of Equipment (includes <u>ONLY</u> oxygen, IV/Infusion therapy, enteral/ parenteral nutrition equipment or supplies):** <u>Patient's ability</u> to set up, monitor and change equipment reliably and safely, add appropriate fluids or medication, clean/store/dispose of equipment or supplies using proper technique. **(NOTE: This refers to ability, not compliance or willingness.)**

- ☐ 0 - Patient manages all tasks related to equipment completely independently.
- ☐ 1 - If someone else sets up equipment (i.e., fills portable oxygen tank, provides patient with prepared solutions), patient is able to manage all other aspects of equipment.
- ☐ 2 - Patient requires considerable assistance from another person to manage equipment, but independently completes portions of the task.
- ☐ 3 - Patient is only able to monitor equipment (e.g., liter flow, fluid in bag) and must call someone else to manage the equipment.
- ☐ 4 - Patient is completely dependent on someone else to manage all equipment.
- ☐ NA - No equipment of this type used in care **[If NA, go to *M0830*]**

79. **(M0820) Caregiver Management of Equipment (includes <u>ONLY</u> oxygen, IV/Infusion equipment, enteral/parenteral nutrition, ventilator therapy equipment or supplies):** <u>Caregiver's ability</u> to set up, monitor, and change equipment reliably and safely, add appropriate fluids or medication, clean/store/dispose of equipment or supplies using proper technique. **(NOTE: This refers to ability, not compliance or willingness.)**

- ☐ 0 - Caregiver manages all tasks related to equipment completely independently.
- ☐ 1 - If someone else sets up equipment, caregiver is able to manage all other aspects.
- ☐ 2 - Caregiver requires considerable assistance from another person to manage equipment, but independently completes significant portions of task.
- ☐ 3 - Caregiver is only able to complete small portions of task (e.g., administer nebulizer treatment, clean/store/dispose of equipment or supplies).
- ☐ 4 - Caregiver is completely dependent on someone else to manage all equipment.
- ☐ NA - No caregiver
- ☐ UK - Unknown

EMERGENT CARE

80. **(M0830) Emergent Care:** Since the last time OASIS data were collected, has the patient utilized any of the following services for emergent care (other than home care agency services)? **(Mark all that apply.)**

- ☐ 0 - No emergent care services [**If No emergent care and patient discharged, go to** *M0855*]
- ☐ 1 - Hospital emergency room (includes 23-hour holding)
- ☐ 2 - Doctor's office emergency visit/house call
- ☐ 3 - Outpatient department/clinic emergency (includes urgicenter sites)
- ☐ UK - Unknown

81. **(M0840) Emergent Care Reason:** For what reason(s) did the patient/family seek emergent care? **(Mark all that apply.)**

- ☐ 1 - Improper medication administration, medication side effects, toxicity, anaphylaxis
- ☐ 2 - Nausea, dehydration, malnutrition, constipation, impaction
- ☐ 3 - Injury caused by fall or accident at home
- ☐ 4 - Respiratory problems (e.g., shortness of breath, respiratory infection, tracheobronchial obstruction)
- ☐ 5 - Wound infection, deteriorating wound status, new lesion/ulcer
- ☐ 6 - Cardiac problems (e.g., fluid overload, exacerbation of CHF, chest pain)
- ☐ 7 - Hypo/Hyperglycemia, diabetes out of control
- ☐ 8 - GI bleeding, obstruction
- ☐ 9 - Other than above reasons
- ☐ UK - Reason unknown

DATA ITEMS COLLECTED AT INPATIENT FACILITY ADMISSION OR DISCHARGE ONLY

82. **(M0855)** To which **Inpatient Facility** has the patient been admitted?

- ☐ 1 - Hospital [**Go to** *M0890*]
- ☐ 2 - Rehabilitation facility [**Go to** *M0903*]
- ☐ 3 - Nursing home [**Go to** *M0900*]
- ☐ 4 - Hospice [**Go to** *M0903*]
- ☐ NA - No inpatient facility admission

83. **(M0870) Discharge Disposition:** Where is the patient after discharge from your agency? **(Choose only one answer.)**

- ☐ 1 - Patient remained in the community (not in hospital, nursing home, or rehab facility)
- ☐ 2 - Patient transferred to a noninstitutional hospice [**Go to** *M0903*]
- ☐ 3 - Unknown because patient moved to a geographic location not served by this agency [**Go to** *M0903*]
- ☐ UK - Other unknown [**Go to** *M0903*]

84. **(M0880)** After discharge, does the patient receive health, personal, or support **Services or Assistance?** (Mark all that apply.)

 ☐ 1 - No assistance or services received
 ☐ 2 - Yes, assistance or services provided by family or friends
 ☐ 3 - Yes, assistance or services provided by other community resources (e.g., Meals-on-Wheels, home health services, homemaker assistance, transportation assistance, assisted living, board and care)

 > Go to *M0903*

85. **(M0890)** If the patient was admitted to an acute care **Hospital**, for what **Reason** was he/she admitted?

 ☐ 1 - Hospitalization for <u>emergent</u> (unscheduled) care
 ☐ 2 - Hospitalization for <u>urgent</u> (scheduled within 24 hours of admission) care
 ☐ 3 - Hospitalization for <u>elective</u> (scheduled more than 24 hours before admission) care
 ☐ UK - Unknown

86. **(M0895)** Reason for Hospitalization: (Mark all that apply.)

 ☐ 1 - Improper medication administration, medication side effects, toxicity, anaphylaxis
 ☐ 2 - Injury caused by fall or accident at home
 ☐ 3 - Respiratory problems (SOB, infection, obstruction)
 ☐ 4 - Wound or tube site infection, deteriorating wound status, new lesion/ulcer
 ☐ 5 - Hypo/Hyperglycemia, diabetes out of control
 ☐ 6 - GI bleeding, obstruction
 ☐ 7 - Exacerbation of CHF, fluid overload, heart failure
 ☐ 8 - Myocardial infarction, stroke
 ☐ 9 - Chemotherapy
 ☐ 10 - Scheduled surgical procedure
 ☐ 11 - Urinary tract infection
 ☐ 12 - IV catheter-related infection
 ☐ 13 - Deep vein thrombosis, pulmonary embolus
 ☐ 14 - Uncontrolled pain
 ☐ 15 - Psychotic episode
 ☐ 16 - Other than above reasons

 > Go to *M0903*

87. **(M0900)** For what **Reason(s)** was the patient **Admitted** to a **Nursing Home?** (Mark all that apply.)

 ☐ 1 - Therapy services
 ☐ 2 - Respite care
 ☐ 3 - Hospice care
 ☐ 4 - Permanent placement
 ☐ 5 - Unsafe for care at home
 ☐ 6 - Other
 ☐ UK - Unknown

 > Go to *M0903*

88. **(M0903)** Date of Last (Most Recent) Home Visit:

 __ __/__ __/__ __ __ __
 month day year

89. (M0906) Discharge/Transfer/Death Date: Enter the date of the discharge, transfer, or death (at home) of the patient.

__ __/__ __/__ __ __ __
month day year

☐ UK - Unknown

Access   The availability and ability of an individual to receive health care, including all factors related to cost, location, and transportation.

Accountable health plan (AHP)   A health insurance plan that would be recognized by a government entity as being qualified to provide total health services to a specific population in a geographical area and that is responsible for reporting medical outcomes.

Accreditation   A rigorous process that examines various components of home care operations and clinical practice. The achievement of accreditation designates that the organization has gone through the accreditation process and meets predetermined standards as measured by on-site nurses and other survey team "visitors."

A process that an organization or program undertakes to demonstrate it has met established standards or requirements (e.g., the Joint Commission for Accreditation of Health Care Organizations [JCAHO] Standards for Home Health and the Community Health Accreditation Program [CHAP]).

Activities of daily living (ADLs)   Basic, usually self-care activities that must be done daily to care for our bodies and overall health maintenance. These activities include personal hygiene tasks such as bathing and grooming and obtaining and preparing food. Others include toileting and transferring in and out of bed. These activities are important indicators because they demonstrate or show the patient's functional status or health care needs.

Basic self-care activities, such as eating, bathing, dressing, transferring in and out of bed, and toileting, that are widely used to assess individual functional status. See also instrumental care.

Acuity   The degree of disease or injury before a patient receives treatment. The measurement of this degree determines the amount of health care resources projected to be expended on this patient (e.g., nursing care or placement in a specialized care unit).

Adjusted average per capita cost (AAPCC)   An estimate of the total payment for services a managed care payor would make for a unique category of services, divided by the number of beneficiaries eligible for the services. This estimate is usually used in negotiating capitated agreements.

Advocacy   A role assumed by a health care professional designed to maximize patient self-determination through education, support, and affirmation of patient health care decisions.

Agency for Health Care Policy and Research (AHCPR)   An agency of the U.S. Department of Health and Human Services that sponsors research projects and develops clinical practice guidelines related to the delivery of health care services.

Autonomy   Respect for clients as individuals who are capable of making their own choices about health care and life-style options.

Benchmark   A systematic process to measure or quantify; a standard for comparing two similar types of products and services when trying to identify areas for improvement in an organization.

Capitated risk The financial risk involved in not being able to accurately estimate the cost of and contract appropriately for care or services to a capitated population.

Capitation A set dollar amount established to cover the cost of health care services delivered to an individual. The amount is based on the number of members in the plan, not the amount of services used.

Capitation management The process of gathering as much information on the population to be capitated and understanding the key characteristics of that population in order to manage the financial risk involved in providing care or services.

Caregiver Anyone who provides care or services to or for a patient.

Care plan A plan of action for care that is developed, delivered, and evaluated by the nurse and other team members. This may also be called the plan of care and varies among organizations.

Case management A system for overseeing a patient's care usually across health care systems. For example, a nurse or therapist case manager may coordinate care and services from the hospital, to the nursing home, and in the patient's home.

System of patient care delivery that focuses on the achievement of outcomes within effective and appropriate time frames and use of resources. Case management attempts to control the quality and cost of patient care and focuses on an entire episode of illness, crossing all settings in which the patient receives care. Case management incorporates the principles of managed care.

Case (care) manager One person who is responsible for the overall care of the patient and use of resources for that care. The case (or care) manager may be a nurse, a social worker, or a therapist.

The primary person (registered nurse or other health care professional) responsible for developing patient care outcomes for his or her case load. A case manager is accountable for meeting outcomes within an appropriate length of stay, the effective use of resources, and preestablished standards. A case manager collaborates with the health care team and the patient to accomplish those outcomes.

Case mix The distribution of different types of patients seen at a setting; collection of case types. The diagnosis-specific makeup of acute care settings patients.

Case type A system that groups patients based on the different types (mix) of diagnoses (cases) for which its patients are treated.

Catheter Any rounded or tubular medical device that is inserted into veins, cavities, or other body passages. The purpose of a catheter is to improve or replace function. Examples include a urinary Foley catheter in the bladder from which urine drains into a collection bag, suction catheters, and intravenous catheters inserted into the vein which allow for the delivery of fluids.

Chronic A slow or persistent illness or health problem that must be cared for throughout life. Examples include diabetes, glaucoma, and some chronic lung conditions.

Classification system A system of categorizing elements of similar groups using preestablished criteria.

Client The one who receives care. Also called the patient, customer, or consumer of health care services or products.

An individual, customer, consumer, or patient who received care or services.

Clinical care All of the events that encompass the diagnosis and treatment of illness and the attainment of specific patient outcomes; it is the visualization of the health care team member and the physician working closely with the patient and the patient's family to meet predetermined clinical outcomes.

Clinical path (CP)   A structured plan for care, often categorized by diagnosis or patient problem, that defines specific care interventions, team members, and other information across a time line.

Clinical management tools that organize, sequence, and time the major interventions of nursing staff, physicians, rehabilitation therapists, and other health professionals for a particular case type of condition. The pathways describe a standard of practice and are, in essence, a clinical budget.

Coinsurance   The amount or percentage of the cost of services that consumers may be required to pay under a cost-sharing agreement with their insurance plan or program. It may also be called a copayment.

Collaboration   The active process of working together and valuing another's input toward reaching patient goals.

The act of working together to achieve a common goal(s). In health care, collaboration is a joint effort of staff from many disciplines planning together to improve the processes, leading to improved patient care.

Community health nursing   A synthesis of nursing practice and public health practice applied to promoting and preserving the health of the population. Health promotion, health maintenance, health education and management, and the coordination and continuity of care contribute to a holistic approach to the management of the health care of individuals, families, and groups within a community.

Continuous quality improvement (CQI)   An ongoing process that seeks to continuously improve patient care, delivery of services, staff education, and other important parts of operations or other parts of an organization. Accreditation standards demand continuous quality improvement.

A conceptual framework for evaluating the quality of care that emphasizes an analytical approach to understanding the contributions of all components of the health care system in achieving results and constantly incorporating improvements into the system.

Cost-based reimbursement   Reimbursement to health care providers based on the aggregation of allowable costs, up to a certain limit (e.g., cost caps). This system of reimbursement was originally established for Medicare program providers and is quickly disappearing.

Cost containment   Those measures or requirements established by organizations involved in the delivery of health care to control the increases in use or expenditures.

Cost per case   A Medicare reimbursement methodology that pays a single cost per discharge, regardless of the actual cost per treatment. The cost per case is an average amount based on total costs divided by total discharges.

Cost reimbursement   The methodology historically used by the Health Care Financing Administration to pay providers for Medicare home health benefits. The reimbursement is based on the cost of care, and profit is not included. Settlement is accomplished through the submission of a cost report to the organization's fiscal intermediary.

Cost shifting   The act of increasing rates to one segment of the patient population to offset losses incurred by another segment such as Medicaid recipients.

Critical path   A tool for case management and managed care where the physician, nurse, rehabilitation therapist, and others provide care in a timely fashion to achieve patient-centered outcomes. Those key incidents may be categorized according to tests, activities, treatment, medication, diet, discharge planning, teaching, and outcomes. This can also be referred to as a clinical path. (See Clinical paths.)

Data Products of measurement (singular form: datum) compiled in such a fashion that discussion can be formulated or inference can be obtained.

Decubitus ulcer An area or redness or skin breakdown possibly affecting surrounding tissues, usually over a bony prominence and related to immobility. The new term is pressure ulcer.

Dementia Changes in brain function that cause memory loss, confusion, or the loss or ability to safely function independently.

Deviation In mathematics, deviation is an abnormality or departure from the norm; statistically a deviation is the difference in absolute numbers between one number in the set and the calculated mean of the set.

Diagnoses The identification of problems or diseases. The word for one or a single diagnoses is diagnosis.

Diagnostic-related group (DRG) optimization A logical approach for ensuring full reimbursement for all services and care rendered to the patient.

Diagnostic-related groups (DRGs) A code of classifying patient illnesses according to principal diagnosis and treatment requirements. Under Medicare each DRG has its own price (weight) that a hospital is paid, regardless of the actual cost of treatment.

Dietitian A member of the health care team who promotes optimal nutrition, based on the patient's individual needs. The dietitian may be called an R.D., a registered dietician, or an L.D., a licensed dietitian. The dietitian may make home visits or teach the other team members about dietary related issues such as effective nutrition, meal preparation, and special diets.

Documentation The writing of clinical notes that contains information needed for communication, legal, and other reasons.

Effective management A health care management style that shares the focus of patient care with administration of the program and effectively seeks improvement through the simplification and review of all systems involved in care or service delivery.

Encounter data Data on the utilization of products or services (usually expressed in units or a dollar value) by a given population.

End-result feedback A review of a specific process or series of processes; the end results are integrated into the input information to effect a change in the ongoing process.

Enteral nutrition Provision of nourishment via a tube inserted into the nose and down to the stomach or through a surgical site through the stomach. A G-tube is an example of enteral nutrition.

Enterostomal therapy nurse (ET nurse) A nurse specialist with special education and training who cares for patients with wounds or assists other nurses and team members to care for these patients. The ET nurse may also visit patients with an ostomy, a urinary or fecal diversion from usual function, as well as other skin care challenges.

Equity of care A health care system that differentiates levels of care based on assessed patient needs, not individual or group characteristics (e.g., ability to pay).

Extended care services Patient care services provided as an alternative to inpatient hospitalization in a skilled nursing facility, rehabilitation facility, or subacute facility offered after an acute illness or injury.

Fee for service A health plan in which beneficiaries choose their health care provider and the health plan pays the provider charge for services. This type of plan usually includes some element of utilization review or prior approval by the plan for certain, if not all, services.

Gatekeeper   One who has the overall responsibility for a patient's course of care and reviews and approves or disapproves all requests for health care services. This role has traditionally been held by a physician, but may be a managed care provider, a payor, or a subcontracted utilization review group.

Geriatrics   Services or care related or provided to the elderly, related to the process or aging.

Goals   The end point of care or the desired results for care. For example, if the goal is to provide safe mobility, everything done should support that goal. The team members work together to achieve the patient goals.

   The desired result of an action or series of actions an individual or organization might strive for; a goal is different from an objective in that a goal is more broad based, and objectives are more quantifiable and specific and are derived from a goal statement.

Health Care Financing Administration (HCFA)   An agency of the U.S. Government under the Department of Health and Human Services (HHS) responsible for the Medicare and Medicaid programs. This direction includes various requirements, policies, payment for services, and many other operational aspects of the programs.

   HCFA sets the coverage policy, payment, and other guidelines and directs the activities of government contractors (e.g., carriers and fiscal intermediaries).

Health education   Training or education activities provided to patients to encourage life-style modifications, thereby reducing behavioral risk factors and improving healthy activities.

Health maintenance organization (HMO)   A health care provider organization that offers a comprehensive health service plan to its beneficiaries through an established network of primary care physicians, specialists, clinics, and hospitals. It provides these services on a prepaid, fixed-cost basis.

Homebound   A term used in the Medicare home care program that means the patient cannot leave the home without assistance and that leaving the home is a considerable and taxing effort and occurs infrequently and lasts for a short duration. Homebound means primarily confined to the home for medical reasons. Homebound is one of the admitting criteria for patients admitted to a Medicare-certified home care program. For this reason, when patients are "no longer homebound," they are discharged from Medicare home care.

Home care/home health   The provision of a range of health services, products, supplies, and equipment to patients in their homes.

   A range of health care services and products provided to a patient in his or her place of residence. Medicare currently reimburses skilled nursing, speech-language pathology, physical and occupational therapy, medical social work, and home health aide services.

Home health agency (HHA)   An organization that provides health care to patients in their homes. They may or may not be licensed, depending on the state and requirements. Medicare-certified agencies must have a survey or a special review to be certified to accept Medicare patients and receive government payment for those services.

Hospice   A special way of caring for patients with a terminal illness or a limited life expectancy. Hospice cares for the patient and his or her family and tries to make every remaining day the best that they can be. Hospice team members include specially trained hospice volunteers, bereavement counselors, certified nursing assistants (CNAs) or hospice aides, spiritual counselors, nurses, and other services. Hospice is a philosophy, not a place, but the bulk of hospice care is provided at home.

Services provided to patients with a documented terminal illness in which the focus changes from curative intervention to palliative care. The service implies patient knowledge and acceptance of disease prognosis and life expectancy. Medicare coverage includes nursing care under the supervision of a registered nurse; medical social services under the direction of a physician; physician services, counseling services for the individual and caregivers; medical supplies, home health aide and homemaker services; and physical, occupational, and speech language pathology therapy services. Other core hospice services include volunteer support and bereavement counseling.

ICD-9 code A coding methodology developed to identify specific clinical diagnoses for the purpose of data collection and payment.

Indemnity plan An insurance plan that allows members to choose their own health care providers who are paid on a fee-for-service basis and are not usually controlled through prior authorization or utilization controls.

Individual practice (independent physician) association A legal entity formed by a group of physicians, dentists, or other health care professionals to provide contracted services to a group of beneficiaries or members of a managed care plan.

Instrumental care (instrumental activities of daily living [IADLs]) The provision of assistance with IADLs such as shopping, cooking, transportation, financial management, homemaking, and home maintenance.

Integrated delivery network A provider of health care services that offers a wide continuum of services to its customer population. It usually comprises one or more acute care hospital(s), skilled and intermediate nursing facilities, outpatient and ambulatory surgery centers, home health care agency(ies), hospices, and physicians who are either employees of the group or tightly controlled by utilization management techniques.

Intermediate care facility (ICF) An organization licensed by state law and recognized under the Medicaid program to provide care to those individuals whose treatment regimen does not require the degree or skills necessary to justify placement in an acute or skilled care facility.

Intervention Any happening or event that interrupts or changes events in progress.

Length of stay (LOS) The number of hospital or home care days for each patient. Each patient's hospitalization is subject to review to determine the appropriateness of the length of stay (ALOS, average length of stay).

Long-term care A variety of health services provided to individuals with physical or mental disabilities needing assistance on a continuing basis. These services can be provided in a multitude of settings (e.g., homes, subacute skilled nursing facilities, retirement facilities, assistive living centers, intermediate care facilities, and senior day care).

Managed care Care that is organized to provide care to patients using financial and people resources effectively throughout care.

Care that is organized to achieve specific patient outcomes within fiscally responsible time frames (length of stay) using resources that are appropriate in amount and sequenced to the specific case type and population of the individual patient. Care is structured by case management care plans and clinical paths that are based on knowledge by case type regarding usual length of stay, critical events and their timing, anticipated outcomes, and resource utilization.

Managed care plan or organization (MCP or MCO)   Any organization providing a network of patient care services, including physician, clinic, home care, or hospital care, for a set, agreed-on payment. These plans use a variety of cost-containment measures, discounts, and utilization review services in an effort to control or manage the risk of providing health care.

Master capitation   The primary holder of a capitated contract who may subcontract to other providers for services, but remains financially at risk for the capitated contract.

Medicaid   A health program that is administered at the state level for patients who qualify. The qualification is financial. Medicaid coverage varies by state. Sometimes even the name is different. For example, in California it is called Medical.

Medicare   A federal program for people over age 65, who are disabled, or who have end-stage renal disease (ESRD). Medicare is complex but has two parts, A and B, that cover different services such as inpatient hospitalization (after the Medicare beneficiary pays a deductible), home care, hospice, and other services. Medicare is a medical insurance program; and like all insurance programs, there are exclusions, eligibility, and coverage rules.

Medicare health maintenance organization   An alternative insurance product for Medicare beneficiaries that allows commercial insurers to contract with the Health Care Financing Administration to provide similar Medicare-covered services. Providers must have a contract with such insurers to provide beneficiary care. The advantages of such a program are that beneficiaries do not have to submit paperwork for payment, do not have to pay a copayment or deductible, and may have a richer benefit package. However, beneficiaries are limited in the number of providers to whom they may go for services and the number or types of services allowed.

Normal cause variance   Normal variation caused by the system. For example, the variation of plus or minus 15 minutes for the results of a particular laboratory test.

Nursing care plan   A plan of action developed by a professional nurse for a specific patient that involves all the nursing activities required to effect a positive outcome in the patients recovery period. This plan may include prescriptive plans of other disciplines.

Occupational Safety and Health Administration (OSHA)   The part of the U.S. Government that regulates employee or worker safety. OSHA requires various standard be maintained related to health care.

Occupational therapy   Occupational therapy (OT) focuses on quality of life and making the patient more independent in functions. The OT may be called in for a home safety assessment, to identify needed adaptive or assistive devices that make the patient safer at home, to teach energy conservation techniques to patients with shortness of breath, or for many other reasons.

Outcomes   Outcomes are quantifiable or measurable goals of care. An example is that the patient, by a certain date, can name all of his or her medications and the times to take them.

Outcomes, clinical   The results or effects of clinical processes on patients. The results may be described by outcome criteria.

Outcomes criteria   The ends to be achieved. From a knowledge of the usual course of events and the factors relevant to the patient group involved, the clinician should be able to determine the desired results that, in a given patient at the end of a program or service of care, are based on knowledge about the needs of this group of patients and carried out in a fashion adequate to achieve its purpose.

Outliers Cases in which a patient's length of stay exceeds the national average by 20 days or a 1.94% standard deviation, or in which the cost of treatment exceeds the national average diagnostic-related group rate by $12,000 or 150%, whichever is greater.

Payor The payor or insurance company financially responsible for the services or care provided to patients. Example include Medicare or other insurance companies.

The organization responsible for paying a health care provider for the health care products and/or services provided to a patient or beneficiary.

Performance measure A quantifiable standard or measurement to determine how successful a health care provider has been in meeting established outcomes or goals of care.

Personal emergency response system (PERS) PERS is a technology that links the frail, elderly or homebound to community resources in the case of a fall or other emergency. PERS usually has a personal help button that, when activated, calls for help. To be effective, the PERS personal help button must be worn or within reach at all times.

Physical therapy (PT) A specialty of the rehabilitative services that focuses on loss of mobility and function of patients due to illness or injury. PTs work with stroke patients, muscular dystrophy patients, and others who needs home exercises or home exercise programs to restore safe mobility and function.

Physician hospital organization (PHO) A legal organization jointly owned by a hospital and a group of physicians to collectively pool their resources to negotiate contracts and provide services to a managed care organization. This is also known as a physician hospital network (PHN).

Preferred provider organization (PPO) A health services program that provides its members with services from contracted providers of care. Beneficiaries receive better cost coverage by using a contracted provider; they can use a noncontracted provider, but will be responsible for a copayment or additional fee for service.

Primary prevention Measures that actively promote health, prevent illness, and provide specific protection.

Process A series of activities or events that are related and sequenced in such a faction as to effect a prescribed or established patient outcome.

Professional care Home health services in which the boundaries of practice are determined by professional standards with a basis in scientific theory and research.

Prospective payment system (PPS) The third-party payment system that establishes certain payment rates for services, regardless of the actual cost of care provided. The Medicare diagnostic-related group system for inpatient acute care services is the most widely known example of this type of payment. The prospective payment system was established in 1981 under the Tax Equity and Fiscal Responsibility Act (TEFRA).

Quality A degree of excellence. The achievement of individualized outcomes. Organizationally defined.

Quality assessment The measurement or assessment of care provided to an individual or a group.

Quality assurance The systematic review of all activities included in the provision of services or the production of a product that meets preestablished criteria, thereby providing a sense of confidence that a certain level of quality has been achieved. The achievement of a level of performance or quality status that has not been met before in this process.

Ratio of cost to charges (RCC)   Method of estimating the cost of care. Cost includes fixed (administrative) and variable (supplies). Ratio = cost/charges.

Rehabilitation   The term used to describe the care and efforts of team members to restore function and mobility after illness or injury. Members of the rehabilitation team include the physical therapist, occupational therapist, nurse, speech-language pathologist, and others, based on the patient's individualized rehabilitation program and other needs.

Resource utilization   The using up of assets; the kinds and number of items (e.g., nursing hours, visits, supplies) used in performing patient care.

Respiratory therapy   The respiratory therapist is a specialist usually involved with patients who need oxygen or have other respiratory problems or illnesses.

Risk bands   The level of protection guaranteed in a capitated agreement that fluctuates between the risk "floor" and risk "ceiling." Service providers receive refunds if costs do not reach the floor and provide additional payments if the costs go above the ceiling.

Risk pool   An incentive pool of monies, over and above the direct payment made to a service provider, that is distributed to a determined number of providers if certain predetermined financial outcomes are met.

Secondary care   Early diagnosis measures and prompt interventions to limit disabilities.

Sentinel event   Significant or serious patient event or outcome that needs to be evaluated immediately. Sentinel events are commonly risk management issues.

Social work services (SWS)   Social work services, also called medical social services (MSS), are valuable services to patients and their families for a number of reasons. The social worker may be involved when there are problems that prevent the plan of care from being implemented. For example, if the patient has diabetes and cannot afford food or insulin or if there are family or other problems that are causing the patient not to improve or be in unsafe conditions.

Special cause variance   Variation not common to the system. For example, a variation from an established parameter caused by machine malfunction.

Speech-language pathology (SLP)   The speech-language pathologist is involved primarily with patients who have swallowing or communication problems after surgery or due to other problems such as a stroke.

Standard   A level of performance or a set of conditions considered acceptable by some authority or by the individual or individuals engaged in performing or maintaining the set of conditions in question.

Structure   The framework of an organization that supports and defines how the components of a process are bound together to meet or achieve a given outcome (e.g., in home health agencies, the policies, procedures, and clinical competency checklists and standards define in part how patient care will be delivered).

Subcapitation   A subset of capitated monies set aside for a particular group of services (e.g., home care services under a hospital plan or home medical equipment as a subcapitation to a home care organization).

Supervisory visit   Supervisory visits are requirements of Medicare. The nurse may visit sometimes when the home health aide is providing care in the home and other times when the aide is not at the home. Supervision is a standard practice in home and hospice care and assists in ensuring quality of care for patients.

Support services   Includes all the departments and service areas within the hospital or health care organization that provide the necessary structure to support care delivery. Controls are applied through administrative or managerial channels and involve continual monitoring of the case management system.

Tertiary prevention   Rehabilitative activities and measures that reduce impairments and disabilities, minimize suffering caused by departures from good health, and promote the patient's adjustment to immediate conditions.

Time line   Identifies when an event or a series of events should occur, following a preestablished and agreed on framework for those events to happen or specific outcomes to be achieved.

Total quality management   A system of continuous quality improvement that empowers employees to review and concentrate on the systems or processes affecting group achievements and is directed from senior management.

Uniform clinical data set   A mandate from the Health Care Financing Administration (HCFA) that is a part of the peer review organization's scope of work to ultimately provide HCFA with the data necessary to start defining Medicare research activities.

Utilization management (UM)   A program established by health care providers to assess efficiency and quality of patient care based on established criteria.

Validity   The amount or degree to which an observed outcome or event correlates with what really happens.

Variance   The difference between what is expected and what actually happens. Variances are differentiated by system (internal or external), practitioner, and patient.

Venipuncture   A puncture into the vein to draw blood. The nurse or laboratory technician obtains blood through venipuncture for laboratory analysis.

INDEX